Mana

Issues in services for people with learning difficulties

Peter Gilbert and Terry Scragg

COMMUNITY CARE
THE INDEPENDENT VOICE OF SOCIAL WORK

1992

Published in 1992 by
Community Care/Reed Business Publishing Group
Quadrant House, The Quadrant, Sutton
Surrey SM2 5AS

ISBN 0 617 01006 4

Set in 11/11 Souvenir Light and printed in Great Britain
by The Printing Unit, University of Sheffield

This book is
for the two Sues, our children, and all
our friends and colleagues over many years

and dedicated to Professor Joan Bicknell, who has
done so much to stimulate quality services
for people with learning difficulties and their families.

PETER GILBERT was educated at Worth Abbey School, Sussex. Following two years at the Royal Military Academy, Sandhurst, and three years in the army, he went to Oxford. He joined West Sussex SSD as a trainee. He completed a master's degree in social work at Sussex University and spent four years as a generic social worker. In 1981 he became team leader at the Forest Hospital, Horsham.

He is the author of *Mental Handicap: A Practical Guide for Social Workers* and is the co-author of a number of information books for parents, including the West Sussex SSD *Coping with Mental Handicap* series and *We are One People* for the Diocese of Arundel and Brighton. He wrote the chapter on the role of the social worker for *Mental Handicap: A Multi-Disciplinary Approach* (the successor to *Tredgold's*) and has also contributed to *Social Work: A Christian Perspective* and *The Residential Opportunity?* He is co-author (with Peter Dickens) of the *State and the Housing Question* and is a regular contributor to *Community Care.*

Peter Gilbert co-founded the first community mental handicap team in West Sussex, became the social work representative on the English National Board's specialist panel for post-qualifying nurse training in learning difficulties, and contributed to the English National Board training pack for Registered Mental Handicap Nurses, *Caring for People with Mental Handicap.*

With Terry Scragg, he was a member of the consultative committee of the Cental Council for Education and Training in Social Work and is currently a member of the social welfare committee for the National Bishops Conference for England and Wales.

After a period as a manager of services for people with learning difficulties with the London Borough of Merton, he moved to Kent in 1989 as area manager for specialist services (physical disability, mental health and learning difficulties) in West Kent. In 1990 he was appointed general manager for service provision with the same authority and in May this year became director of operations (adult services), Staffordshire SSD. He is a visiting fellow in social work and social administration at Sussex University.

TERRY SCRAGG has qualifications in nursing (learning difficulties), social work, social services planning, and rehabilitation. He has worked in a long-stay hospital, and as mental health social worker, team manager and senior training officer in a social services department.

For the last 12 years he has been in social work education and is currently head of social work studies at the West Sussex Institute of Higher Education. He was responsible for one of the first post-qualifying courses for social workers in the field of disability and has worked on the Certificate in Social Service course, teaching on modules for staff working in services for people with learning difficulties, and staff with management responsibilities. He is a member of the joint management committee of the Sussex CSS scheme. He is also involved in extensive consultancy and training in social services departments, health authorities and voluntary organisations.

In 1980 he was awarded a Council of Europe fellowship to study services for people with long-term disabilities in Denmark and Sweden. He is currently working with a number of voluntary organisations on preparing staff for roles in community-based services, and on quality assurance in the context of the White Paper, *Caring for People*. He is also undertaking a research project funded by CCETSW and Kent SSD on change in social education centres and the implications for staff development.

He was a member of Worthing Health Authority 1987-1990.

DAVID CLARIDGE is assistant director (adult services), London borough of Croydon.

ALEXIS WAITMAN is a freelance consultant and trainer.

Acknowledgements

In a publication about leadership and service delivery, authors gain fresh insights from almost everyone they meet and work with. The authors would like to thank all their colleagues over many years for their inspiration, but would especially like to thank the following:

Alexis Waitman, freelance consultant and trainer, for chapter 12. David Claridge, assistant director, Croydon SSD, for chapter 13.

Teresa Temple and Sue Marks for patiently typing the text and battling successfully with Peter Gilbert's handwriting (!) and Sandra Perrin for additional work.

Terry Philpot, editor of *Community Care*, who edited the manuscript for publication, was a constant support in the writing of this book.

For their general support and encouragement we would like to thank:

Hugh England of Sussex University; Dr Christine Russell-Hodgson of Kent SSD; Colin Whittington and Jenny Weinstein of the Central Council for Education and Training in Social Work; Alistair Bell and Jill Woolf from Merton Personal Services Department; Ray Stephens, David Grant, Fay Wedlake, Paul Fisher and Andy Lane from Kent SSD; Wayne Osbond of St Raphaels; Joyce Beak and Brian Goacher of Tunbridge Wells Health Authority; Phyllis Mackenzie of the Leybourne Grange library; Professor Chris Cullen of the University of St Andrews; Liz Foster, Neil Perkins, John Munro and Nick Longdon from West Sussex SSD; Professor Sheila Hollins of St George's Hospital Medical School; Hilary Brown of the University of Kent; Sally Fraser of the South East Thames Regional Health Authority; Dr Sophie Thompson and Rosemary Armstrong of Merton and Sutton DHA; Morag Plank of Merton MENCAP and Campaign for Mentally Handicapped People (now Values in Action); all in service Group 13; Gery Murphy of ITCR; Trevor Bennett of the Isle of Wight SSD; David Browning of the Audit Commission; Chris and Jo Dobson; Gary Bourlet of People First; Stephen Bayliss; Edna Wallace formerly of Wandsworth CMHT; Jenny Lumley; Trevor Vigar of the English National Board; and Enrique Valles and Sally Coren of the old Mid Downs CMHT group.

For their help with specific chapters we would like to thank: Carol Witherspoon, Surrey SSD (chapter 3); Gery Murphy of ITCR, Hilary Brown, senior training adviser, UKC and SETRHA (chapter 8); David Wright and Jill Woolf, development and inspection unit, London Borough of Merton and Colin Whittington from CCETSW (chapter 15); Dr Christine Russell-Hodgson, former head of policy planning, Kent SSD; Trevor Bennett, deputy director and Bob Steele, community services manager, Isle of Wight SSD and DHA respectively; and John Spargo, divisional manager, Hillingdon SSD (chapter 19); and Norman Warner, director of social services, Kent SSD, and Trevor Knowles, director of personal services, Merton PSD, for permission to use information regarding their organisational structures; Enrique Valles, principal psychologist, Tunbridge Wells DHA and David Grant, former senior manager, Kent SSD (chapter 20); and to acknowledge the inspiration of Barry Spooner, without whom the Mid Downs CMHT would not have been created; Sophia Chung, David Grant and Kath Strange, Kent SSD, and Linda Hay, Hampshire SSD; (chapter 21); Brian Dumbrell, Kent County Council, Joe Graham, Canterbury Oast Trust, Richard Perry, assistant director, West Sussex County SSD, and Jill Woolf, London Borough of Merton (chapter 22); and Carol Batchelor, manager (recruitment and appraisal), Kent SSD (chapter 11).

The opinions expressed in this book are entirely those of the authors and do not necessarily reflect the views of their authorities.

The Authors and publishers wish to thank the following for their permission to use published material:
Harper and Row and NISW for the diagrams in Chapter 1; The Audit Commission for diagrams in various chapters; Human Policy Press for the diagram from Wolfensberger in Chapter 2; *CMH* for Table 2.12; *Community Living* for permission to reprint David Barron's story; Souvenir Press and Falmer Press for the diagrams in Chapter 3; West Sussex SSD for permission to reprint "Brian Johnson's" Story; Crown Books for Table 6.1.1.; Pan for the diagram in Chapter 6; *MARC* for the resources checklist in Chapter 7; Collins for the table and diagram and Wandsworth SSD for the diagram in Chapter 8; *Community Care* for Table 11.1.1 and the Industrial Society for Table 11.1.2; Kent SSD for the diagram in Chapter 10; The Audit Commission for the diagram in Chapter 19; CMH for Table 20.1.1.; *The Observer* for 'A Life of One's own'; *Community Care* for 'I Enjoy Life'.

PETER GILBERT and TERRY SCRAGG
January 1992

"When one person dreams alone it is only a dream.
When we dream together it is the beginning of reality."

Helder Camara

"The organisation which treats people like assets, requiring maintenance, hire and investment, can behave quite differently from the organisation which looks upon them as costs . . . Upside-down thinking changes nothing save the way we think, but that can make all the difference."

Charles Handy, *The Age of Unreason*, (1989)

Contents

PART III SERVICE MODELS

APPENDIX

Introduction

"Let us teach ourselves and others that politics can be not only the art of the possible, especially if this means the art of speculation, calculation, intrigue, secret deals and pragmatic manoeuvering, but that it can even be the art of the impossible, namely the art of improving ourselves and the world."

Vaclav Havel, president of Czechoslovakia

Introducing the issues

"Leadership is the sheer abililty to influence people and events . . . this ability is needed more than ever in local government if it is to move quickly enough to meet the challenges facing it".
Leadership in Local Government

"They are decided only to be undecided, resolved to be irresolute, adamant for drift, all-powerful for impotence".
Winston Churchill on the government of 1936.

Churchill's philippic against the British government of 1936 could be equally well applied to a number of top managers in the public services during two troubled decades. Too many tried to please and appease politicians, press, unions, pressure groups and powerful staff interests, and ended by pleasing no-one, while producing only an etiolated service. As senior managers have too often been like the girl in *Oklahoma* "who can't say 'no' ", it has fallen on the middle and front line managers to set objectives, standards and priorities in an era of competing pressures. The middle manager's life is not an easy one. He or she is "the piggy in the middle" (See Figure 1). As an experienced establishment manager once said to one of the authors: "You must be mad to take a job like this. If you do what the bosses want then you'll alienate the staff; if you do what the staff are pressing for then you'll be in trouble with 'Them!'."

Well, managing in the frontline may be a form of madness, but it is exhilarating too if you can control the middle ground, set your goals and go for them.

Figure 1: *The frontline manager: piggy in the middle or creative central force?*

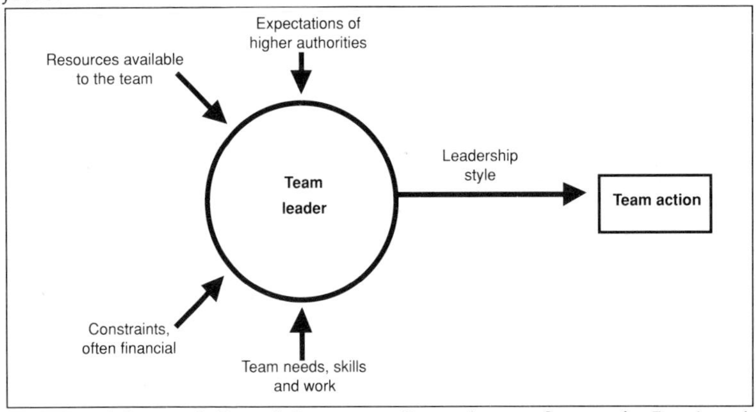

(From David Sines, ed, *Towards Integration: Comprehensive Services for People with Mental Handicaps*, Harper and Row, 1988).

Just as Peter Gilbert's book, *Mental Handicap: A Practical Guide for Social Workers,* was written as a primer for staff attracted to an increasingly specialised area of work, so this book is intended to be a down-to-earth manual, not only for the women and men in the middle, as team, establishment or service managers, but also practitioners who wish for a window on management; consumers of management or services who would like to see what they should be getting; and even senior managers with an eye on the horizons of the NHS and Community Care Act.

If there was ever a time when managers could rest on their laurels, it certainly isn't now. Impending changes include:

- The NHS and Community Care Act stemming from the Griffiths report, which many believe is more far-reaching than the Seebohm reorganisation of 1971.
- The increasing use of information technology to give and receive adequate information.
- The devolving of budgetary responsibility to frontline managers.
- "Multiple lines of accountability" in many new multi-agency projects, which require managers to have "double vision to see all steps in a project, both in tactical and strategic lights" (J Renshaw *et al,* 1988).
- An increasing pace of change, both within organisations and external to them.
- A stress on the business aspect of social care, rather than just professional practice.
- Managing within a cultural sea change of an increasing business imperative, while still coping with the demands of the political process and politicians who sometimes combine the mental acuity of J Danforth Quayle, the personal humility of Charles Dickens' Mayor Sapsea, and the veracity of Pinocchio.

Over the past decade managers have been attempting to improve the delivery of services through applying systems designed to increase integration and co-operation. The *Caring for People* White Paper (DOH 1989) has introduced a change of orientation towards a purposeful separation of services into care provision and care purchase, so as to enable consumers to have "a greater individual say in how they live their lives and the services they need to help them to do so". Part I of this book is designed to give the reader the historical and social context in which they have to operate.

While engaged in these transmutations, managers will be painfully aware that in social care we are still not getting the basics right. The Social Services Inspectorate report on day services (1989) made the following criticisms:

- Inadequate information for service planning.
- A lack of clarity on what the service should be about and knowledge about how it should be done.
- Senior and middle managers lacking specialist knowledge and unable to give proper support to the units.
- Staff left uncertain of their roles and tasks.
- A lack of understanding as to the nature of the educational process: how assessment leads to individual plans, activity and then review.
- Day services with no established tradition of staff supervision.
- Few unit managers have control over their budget or even knowledge as to the budget heads to which they should work.
- A general lack of formal induction to the organisation, leading to "sense of isolation" and " professional estrangement" from their department.
- Inadequate training.
- Parents and clients rarely involved in planning, which isn't very surprising as the staff themselves appear to have been marginalised.

In residential care the December 1989 independent enquiry by the Social Care Association into Patmos Lodge, spoke of "no effective leadership from those paid to manage", and when an NHS unit wished to introduce a leadership course it found the strengths and weaknesses in its staff group as follows:

Strengths	*Weaknesses*
Enormous goodwill.	Traditional attitudes and approach.
An intense desire to learn.	Inhibition.
Nursing training and qualifications.	Lack of imagination.
Comparable experience at ward level.	Ill-defined tasks and responsibilities.
Maturity.	Ineffectiveness because the students had not been encouraged to use their own initiative.

(see J Adair, 1973)

Ineffective management, unclear responsibilities and an inability to say "no" to impossible demands from above is not the perogative of social care. The Clapham rail disaster report of 8 November 1989, speaks of a "lack of communication which pervaded the department"; inadequate planning and supervision; a crippling recruitment and retention crisis; examples of "management by inactivity and inertia"; a slipshod style which led to crash errors". The report painted a picture of a middle management disorientated and demoralised by reorganisations and unable or unwilling to promote good standards below while resisting unrealistic demands from above.

A most ingenious paradox

"Expert management", states the Wagner committee "is essential for staff to be able to give of their best and ensure that quality services are achieved" (NISW, 1988 and Kelly and Beck, 1989). The challenge is to get expert management and real expertise, not just what Alistair Mant describes as "the risers . . . focused on competition and movement rather than the verities of life" (Mant, 1983). In Chapters 5 and 6 we discuss the essentials of management and how to be effective without losing your soul!

One director of social services has written that it is "the ability to cope with ambiguity and paradox" ("Open Forum" *Insight*, 24 May 1989), which marks out the successful manager, who, to misquote Stevie Smith, is waving not drowning. Mant describes two basic kinds of managers: "Binary", who are in a cut-throat survival mode, and "Ternary", whose power is regulated by some third force. These latter are people who ask for or develop a sense of purpose, who can cope with paradox and turn it to good ends.

To cope creatively, organisations and the individuals within them require a sense of direction and training to follow that road and subsequent avenues which present themselves. Professor Charles Handy and others have pointed out that Britain has far less top managers with qualifications than their main industrial rivals, and that we are only just beginning to take training for managers seriously. As organisations push accountability down the line there is an increased "need for more people to know the rudiments of business and to acquire the skills of management" (Handy *et al*, 1988).

In 1988 the Social Services Inspectorate published a study report on frontline managers (SSI, 1988). It found, in the words of one inspector, that "most of the management was intuitive with very able people managing against formidable odds". Such managers were not trained to fulfill their roles and operated in a policy vacuum. It is just this sort of lacuna which John Kelsall (1987) humorously describes as three styles of middle management for residential homes:

- The manager who only appears when something goes wrong.
- The VIP manager: "Direct contact with residents is as uncomfortable for him as a coffee stain on his new suit".
- The drop-in manager: "Should you . . . discuss your latest ideas about a residents' committee? . . . No, let him be, it would be unkind to disturb his game of snooker with the residents".

To do a good management job does not require someone to be Napoleon. Mant found that the bosses most people rate the best are those "who simply keep their eye on the ball, with a certain humility, but nonetheless grow in the fullness of time and in the eyes of others into charismatic giants". The manager today needs some guidelines on what they have to do, and some pointers on how to do it. This is what we have tried to set out in chapters 7 to 17. When Peter Gilbert was co-leading a diagnostic workshop on training with junior day and residential staff, they rated "supervision" as one of the prime requirements so that they could both receive and give a clearer lead and development. Middle managers will be the key people in initiating staff development programmes (see Figure 2, and chapters 8, 15 and 16).

Models of good practice are increasingly needed (eg Audit Commission, 1985, LGTB, 1984, and Renshaw *et al,* 1988) to stimulate a creative approach and to point the way forward. In Part III we have put forward a number of service models which we feel have made a contribution to the debate on service evolution, while highlighting some of the progress they themselves feel they need to make.

Redeeming defects

"Trust and credibility come through everyone's observation of the manager's symbolic integrity, not his or her 'policy document'". Tom Peters, *Thriving on Chaos.*

What type of manager, then, is required at such a time? In the '70s both the health and social services were proponents and victims of consensus management. In the '80s, the need for a more task-centred approach also let in the individual "raiders", at a time when business was prey to corporate raiders, and denegrated the patient "builders". Now, at a time when industry and commerce, and even government are attempting to rediscover values, social care is often found attempting to throw values overboard in a search for efficiency without effectiveness.

What good is it to talk to staff about "quality", if we ourselves, in the words of Oscar Wilde, "know the price of everything and the value of nothing"? Staff are not automatons and neither should managers be. The philosopher Friedrich Neitzsche wrote that "he who has a why to live by can bear almost any how". Harold MacMillan, speaking about the burden of office amidst private anguish, said that he saw a need for everyone bearing responsibility to have a strong belief system for "if you don't believe . . . you can't solve these problems and you can't even then survive them" (Alistair Horne, 1989). More recently, an NHS district general manager, on appointing someone to run his mental health service, remarked not only on the man's competence but on his value system — "a value system articulates the manager. Without it he becomes only a pragmatist" ("NHS stands on its own feet", Murray, 1988).

In the future a new form of consensus may emerge (Handy, 1989) where the "post-heroic" leader enables problems to be solved in a way that develops *other people's* capacity to function effectively and cope with future challenges, rather than build his

Figure 2: *The basic elements of a more coherent approach to staff development and training*

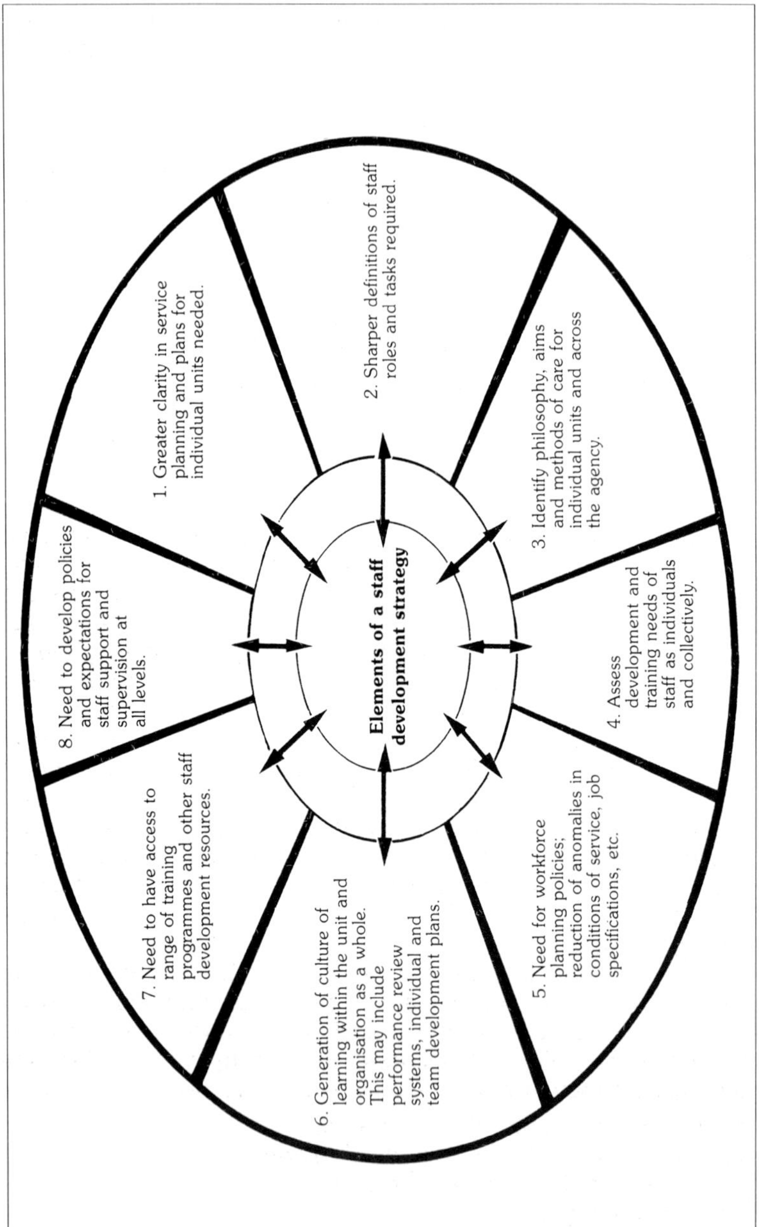

(From R Douglas and C Payne, 1988)

or her own ego. The Japanese successful form of bottom-up planning and quality circles has begun to exercise some leverage, and the SRU's *The Search for the Euro-Executive* indicates that flatter hierarchies and increasing communication through information technology may make co-operation, an understanding of different cultures, and the ability to move between cultures the dominant qualities in the 1990s. In this sense the "male" attributes expressed in Action-Centred Leadership (chapter 6) will need to be complemented and transformed by the "female" essence (chapter 12). Humaneness and humanness may once again become virtues. We may not wish to be the sort of person that Disraeli characterised Gladstone — having "not a single redeeming defect"!

Some of our barbarians are missing

"And some men have arrived from the frontiers
And they say that barbarians don't exist any longer.
And now, what will become of us without barbarians?
They were a kind of solution".
C P Cavafy

The history of mankind appears to demonstrate that we need enemies. In social care it has been easier to indulge in the collusion of NHS versus social services, and social services versus the independent sector, rather than engage in issues of quality (Russell, 1986). The White Paper, *Caring for People,* is aimed at freeing consumers of services from the "this is the menu, take it or leave it" attitude that has so often bedevilled social care. If consumers are freed then so must staff be in the sense that to stick to tasks in difficult times and come up with imaginative solutions to challenges, they must feel in control of their destinies. As one director remarked: "You have to push down enterprise in organisations as far as possible" (Murray, 1988). To remind us that services are there for the benefit of the users, not ourselves, we have interspersed the personal views of service users throughout the text.

In the volcanic changes that occur over the next decade and beyond, we will need a sense of history (see chapters 1 and 2), and yet, as Eugene Dillenbury preached, we must "make nostalgia a thing of the past". We will have to build up and build on the people we depend on, to make the social care which we espouse.

"Tell me where is the limit of the sea,
Tell me where is the limit of the horizon,
Tell me where is the limit of the sky,
And I will tell you
Where is the limit of the courage
Of my people".
Arnaldo Zenteno

John Adair (1973), *Action-Centred Leadership,* Gower.

DOH (1989), *Caring for People: Community Care in the Next Decade and Beyond,* HMSO, CM849.

Charles Dickens (1870), *The Mystery of Edwin Drood.*

Robin Douglas and Chris Payne (1988), *Organising for Learning,* NISW.

Peter Gilbert, *Mental Handicap: A Practical Guide for Social Workers, Community Care* (1985).

Sir Roy Griffiths (1988), *Community Care: Agenda for Action,* HMSO.

C Handy, C Gordon, I Gow and C Randlesome (1988), *Making Managers,* Pitman.

Charles Handy (1989), *The Age of Unreason,* Hutchinson.

Alistair Horne (1989), *MacMillan 1957-1986,* Macmillan.

Des Kelly and Martin Beck, "Pushed and pulled in all directions", "Home Front", *Community Care,* 3 August 1989.

John Kelsall, "Three styles of homes management", *Social Work Today,* 6 April 1987.

Local Government Training Board (1984), *Leadership in Local Government,* LGTB.

Alistair Mant (1983), *Leaders we Deserve,* Blackwell.

Nicholas Murray, "Encouraging enterprise", *Insight,* 29 November 1988.

NISW (1988), *Residential Care: A Positive Choice* (The Wagner report), HMSO.

Tom Peters (1987), *Thriving on Chaos,* Pan.

J Renshaw *et al* (1988), *Care in the Community: The First Steps,* PSSRU/Gower.

Oliver Russell, "Planning for quality" in Linda Ward ed. (1986), *Getting Better All The Time?,* Kings Fund Project Paper No.66.

SSI (1988), *Managing to Care: A Study of Firstline Managers in Social Services Departments in Day and Domiciliary Care,* Department of Social Services (Now Health).

SSI (1989), *Inspection of Day Services for People with a Mental Handicap,* Department of Health.

PART I
Social policy and social trends

"When I consider any social system that prevails in the modern world, I can't . . . see it as anything but a conspiracy of the rich to advance their interests under the pretext of organising society."
Thomas More, *Utopia*

"This is strategic management. You have to change the environment — otherwise the environment changes you!"
Professor Magdolna Csath, University of Budapest.

1

Bricks without straw: An historical perspective

"Many social services departments and voluntary groups grappling with the problems at local level certainly felt that the Israelites, faced with the requirement to make bricks without straw, had a comparatively routine and possible task."
Sir Roy Griffiths, *Community Care: Agenda for Action,* (1988)

"More than at any time in history, mankind faces a crossroads. One path leads to despair and utter hopelessness, the other to total extinction. Let us pray we have the wisdom to choose correctly."
Woody Allen

"A civilisation or society must be judged by the care it gives to its weakest and most under-priviledged members."
Mahatma Ghandi

"Those who forget the past are condemned to repeat it."
George Santayana

In January 1984 the influential House of Commons Select Committee on Social Services decided "to undertake an enquiry into community care". As the committee pointed out the phrase "Community Care" had "come to have such general reference as to be virtually meaningless".

The committee, chaired by Renée Short, received evidence from a wide variety of individuals and organisations, and also visited operational projects both at home and abroad. In a wide-ranging and hard-hitting, if at times rather impressionistic document, the committee placed community care policies accurately at a crossroads and exposed some of the platitudes surrounding it.

Assumptions had been made, for whatever reason, and on whatever grounds, that the closure of the Victorian hospitals and the transfer of care elsewhere would save money. The committee used a simple logic to demonstrate that an underfunded "mental disability service" could not be improved in any location without an injection of finance. "Proceeding with a policy of community care on a cost-neutral assumption", stated the committee, "is not simply naive it is positively inhuman". The Minister of Health himself admitted that "if you have some hospital facility in the past which has been greatly under-funded, if you transfer the function to community care, the cost will go up" (Para.21).

As the report makes clear "the almost obsessive concentration in public policy" on closing the institutions in the years since the implicit launch of that policy in 1961 (see below), had obscured the fact that about 80 per cent of children, and at least 40 per cent of adults with learning disabilities lived with their parents, with another significant proportion of adults living in their own homes or alternative non-hospital provision.

The committee recorded a "ground swell of opinion" expressing concern as to how the reality, as opposed to the rhetoric, was progressing. One representative of a voluntary body spoke graphically of the gulf between hospital and community services: "It seems to me it is like asking a passenger to jump off an elderly ship into the stormy sea with the assurance that the lifeboat will be along in a few months' time."

In the following year, the increasingly authoritative Audit Commission published *Making a Reality of Community Care.* With remorseless precision the commission put the bones on the flesh of the select committee's report and pinpointed a number of problems which constitute formidable obstacles to be overcome.

Funding

- Inadequate account taken of the shift in responsibilities from the NHS to social services.
- The Rate Support Grant system determines the expansion of community-based services by local authorities.
- Arrangements for jointly funding services by NHS and social services are flawed.
- The social security Income Support system pushes money towards the funding of residential care rather than care in people's own homes.
- Lack of "bridging finance" to allow community facilities to be built up as the hospital service ebbs.

Ironically the decrease in patient numbers in the old long-stay hospitals has seen a dramatic rise in both staff and costs and a high proportion of funds still tied up in the institutions, although anyone who worked in such hospitals will testify to the fact that staffing levels were very low. The lack of any national co-ordination of resource transfer for a relatively small number of people — 34,180 (in England and Wales) in 1986 — meant that resource allocation was always going to be uneven.

Organisational

- The structure of local community-based services is confused,

Figure 1.3.1: *Numbers and total public expenditure*

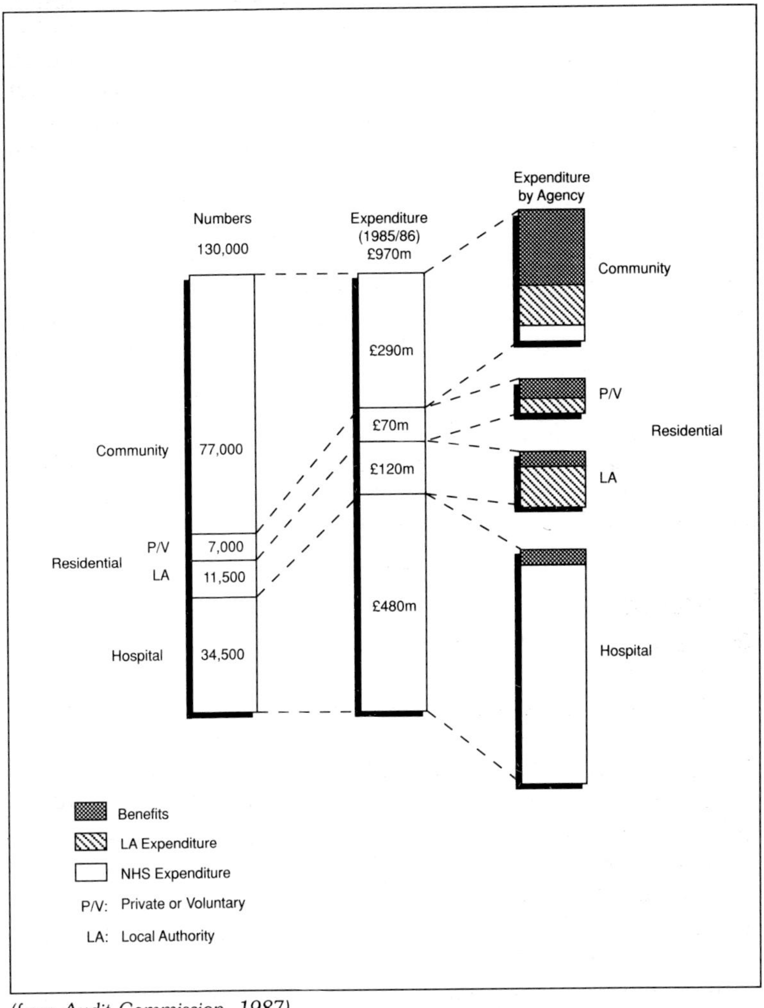

(from Audit Commission, 1987)

with responsibility and accountability for elements of the services fragmented between tiers of the NHS and within local government.

- The different planning cycles and styles of management between the NHS and social services.
- Competing priorities within the organisations, for example, child protection for SSDS and acute services for the NHS.

Inadequate Staffing

- Lack of a proper staff development and deployment policy.

Figure 1.3.2: *Principal agencies involved in community care*

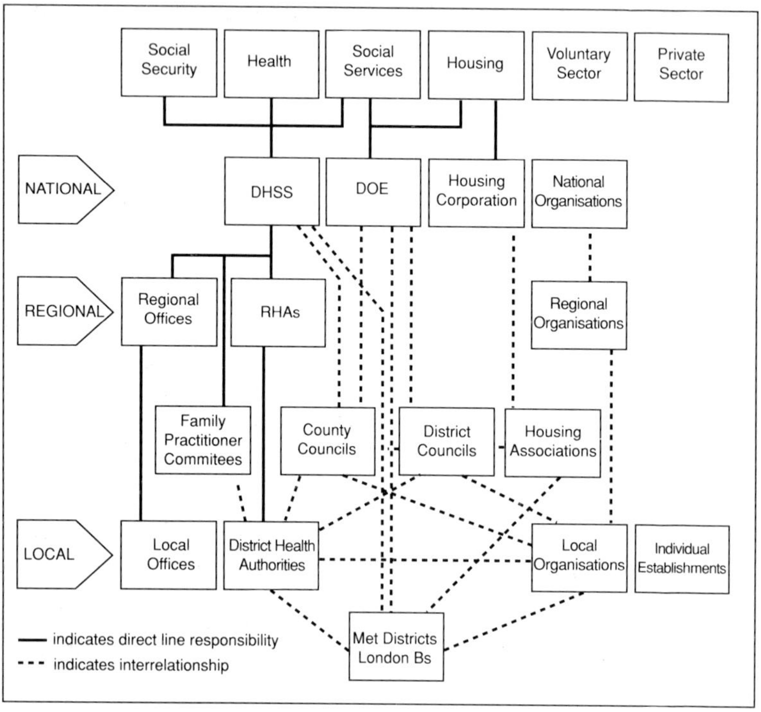

(The Audit Commission for Local Authorities in England and Wales, *Making a Reality of Community Care*, HMSO, 1986)

- Inattention to the number of remedial therapists required in the future.
- Difficulties in transferring groups of staff with one set of pay and conditions of service into a new service (see also Audit Commission, 1989, page 7).

The results of these barriers were threefold the Commission concluded. They were slow progress in developments, especially for people with a mental illness. An uneven response across the country — people receive a service based on the lottery of where they happen to live, not on what they need. And an unattractive prospect for the future — long-stay hospital provision is being reduced "at a significant rate"; community-based services are slow to expand; and in the resulting hiatus "there has been a shift in services from old, remote, long-stay hospitals to new long-stay residential homes, missing out a wider range of more flexible, more cost-effective forms of community care on the way".

The Audit Commission clearly felt that people with learning difficulties were a large enough and identifiable enough group for social policy in the late twentieth century to meet their requirements, but it had to admit: "The conclusion is inescapable: many authorities have a considerable distance yet to travel before community care becomes a local reality for mentally handicapped people".

The Ancient World

"When we attempt to answer the question 'what is history?' our answer, consciously or unconsciously, reflects our own position in time."

E.H. Carr, *What is History?*

When speaking of the ancient world it is all too easy to idealise or condemn. The reality is that in all societies throughout history the treatment of vulnerable people has depended on the prevailing philosophy of the time and the economic strength of the society involved. Classical texts are sometimes difficult to interpret whether mental illness or learning difficulty is meant, as most unusual behaviour is classed as "madness".

The Spartans, a warrior society, exposed all infants with disabilities on the hillside to die. The writings of Plato in Athens indicated a tolerance for unusual behaviour and a desire to retain the coherence of the family unit (see V. Ehrenberg, *From Solon to Socrates,* Methuen, 1968). Those who suffered from a mental disorder had their property safeguarded by the courts, and many citizens regarded strange utterings as a gift of the gods. Plato quotes Socrates as preaching that "the greatest blessings come by way of madness, indeed of madness that is heaven sent" (Plato, *Phaedrus*). By the fifth century BC however, the challenging of the old religious beliefs and a greater accent on personal power, wealth and display as the demonstration of virtue, meant that the mentally disordered lost their role in society and became objects of ridicule.

Jewish society also accorded some respect, even reverence, to those who were deemed to be uttering what might be prophecies. Mosaic Law recognised the appointment of guardians for those who were not in full possession of their faculties. A study of Jewish law shows how careful this society was to examine motives. For example, it was proposed that a man who tore his garments in public must be deranged, but it was pointed out that the person might be displaying grief, or be a cynic philosopher, exhibiting his contempt for material things?

The more utilitarian Romans appear to have kept "idiots" for amusement. (The word "idiot" is derived from the ancient Greek *idios,* meaning private or separate, signifying a person who could not converse and take part in public life in Greek society, but became *idiota* — an ignorant person — under the Roman state.)

The Koran states explicitly that adherents to the Muslim faith should "maintain them (those of weak understanding) and clothe them and speak kindly unto them". Recent archeological finds in Mexico indicate that the Olmec people, who inhabited that region from about 1500 BC to 300 AD may have viewed people with Down's Syndrome as bearing a mystical significance.

The findings from the ancient world are confusing, but appear to signify that in some societies people with learning difficulties were valued, if not for themselves, then for mystical properties attributed to them.

The Middle Ages and the Renaissance

"The age which gave European civilisation its impetus. Our intellectual energy, our contact with the great minds of Greece, our ability to move and change, our belief that God may be approached through beauty, our feeling of compassion, our sense of the unity of Christendom . . . . ."
Kenneth Clark, *Civilisation*

The synthesis of thought and purpose, described by Lord Clark, made the Middle Ages an unusually homogeneous age. "A common Latin culture and common religious beliefs, both inheritances of the past, brought men together" as Maurice Keen described it in *The History of Medieval Europe,* (Pelican, 1969).

Attitudes to people with learning difficulties were informed by New Testament precepts: "God's foolishness is wiser than human wisdom and God's weakness is stronger than human strength" (I Corinthinians 1, 25). Michael Bayley (1989) described the world view of the Middle Ages as "essentially corporative and co-operative". Society was meant, as in Biblical times, to care for the widow and orphan.

Stratford (1989) pointed to archaeological evidence that people with learning difficulties were cared for by the monasteries, which provided a national, or even international network of care. Those who were not able to live within their own communities were catered for by the monastic houses. (Villages in the surrounding countryside referred to these people as *Les Cretien* (Christians), hence the origin of the word cretins. Just as with "idiot", a term can so easily be transmuted from being neutral, or even approbatory, to the derogatory.)

This attitude, which was generally positive, though often tinged with superstition, continued on into the Rennaisance and beyond. Legal measures were taken to distinguish between mental illness (lunatics) and learning difficulty (idiots or natural fools) and protect their property in laws such as Edward II's *De Praerogativa Regis,* in England (see Appendix I). Paracelsus, a Swiss physician of the early sixteenth century, wrote that the "fool" might well not only be equal to other people in the eyes of God, but even superior, as their spontaneity could bring them nearer to God — "the wisdom that is also in fools, like light in a fog can shine through more clearly" (quoted in Ryan and Thomas, 1987). During the Renaissance a number of celebrated paintings with religious themes, feature children with learning difficulties; such a one is Mantegna's *Madonna and Child*, where the Christchild, Stratford remarks, is "undoubtedly a child with Down's Syndrome". As the author goes on to say, "the fact that such a painting could be produced says something about the prevailing attitudes at the time" (Stratford, 1989).

The Reformation – The Birth of Privatisation?

"A narrow line divides the Protestant ethic from the unacceptable face of capitalism".
Christopher Hill, *John Bunyan and his Church*

Table 1.1.1 *Historical attitudes and responses*

Images and attitudes	*Response*
Sub human Lacks the emotional and physical needs of normal people. Primitive and unpredictable behavour.	No rights. People with learning difficulties segregated and controlled.
Threat to society A weak mind in a strong body with potential for unpredictable behaviour and procreation	Control and segregation leading to a denial of freedom and possibly destruction.
The eternal child Catered for as children with no responsibilities and no rights.	Stress on care but not development.
Scapegoat Tolerated and cared for until society comes under pressure.	Segregated and perhaps killed at times of societal stress.
The uneconomic unit A burden on society.	Segregation into units to fit economics of scale and exploitation.
Burden on charity Judgement of weakness from a strong moralistic standpoint.	Basic needs are met in return for submission and gratitude.
Objects of pity Suffering individuals of whom no demands should be made.	Paternalistic. Shelter against risk. Low expectations.
Sick person Seen as sick and the passive recipient of medical care.	Hospital model of care with emphasis on diagnosis and prognosis.
Developing individual An optimistic view of the individual with potential for growth.	Stress on individuality, dignity and personal responsibility.
The unfulfilled hope Seen as not having met society's expectations after increased expenditure on education and training.	Return to antagonistic or paternalistic ideology.

As we have already noted, the treatment of vulnerable individuals is dependent on how society views them. In the sixteenth century the dominant world view of Christian philosophers such as Thomas Acquinas, what G.K. Chesterton, on his *A Meditation on the Manichees*, called a philosophy which is "entirely the praise of Life, the praise of Being", gave way to a fundamentally pessimistic view of mankind and the natural world, derived from a misuse of Augustinian doctrine and the heritage of Manichean heresy and neoplatonism. The Reformation period, while sweeping away much that was corrupt and repressive, set-up two new and contradictory gods of individualism and distrust of the material world.

In this context it is not surprising that, far from believing, as Paracelsus did, that childlikeness could be near to godliness, reformers such as Luther and Calvin preached that people with learning difficulties were filled with Satan, and that their birth was derived from sin by the parents, more particularly the mother. "The devil sits in changelings" proclaimed Luther, "where the soul should have been". He recommended drowning them at birth, and his attitude to the disabled and the burning of learned books looked forward to another cataclysmic movement in Germany some four centuries later (see Hallas, 1982 and Abbott and Sapsford, 1987).

All ideologists have a tendency to exaggerate their case, and all reform movements have unforeseen consequences. Shocked by the social upheaval in Germany, which was in part the parent and in part the child of his teaching, Luther retreated more and more to a privatised form of religion: "Therefore the first care of every Christian ought to be to lay aside all reliance on works, and to strengthen his faith alone more and more." As R.H. Tawney wrote, in his influential *Religion and the Rise of Capitalism*, this approach deepened faith "but it riveted on the social thought of Protestantism a dualism which, as its implications were developed, emptied religion of its social content and society of its soul".

Paupers and Poor Law

"The sluggard shall be clothed in Raggs. He that will not work shall not eat."
John Beller, 1696.

The dissolution of the monasteries destroyed the medieval welfare system at a time when the embryonic secular society was unable to provide a humane alternative. Monastic lands went in spoil to great landowners and the Crown, and increased the power of a wealthy élite. At the same time, the sixteenth and seventeenth centuries saw a pincer movement on the poor. On the one hand the great landowners started to enclose the common lands which deprived many cottagers of their means of living. This was presented as a religious duty to "save" the poor from themselves.

Concurrently the Vagrancy Acts attempted to stop these "masterless men" travelling to other parts of the country, but forced them to work for the great landowners — "getting on your bike" was not a virtue in the days of the Elizabethan Poor Law!

There was some toleration of unusual behaviour during the Civil War and Commonwealth, partly because religious and political groups often made their points in a demonstrative way. These groups often returned to a pre-Reformation view of the world in direct contradiction to the Puritans' normative stance. John Lilburne, the Leveller, suggested in 1646 that God "doth not choose many rich, nor many wise . . . but the fools, idiots, base and contemptable poor men and women in the esteem of the world".

When the Restoration came in 1660, however, "mental disorder" was classified with "social disorder" and shunned. The great landowners who had enclosed the land in the last hundred years now began to build their sculptured parks to impose order on nature.

A new institutional model for treating the poor and deviant was born out of a number of factors. There were the industrial and technological changes in agriculture, increased mobility of the population, and the unplanned growth in the major population centres — London grew eightfold between 1500 and 1650. There was also the breakdown of the old paternalistic relationships and an increase in "masterless men", as well as an underclass more visibly poor and more desperate. Then came the rising costs of parish welfare benefits, and a belief that these encouraged idleness. Lastly, there was the growth of the capitalist market system with its requirement for disciplined labour and its change in the nature of relationships, which, as Karl Marx put it "left no other nexus between man and man than naked self-interest" *(Critique of Political Economy)*.

The construction of the workhouses throughout Britain and America were meant to deter people from seeking assistance or, if they should seek it, then as Jeremy Bentham, the Utilitarian, put it a century later, it would act as a "mill to grind rogues honest and idle men industrious".

The regime was so harsh, that some, like the famous "Elephant Man" chose to exhibit themselves in touring fairs rather than remain in the institution. Many were swept up however, to languish within the workhouse walls. In the New York City institution in 1795, there were 622 inmates for a capacity of 300. Besides the poor and orphans there were 14 blind, "28 affected with lunacy, insanity and idiotism", as well as many with senile dementia (Skull, 1984).

Families with a dependent member came under increasing strain in the 18th century, despite its depiction as a "Golden Age". The novelist, Jane Austen, lived in an archetypal Georgian family, yet her biographer, David Cecil, tells us that she had a brother,

George, who "does not come into this story; he was mentally defective, and from an early age spent his life away from home". One Austen expert, Judith Tomlin, is of the opinion that "pre-Victorian practical attitudes would prevail. They would not conceal George, but he would drop out of family life at the moment it was realised he could not be trained to rigid social behaviour, or benefit from a classical education" (correspondence with the authors). George was fostered out, but the family kept in contact with him till he died. Charles Dickens, in *David Copperfield*, describes the character, Mr Dick, as a "natural" (that is, a "natural fool" from birth). It is David's aunt who steps in when "his own brother would have him shut up for life", in a "private asylum" (chapter 14 of the novel).

The crowding of workhouses with such a wide variety of dependent people led, in the view of Parry-Jones (1972), "to an increasing dependence on the system of contracting-out by parishes to private madhouses". Concern over the treatment of the "insane poor" and "idiots" led to the appointment in 1807 of a Parliamentary select committee. The opinion of this body was that the treatment of inmates of these private establishsments was dependent "wholly upon the good conduct of the keeper" as there was no system of inspection (quoted in Parry-Jones, 1972). In America, people with a learning difficulty were often auctioned off to the highest bidder amongst the private home owners.

One concerned proprietor, Thomas Bakewell, reflected on his experiences thus:

"Tis there that wasting age retires
To wait till painful life expires.
Go, look within the ample space
Where cold damp vapours fill the place.
There see the idiots vacant stare, and th' wild maniacs frantic glare
Where tho' strong chains the body bind
No fetters can restrain the mind".

The rise of the asylum

"The beauty also of the sight of the asylum looking out on the free downs which are ever changing their distance and their shape as the lights and cloud-shadows sail on them, and over the graceful forms of those endless variety of slopes, the eye wanders . . . within an entrancing feeling of fullness and a restful satisfaction of the pure sense of form".
The superintendent of St Francis' Hospital (The Sussex Asylum) Report dated Christmas Day 1859 (East Sussex county archives).

The superintendent's "sense of form" is very much a reflection of the then prevalent Chartesian philosophy. Descartes viewed the world and human beings as mechanisms subject to scientific laws. As Rothman (1971) evinces, the great asylums were designed to be curative by their very architectural conception.

It was Lord Shaftesbury who led a sustained campaign in Parliament for a reform of the mental health laws and for proper provision to be made. Since the County Asylum Act of 1808 only nine counties had built specialist institutions. In 1845 Shaftesbury urged Parliament that such vulnerable people "should not be the subjects of financial speculation" and again in 1859, he told the House of Commons Select Committee that private asylums were "utterly abominable and indefensible", and that "the principle of profit vitiates the whole thing". He looked to grant-supported asylums that would create an "admirable, sound and efficient system" (quoted in T. Philpot, "Lord Shaftesbury, and the reform of the lunacy laws", *Nursing Mirror,* 2 November 1973).

The 1845 Lunatics Act made it mandatory for each county to have its own asylum and brought in procedures for certification of patients and inspection of establishments. While many people with learning difficulties took places in the new asylums, a parallel movement was developing to provide specific facilities for "idiots". In 1801 Jean Marie Itard published his treatise on the education of the "wild boy of Aveyron". His pupil Edouard Seguin took these educational methods forward in his work as physician at the Vicetre Hospital in Paris, and in the publication of his *The Moral Treatment, Hygiene and Education of Idiots and Other Backward Children* (1846). Seguin emigrated to the USA in 1848, and carried on his pioneering works. In one of his later publications can be found an echo of earlier Christian writings: "An idiot is endowed with moral nature and is influenced by the same things as the rest of humanity." And one enduring statement: "Before entering further into the generalities of training, the individuality of the child is to be secured; for respect of individuality is the first test of the fitness of a teacher" *(Idiocy and its Treatment by the Physiological Method,* 1866).

Table 1.1.2: *Total patients in public asylums in England and Wales, 1850-1930 and rate/10,000 People*

Year	*Patients*	*Rate/10,000*
1850	7,140	4.03
1860	15,845	7.96
1870	27,109	12.05
1880	40,088	15.73
1890	52,937	18.34
1900	74,004	23.05
1910	97,580	27.49
1920	93,648	24.84
1930	119,659	30.14

(*Annual Reports of the Lunacy Commissioners* (1850-1910); *Annual Reports of the Board of Control* (1920-1930). London:/Skull, 1984)

In Britain a small "school for idiots" was set up in Bath in 1846, and the following year an "asylum for idiots" was founded in

Highgate under influential patronage. A report in 1850 on its progress compares the neglect often found in home life with no domiciliary help and the benefits of the educational approach (see Ryan and Thomas, 1987, chapter 5).

The county asylums and the new educational establishments aimed to reform and improve, to protect those with disabilities from the rigours of the outside world and shield society from sights it found too grievous to bear close contact with. As Shakespeare says:
"A wretched soul, bruised with adversity,
We bid be quiet when we hear it cry."

Seguin warned that the educational goals he advocated could only be achieved in small groups. The warning was not heeded, and the establishments of all kinds expanded while their isolation from the community at large increased. The Highgate asylum is a good case in point. Moving to an imposing position near Redhill, Surrey, in 1855, and renamed the Royal Earlswood, after being officially opened by Prince Albert, it swelled to 561 inmates by 1881. The charitable "asylums for idiots" such as Starcross in Devon (1864), and the Northern Counties at Lancaster (1868), together with public provision like Darenth (1878), took on a life of their own. Increased public fear of mental disorder exemplified by Charlotte Bronte's *Jane Eyre* and/or those who were their custodians, such as in Wilkie Collins, *The Woman in White*, exercised a mounting influence over the public mind, exemplified in the 1890 Lunacy Act, which Kathleen Jones calls "the triumph of legalism" (Jones, 1972).

As the numbers of people in institutions grew, there occurred in the late 19th and early 20th centuries what Wolfensberger (1975) calls "the loss of rationales" and Rothman (1971) "the enduring institution".

If the old hospitals fill us with horror today, and if asylum has become a perjorative term, it is well to remember the 1984 Select Committee's softer judgement on the past: "So far from representing a denial of care, the great asylums signified Victorian social concern, however misguided it may appear today . . . they also represented what was in retrospect an astonishing commitment of money, on staff and building . . . we are under a moral obligation at least to match the degree of commitment shown by earlier generations."

Eugenics: Segregation and "The Final Solution"

"'It's what any state medical service has sooner or later got to face. If you are going to be kept alive in institutions run by and paid for by the state, you must accept the state's right to economise when necessary . . . '"

The Nazi sympathiser in Graham Greene's, *The Ministry of Fear.*

In 1864 there were approximately 400 people with learning difficulties in specialist establishments. This number grew to 2,000 by 1914 but was dwarfed by the overall number, estimated at 29,452, to be found in all public institutions by 1881. It grew steadily in every year thereafter.

In the latter part of the nineteenth century the eugenics movement became a powerful force, arguing for the segregation and sterilisation of "mental defectives". Not only specialists in the field, but the philosopher Bertrand Russell, and politicians like Winston Churchill, flirted with its tenets. People with learning difficulties were seen as being inherently inferior and bestial, and having heightened criminal and immoral tendencies. In America, similar ideas were expressed between the 1850s and 1930s, with some going so far as to say:

"It is not a pessimistic view of life to wish to see a man get out of the world, who is not fit for it, and who has little or no chance of ever becoming so. To one who anticipates the general upward trend of human life, it is evident that the occasional removal by society of an individual, or even of many individuals, may be necessary for the welfare of the social group".

And:

"A misguided philanthropy is persuading us to expend vast sums of money that have been earned by the capable and worthy in the care and perpetuation of those classes which neither our reason nor out judgement would pronounce to be fitted to survive".

(Karl Schwartz, 1908, quoted in M. Rosen *et al*, ed., *The History of Mental Retardation, Collected Papers*, Volume 2, University Park Press, 1976).

The State of Indiana passed the first sterilisation law in 1907 and by the mid-1940s that law had been upheld by the Supreme Court. More than 20 states permitted such operations, and widescale eugenic sterilisations were performed in California.

In Britain the rationale behind the eugenics movement appears to have been a combination of factors:

- ☐ The Social Darwinism of the mid-eighteenth century, as developed by Darwin's half-cousin, Sir Francis Galton. The latter's theory was that defective genes would produce an increased number of criminals and "moral defectives". In 1908 Galton became president of the Eugenics Education Society.
- ☐ Work by Dr Langdon Down (discoverer of Down's Syndrome), proposed that infants born with "Mongolian" features were evidence of racial degeneracy.
- ☐ With the development of classification procedures, such as the Binet Intelligence Test, and with increased longevity in the population, together with the existence of special institutions, more people with learning difficulties were being identified. The Education Acts of 1870, 1876 and 1880 brought in compulsory education which immediately identified those who could not cope.

- ☐ The Boer War had uncovered a large number of citizens unfit for active service. This coupled with Victorian beliefs in British racial superiority induced a sense of national paranoia.
- ☐ The rising cost of special facilities brought the demands for spending to be controlled by one means or another.

The 1913 Mental Deficiency Act steered a careful course between care and control. It created four classifications, placed a duty on local authorities to ascertain the numbers of "mental defectives" within their area, provide suitable institutions, and set up supervision in the community.

Increased classification resulted in a gradual improvement in services, but also increased visibility. The depression of the 1920s and 1930s put considerable pressure on priorities for spending, and with 50,000 people with learning difficulties in specialist institutions (called colonies), and a further 59,000 in Poor Law and psychiatric establishments (Jones, 1972 and Office of Health Economics/Mencap, 1986), questions were asked about the costs of such care provision.

The eugenics movement reached its apotheosis with the rise of Nazi Germany. In 1933 the Nazi regime had introduced a sterilisation law. Writings by jurists and psychiatrists had already created the moral climate where individuals had to justify their lives as worthwhile, according to criteria imposed by society at large. It was proposed that it should be made legal to kill those with incurable handicaps who were "a burden on the community". The relief from suffering was closely interwoven with the removal of "worthless life". Gas chambers were set up in six mental hospitals, and 72,000 people with mental illness and learning difficulties murdered (Jeremy Noakes, "Social outcasts in the Third Reich", in R. Bessel ed., *Life in the Third Reich*, Oxford University Press, 1987).

Although it would be nice to think that "it couldn't have happened here", the historical evidence of influential opinion; eugenic propaganda films with an explicit message of segregation and extermination; British concerns with rising costs and racial fitness; the American moves on sterilisation and the British invention of the modern concentration camp in the Boer War, give the historian cause for doubt.

Care in the community as a policy

"Mentally handicapped children and adults should not be segregated unnecessarily from other people of similar age, nor from the general life of the local community."
Better Services for the Mentally Handicapped, DHSS, 1971.

The horror of the German experience reinforced an already growing belief that the British way of life was of the whole community — the lion and the lamb — lying down together. *The Times* proclaimed in the weeks after Dunkirk: "If we speak of democracy, we do not mean a democracy which maintains the right to vote but forgets the right to work and the right to live. If we speak of freedom, we do not mean a rugged individualism which excludes social organisation and economic planning."

Films designed to boost morale, such as the Basil Rathbone *Sherlock Holmes* series, always stressed the British care of the poor and weak as compared to Germanic "might is right".

Yet the hospitals, as Pauline Morris' extensive survey *(Put Away,* 1969) showed, were increasingly isolated from their local communities. Less and less residents had contact with their families, and the absorption of the local authority institutions into the NHS in 1949 had done little to bring mental handicap services into the mainstream of medical advances. Most hospitals were of 2000 beds or more, some were in huge clusters such as the Epsom group, with St Ebba's and The Manor, linked in a huge circle with three psychiatric hospitals.

The enquiries into the ill-treatment of patients in Ely Hospital near Cardiff in 1969 showed both individual acts of cruelty and the general failings of the hospital system. Other enquiries followed, notably at Normansfield, South London, and South Ockenden, Essex. A view emerged that, though those with disturbed and psychiatric problems might need hospital treatment, the vast majority of people with learning difficulties could live in more homely settings.

A series of reports, laws and research studies, combined with a gradual movement of talented and dedicated people into the service, induced many people to see a continual path of progress.

- ☐ The Brooklands project, by Professor Jack Tizard, demonstrated what Seguin had maintained a century before that progress was possible for individuals if they were given the right environment.
- ☐ The White Paper, *Better Services for the Mentally Handicapped* (1971), painted a comprehensive picture of services and set down the targets to be achieved for future progress.
- ☐ The Education Act of 1971 brought children with severe learning difficulties into the education system for the first time since the late nineteenth century. The Education Act of 1981 put the onus on education authorities to provide integrated education unless there were pressing reasons not to.
- ☐ The National Development Group was formed to give advice in areas such as services for children and day care (see Appendix I).
- ☐ The Court report (1976), Warnock report (1978) and Jay report (1979), though concerned with specific issues

concerning disability, all spoke of the need to relate to people with severe difficulties as "people first and handicapped second", and that services should reflect this philosophical premise.

- ☐ Influential research such as Michael Bayley's in Sheffield, illustrated the strains on families and gave useful pointers to alleviate such stress (*Mental Handicap and Community Care*, Routledge & Kegan Paul, 1973).
- ☐ The government brought in the All-Wales Strategy in 1982 and showed what political will could do if it really wanted to.
- ☐ The Green Paper on *Care in the Community* (1983) made a number of proposals on funding mechanisms.
- ☐ The work of Nirje in Sweden, Bank-Mikkleson in Denmark, and Wolfensberger in the USA, brought forward a new (or rediscovered) philosophy called "normalisation". This set out to let people with learning difficulties "obtain an existence as close to the normal as possible". "Normalisation means to experience the normal rhythm of the year, with holidays and family days of personal significance . . . Children should have available warmth of atmosphere, rich sensory stimulation and surroundings, and settings of proper proportions" (Bengt Nirje, 1969). Often misunderstood, and now in its reinterpretations giving more stress to "value" than "normality" it has been the dominant ideology of the 1970s and 1980s.
- ☐ Spending by local authorities on capital developments reached a peak in the middle 1970s.

As we saw in the nineteenth century, legislation was usually the result of a 40 or 50 year cycle of social concern. In the late twentieth century this cycle has telescoped, often with wild fluctuations, such as with the case of child protection, between the liberty of the subject, protection of the vulnerable and protection for society.

In the mid 1980s, the dominant consensus was that " care in the community is a good thing". But while the BBC's shocking *Silent Minority* film on conditions in St Lawrence's Hospital, Caterham, Surrey, and other mental handicap hospitals, shattered any remaining illusions that hospital care was beneficial, severe doubts began to creep in about care in the community policy and practice (see figure 1.3.3). Newspaper reports began to focus not on ill-treatment in hospital, but neglect in the community, and a notorious *Brass Tacks* edition in 1986 depicted a completely biased portrait of services and hospital discharge procedures in the North West of England. RESCARE was founded with an aim to convert hospitals into "village communities" (see Tonkin, 1987).

In 1990 the concept of community care is still very much that described by Jones *et al* (1978): "To the politician, community is a useful piece of rhetoric; to the sociologist it is a stick to beat institutional care with; to the civil servant it is a cheap alternative to institutional care which can be passed to the local authorities for action or inaction; to the visionary, it is a dream of the new society in which people really do care; to social services departments it is a nightmare of heightened public expectations and inadequate resources to meet them. We are only beginning to find out what it means to the old, the chronic sick and the handicapped".

Lessons from America

"They're so fond of Liberty in this part of the globe, that they buy her and sell her and carry her to market with 'em. They've such a passion for Liberty, that they can't help taking liberties with her . . . "

Charles Dickens, *Martin Chuzzlewit*

It is often said that ten years after America has pursued a particular path, Britain follows. Certainly the pattern of services for people with a mental illness or learning difficulty is clearly mirrored in its development on both sides of the Atlantic.

Just as in Britain, the American and Canadian hospitals were built in isolated settings because the dominant paradigm was that expressed by Edward Jarvis in his 1855 text, *Insanity and Idiocy in Massachusetts*, that "the Hospital should not be surrounded by and near the stimulating affairs of city life". As Rothman (1971, 1980) has written, reformers during the Jackson presidency in the nineteenth century, believed that everybody could be rehabilitated with a single programme, within the well-ordered routine of the asylum.

In the late 1960s and early 1970s there occurred what Dear and Wolch (1987) have termed "a golden consensus":

"A steam roller policy of deinstitutionalisation occurred without prior development of community-based service systems or proper preparation of communities that were expected to receive and support the flood of clients. Service-dependent clients escaped the undesirable effects of the total institution, but were left to fend for themselves in the community".

As Skull has demonstrated, the need to cut welfare spending as the numbers of dependent people, especially the frail elderly, increased, produced a policy of deinstitutionalisation. Many discharged patients drifted into what has been called the "zone of transition" between the central business district and the more affluent residential areas from which they were excluded. American research appears to show that poorer districts with a more transient population are more likely to be tolerant than well-off and stable communities, which have a NIMBY (not-in-my-back-yard) attitude. In the transitional areas, public and private facilities were set up attracting more vulnerable people and creating "service-dependent population ghettos". As in Britain, a few years later, there was a rapid growth in private placements. Between 1969 and 1974, the private long-term health care sector absorbed an increase of more than 48 per cent in its mentally disabled population. The financing of this was mainly through central government funding, which saved individual states the necessity of refurbishing their facilities. Under President Reagan, however, central funding was cut and benefit rules and responsibilities were transferred so rapidly between federal government, state and county that individuals fell through the net each time the system changed. Changes in income support and housing benefit in Britain, over the past two years, have produced a similar effect here, and the funding changes from April 1991 may well have a further knock-on effect.

As Jones (1988) points out, both professional and public expectations in the 1970s were too high and disappointment invariably followed. The system of board-and-care homes, which developed in response to the availability of federal social security benefits, provided conflicts between the profit motive and individual needs for homely environments. Although there are excellent examples of service systems in the USA; positive consequences of a clear lead agency responsibility in Canada; and effective case management systems, many British visitors speak of an increasing tendency to "warehouse" service users in large private institutions which are more cost effective. A number of American states have no registration and inspection system, while one put the licensing and inspection of board-and-care homes in the hands of its state Department of Agriculture! This aggregation of care is also mirrored in Britain where large conglomerates are increasing their hold on the private sector market, especially in the case of elderly people.

As American inner city areas were gentrified the homeless were moved on and out. In effect, they are only entitled to land which is as vulnerable as they are, and as Frederic Engels pointed out in his tract *The Housing Question* (1887), capitalism does not set out to solve problems but only to move them elsewhere for "the same economic necessity which produced them in the first place produces them in the next place also".

Many mentally disabled people have been deinstitutionalised only to be misassigned to prisons which have become the "poor man's mental hospital". Others drift out of yuppified inner cities and are shunned by the surrounding suburbs. They have become a kind of North American "boat people", a modern version of the Narrenschiff or "ship of fools" seen in medieval times, and probably accorded more dignity in those days.

Larry Gostin, former legal director of MIND, has recently complained that the United States government has taken a conscious decision to provide "no care". Many social scientists in America now see reinstitutionalization as likely to become the new policy. In some states this is already occurring. A shelter for the homeless was built recently on an isolated island in New York City with a service capacity of 180. During 1985 it sheltered more than 800 people daily, in a way reminiscent of the overcrowding of the New York almshouse in the late eighteenth century (see Skull, p37). Dear and Wolch (1987) envisage that at the end of the twentieth century, we will either discover that we have a new "landscape of haunted places", reflecting the rebirth of the institution, or a "landscape of despair" filled with the misery of homeless and rootless people. In their description of California they describe the homeless as sleeping "next to the ocean at the continent's edge, a little distance from a tide that could sweep them away. This portrait of the landscape of despair presages the collapse of the human-service system and an abandonment of those in need. The lucky and resourceful who manage to survive hang on by their fingernails at the edge of society".

Just as the weight of opinion in Britain is firmly against a fully American-style health service, the experience across the water gives some indication of what might be expected if we made a gadarene rush towards a laissez-faire American system of social welfare.

Retreat from responsibility – Central government

"Power without responsibility — the prerogative of the harlot down the ages".
Variously attributed

The long-running ambulance workers' dispute of 1989/90 was a good example of the present government's attitude towards power and responsibility. Ostensibly the NHS management were in control of negotiations with the ambulance unions, but in fact the government pulled the strings. A television programme in 1989 on the dearth of social education centre places in Avon County Council had a similar theme. The panel of officials and politicians facing an angry group of parents managed to hand the blame for the current situation from one to another: the social services officers stated that the provision of places was a political decision; the local politicians pleaded a lack of finance from central government; while the MP neatly evaded responsibility by proclaiming that local politicians always resisted earmarked grants from central government because it restricted their local decision making!

The attitude of the New Right is that, in Nicholas Ridley's words, "the proper role of government is nothing", and this has led to the privatisation of many public utilities and to an increasing accent on private health and social care services. Although there is no enforced contracting out of social services functions in the White Paper *Caring for People,* the implication is clear that unless local authorities take action to encourage "a flourishing independent sector" then further legislation will enforce change.

"Victorian values" are often held up as the true beacon to which one should aspire. It should be remembered, however, that the Victorians themselves may not have viewed their value system in the same light as the Thatcher government. The novelist and traditionalist, Anthony Trollope mused that: "Buying and selling is good and necessary . . . but it cannot be the noblest work of man; and let us hope that it may not in our time be esteemed the noblest work of an Englishman" *(Doctor Thorne)*

The Victorian mayor of Birmingham, Joseph Chamberlain, persuaded the corporation to buy up gas and water from the private contractors and urged government responsibility for the "welfare, the health, the comfort and the lives" of Britain's town dwellers (R. Jay, *Joseph Chamberlain,* Oxford University Press, 1981). It was clear to many local government leaders at the time that private ownership of public utilities, especially when they were monopolies, acted against the public interest, and that philanthropy could not provide the education system which Britain needed to advance technologically, socially or morally. "It is one of the paradoxes of the history of Victorian England", writes Derek Fraser, professor of history at the University of California, "that a society wedded to the principles of self-help, nevertheless created an administrative state with broad social and economic functions" ("Joseph Chamberlain and the municipal ideal", *History Today,* April 1987).

Lord Shaftesbury proclaimed a national responsibility for the mentally ill, while Chamberlain saw it as the "duty of all classes in the community to co-operate for the common good". It is significant that in the 1920s commentators from all shades of political opinion agreed that the nation's housing needs could not be satisfied by the private sector, and in the 1940s it was equally clear that the great charitable hospitals were heading towards bankruptcy. The National Assistance Act of 1948 was hailed by *The Times*: "Today the British people join together in a single national friendly society for mutual support during the common misfortunes of life. The National Assistance Act winds up half a millenium of social history by finally burying the Poor Law" (5 July 1948).

In 1990 the government is keen, like a dog "to a bone" to dig it up again!

In the year's debate following the publication of Sir Roy Griffith's *Agenda for Action* (1988), one of the proposals was that by the right-wing think tank, the Adam Smith Institute. This report proposed a national community care agency which would scrutinise the care manager's assessment, determine entitlement, and then allow the individual to use the internal market to procure the best and most economic form of care available to them (M. Pirie and E. Butler, *Extending Care*, Adam Smith Institute, 1989). This relatively neat solution was not accepted, at least partly because it would have focused too much attention on the decision-making of central government. Much better for government to lay down policy, undertake inspections, but ensure that the responsibility for denying a particular service is left in the hands of local officers and politicians. The spirit of Pontius Pilate is alive and well and living in SW1!

In an apparent contradiction of this trend, the NHS and Community Care Act erodes the voice of local politicians who will no longer have set places on the boards of district health authorities. Those places will now be filled by appointees, presumably those who are "ideologically sound". There were also strong rumours following the 1987 general election that the government was toying with the idea of abolishing the county councils, whose association had too often questioned governmental policies. The trend then is towards a derogation of local democracy with a tightening of central government control; this is camouflaged by a contracting-out of actual services so that credit can be claimed for success and responsibility denied for any failures — the "Who me, Ref?" style of government.

If the present government stays in power well into the 1990s, much will depend on how much more of "the family silver" (as Harold Macmillan called it) it wishes to retain and whether it can transform itself into the "One Nation" party which Disraeli attempted to promote in 1846:

". . . In an age of political materialism, of confused purposes and perplexed intelligence, that aspires only to wealth because it has no other accomplishment . . . Toryism will yet arise from the tomb . . . to bring back strength to the Crown, liberty to the Subject, and to announce that power has only one duty — to secure the social welfare of the people" *(Sybil)*.

Retreat from responsibility – The NHS

"Resources spent caring for people inappropriately in hospital are misapplied and could be put to better use elsewhere. There is however a danger that the resources released will be used for other and more immediately rewarding or "attractive" client groups, and that the most disabled will be neglected".
House of Commons Select Committee, *Community Care*, (1985)

The irony surrounding the so-called "priority services" within the NHS, the people with long-term health needs, is that they do not and never have received priority. The "acute services", especially those requiring high-tech skills such as heart surgery, carry more clout both within the health service and outside it.

The 1974 reorganisation of the NHS "did not provide well-integrated care for clients with long-term needs" (see Renshaw *et al*, 1988) and pressures to develop high-cost acute services; the lower status of doctors in the continuing care field; and the growing realisation that the NHS could not meet all the needs presented to it, led to a gradual retreat from the long-term care of elderly infirm people and those with mental disabilities (see Jones, 1988, chapter 2). New Right thinkers began to urge the nation to "find salvation in the market" in private insurance schemes, as Arthur Seldon had said, but as Titmuss (himself an insurance expert) cautioned, "the evidence, particularly from the United States and Canada", suggested that people with continuing care needs were "categorised as 'bad risks' and treated as second-class consumers" (Titmuss, 1968).

Figure 1.3.3: *Result of hospital non-admission policy*

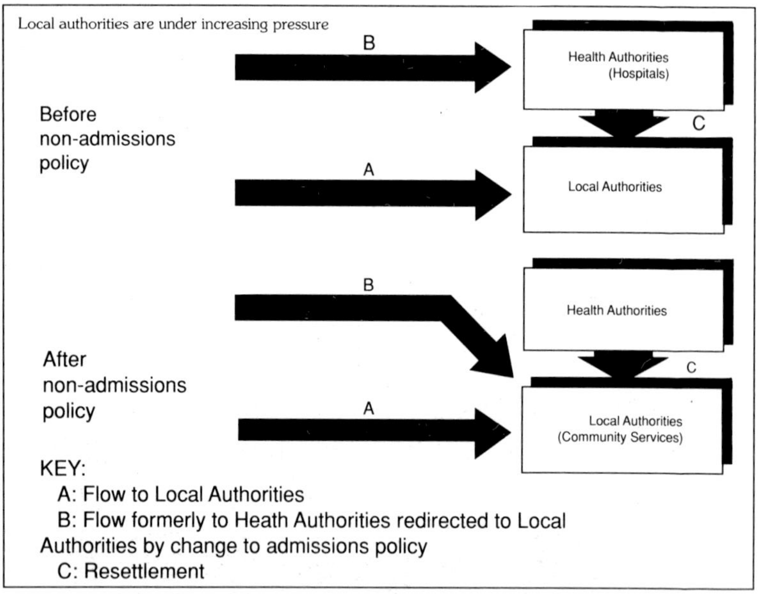

(From Audit Commission, 1987)

The NHS and Community Care Act is driving both hospitals and GP services towards an accent on acute medicine and away from those who have long-term needs. Local authorities have for some time doubted whether the revenue and the capital freed up by the closure of long-stay hospitals would be used for alternative services in the community. Some district health authorities have actually transferred large sums of revenue from community to acute services without consultation with social services colleagues as to its effect (Association of County Councils,

Caring For People — Making a Reality of Community Care, June 1989). Health authority managers in their turn have had to struggle with the government's annual claim that it is pouring money into the NHS but with so-called "cost improvement programmes" in reality biting deep into current services (*Efficiency in the NHS*, Kings Fund, 1989).

As the long-stay hospitals have contracted more clients and carers look to local authority provision. This has placed an "increasing burden" on local authorities (Audit Commission, 1987). This is shown graphically in the diagram below.

Social services have lost out in a number of ways. They have taken on schemes founded on dowries (support payments from a health authority to an SSD to "follow" the former resident into the community) which are either not in perpetuity or not sufficiently inflation-proofed. They are obliged to provide for those people who would have gone into health service care up to a few years ago. Most social services estimate that they now spend hundreds of thousands of pounds each year supporting very disabled people in private and voluntary sector homes "without any extra finance to meet their increased work load" (Audit Commission, 1987).

Figure 1.3.4: *Number of residential places in England*

Community places are not compensating for the loss of hospital beds

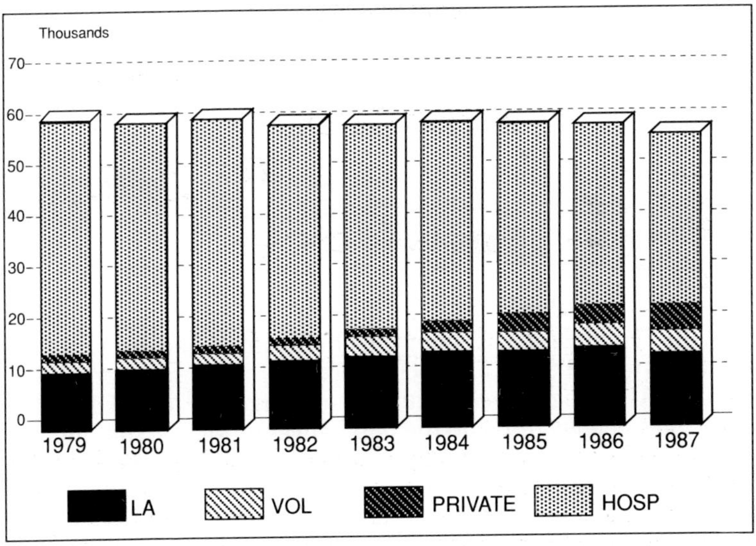

(Audit Commission, 1989)

Some large hospitals, especially those in regions such as South West Thames, where there is an inadequate funding transfer policy, have been placing residents directly into the private sector to obtain lower costs, without any arrangement either with the local authority of origin or of placement. If services are required in the future then the local authorities are left to fight it out as to who picks up the bill.

A number of regional health authorities, such as South East Thames and North Western, have very clear funding policies. Others such as South West Thames are purely opportunistic. In its 1987 regional conference on learning difficulty at Surrey University, the South West Thames Regional Health Authority explained its policies as "chasing the financial loophole".

Many directors of social services are clearly concerned at the combination of the two White Papers, which, as one remarked, will "stack the odds strongly in favour of acute medicine" ("Open Forum", *Insight*, 6 December 1989). Health authorities will no longer have local authority reps on their boards under the new system, and the opportunity to define "health care" and "social care" was missed in *Caring for People.*

The channelling of monies for residential care through local authorities from 1993, however, should at least ensure that health authorities are not able to place residents from long-stay hospitals without the involvement of social services departments.

Rhetoric and reality

"The fortunate and the proud wonder at the insolence of human wretchedness, that it should dare to present itself before them, and with the loathsome aspect of its misery presume to disturb the serenity of their happiness".
Adam Smith, *The Theory of Moral Sentiments.*

"Confronted with such people our natural instinct frequently will be fear, combined possibly also with helplessness . . . Then something is born in us . . . and maybe we discover the great gift of the poor — that they reveal our own poverty".
Jean Vanier

Sir Roy Griffiths, in his letter which accompanied his report to the Secretary of State for Social Services, on 12 February 1989, stated: "At the centre, community care has been talked of for 30 years and in few areas can the gap between political rhetoric and policy on the one hand, or between policy and reality in the field on the other hand, have been so great."

As we have seen throughout this chapter, the welfare of people with learning difficulties has been ever-dependent on the values of a particular society, its economic viability, and the need to identify scapegoats. As Ryan and Thomas assert in the new edition of their thought-provoking book: "The history of mental handicap demonstrates how easily the best-intentioned reforms can turn to repression, especially in conditions of economic stringency and hardening social attitudes, such as those we are witnessing now".

Table 1.1.1 sets out some of the attitudes prevalent in difficult times and the service responses to them. One strand of thought is often a direct reaction to another. In 1990 we can look about us and see some excellent schemes proving conclusively that the most disabled people can be supported in community settings (see P Cambridge and M Knapp ed, 1988). Some of these particular schemes, however, were specially funded by central government grants so the financial implications of their success need careful study.

Community care only becomes a reality if the community cares, as we consider in chapter 3. The most authoritive recent studies by Martin Bulmer (1987) and Ray Snaith's research for the Department of Health (1989), speak of a reality "vacuum" at the heart of community care policies:

"Much of the political rhetoric which surrounds the idea of community or neighbourhood care still assumes, as the 1969 Good Neighbour Campaign did, that there are good neighbours waiting in the social undergrowth and simply needing authoritative call to action" (R Snaith, 1989).

The Snaith study is emphatic, not only that "the highly intensive, tightly knit version of informal help has been lost", but it is right that we don't attempt to return to a rose-coloured version of *Larkrise to Candleford.*

In 1982 Pope John Paul II said in London: "Without the presence of these people in your midst you might be tempted to think of health, strength and power as the only important values to be pursued in life".

Advertising agencies report that "Thatcher's children" are unlikely to want to engage in either voluntary or paid work with "the poor" (Gold, Greenless, Trott, *Spoilt Brats*, January 1990), and a seriously alarmed government has now begun to talk less about individualism and more about "citizenship" — welfare spending can only be controlled and policies implemented if there are people around to care.

If, as John Dunne (1989) reckons, "the central problems in life for the handicapped cannot be resolved until society itself changes to one where community values are paramount", then a philosophical tide must be turned. It has often been said that the Roman Empire fell because of a welfare-style decadence. The most recent study (Ramsey MacMullen, *Corruption and the Decline of Rome,* Yale University Press, 1989) however, places the blame on unhindered individualism:

"Despite its superbly sophisticated system of law, the slow acids of atomised, selfish individualism dissolved larger loyalties and ties on a widening scale until they became, in the manner of the untrammelled market, the rational norm of behaviour, which only the unusually brave and honest could swim against."

Griffiths and after

"It was the best of times, it was the worst of times, it was the age of wisdom, it was the age of foolishness, it was the epoch of belief, it was the epoch of incredulity, it was the season of Light, it was the season of Darkness, it was the spring of hope, the winter of despair, we had everything before us, we had nothing before us."
Charles Dickens, *A Tale of Two Cities*

'"We've got history on our side, Vice Chancellor".
"But we're axing history, Charlie!"'
A Very Peculiar Practice, BBC2

Following the scathing criticisms of community care policy and progress by the Audit Commission in its 1986 report, the government asked Sir Roy Griffiths to: "review the way in which public funds are used to support community care policy and to advise . . . on the options for action that would improve the use of these funds as a contribution to more effective community care".

Sir Roy's credentials, as a doyen of the entrepreneurial spirit from Sainsbury's and the progenitor of general management in the health service were impeccable. Yet the government almost ignored the report, *Community Care: Agenda for Action* when it was published in March 1988. The reason for this lack of glasnost was probably Sir Roy's assertion that: "Elected local authorities are best placed, in my judgement, to assess local needs, set local priorities, and monitor local performance" (Para 5.2). In this the Griffiths report agreed with the Wagner committee on residential care (March 1988) and the Firth committee on public support for residential care (July 1987).

Of course Sir Roy's message was far more subtle than merely trusting everything to local government. At the heart of his succinct report are the themes of:

- Consumer choice
- "Building on informal networks of care"
- Value for money
- Getting rid of the "roadblocks" which obstruct imaginative services based on individual need.
- Local authorities as enablers, not monopolistic providers.

Sir Roy did not argue for fundamental structural change but for a freeing of "the vehicles" so that they could move forward; for measures to clarify the roles of health and social services; the appointment of a government minister to be "seen by the public as being clearly responsible for community care"; making community care monies a specific grant from the centre; and the removal of the "perverse incentives" which led to too many people (mainly those who were elderly) being cared for in residential homes rather than supported in their own home.

In his report, Sir Roy did not explicitly call for more money but he did remark dryly: "The Audit Commission, on the one hand, were satisfied that better value could be obtained from existing resources. On the other hand, many social services departments and voluntary groups, grappling with the problems at local level, certainly felt that the Israelites, faced with the requirement to make bricks without straw, had a comparatively routine and possible task".

Reaction to Griffiths centred for the most part along the lines of the need for a commitment by central government to make the new culture work. Voluntary and parent organisations welcomed the concept of a special minister; the Association of Directors of Social Services suggested the establishment of a community care development agency; the King's Fund Institute drew attention to the All-Wales Strategy, and its derivation from "the explicit commitment" made by the Welsh Office; and the Adam Smith Institute argued for a central independent board to judge individual assessments and allocate funds (M. Pirie and E. Butler, *op cit*).

The White Paper, *Caring For People* (November 1988) followed hard on the heels of the Audit Commission's national review of services. With its accent on consumer choice, promoting domiciliary rather than residential care, and establishing the "right financial and managerial framework", the White Paper is consistent with Griffiths and the Audit Commission. Seven key changes were laid down:

- Local authorities would become responsible for assessing individual need, designing care arrangements and securing their delivery — within available resources.
- Local authorities would be expected to produce and publish clear plans for the development of community care services. These plans were to be consistent with the plans of health authorities and other interested agencies. The government would inspect both the plans and the implementation.
- Local authorities would be expected to make "maximum use of the independent sector".
- After April 1991 local authorities would take responsibility for the financial support of people entering private and voluntary homes (including nursing homes).
- People dependent on DSS benefits would receive the same levels of Income Support and Housing Benefit irrespective of whether they were living in their own homes or in residential homes. (People in local authority homes would not be eligible).
- Local authority inspection and registration units would be at "arm's length" from the management of their own services. They would be responsible for checking standards in both the independent sector *and* local authorities' own homes.
- There would be a new specific grant to promote the development of social care for seriously mentally ill people.

Despite the consistency with previous reports a number of local authority organisations appear to have been taken by surprise, one spokesman described the new responsibilities for local authorities as "a poisoned chalice". Certainly phrases such as promoting "the development of a flourishing independent sector" and "identifying areas of their own work which are sufficiently self-contained to be suitable for 'floating-off' as self-managing units" made it clear the way the tide was running, and every local authority wishing to play a latter day King Canute would be washed away by the funding arrangements which had shifted from the "perverse incentive" towards private residential care to a "perverse disincentive" against care in local authority homes. Other disappointments were the lack of clarification over the issue of social care versus health care, and the avoidance of resource allocation until a few months before the April 1991 start-date. A close reading of chapter six shows that the government expects "the market" to sort out any problems!

As it was, only months before the brave new world was to be embarked upon, the government announced that the legislation would be delayed and implementaion would take place over three years.

The Act takes social care into uncharted waters, with a greater accent on choice than there has ever been before. As one director of social services said, "endless theological debates" about the merits of public versus private provision are "sterile and a waste of management time and energy". Now is an opportunity to specify service requirements and assess the quality of provision against those requirements ("Kent hops to it", *Insight*, 31 January 1990).

As the HMS Community Care launches out, it will have to ensure that real choice does not become undermined by ideology through the emergence of large private care corporations or through a lack of resources. Sir Roy Griffiths remarked on the publication of the White Paper that he had designed a car with four wheels but the government had left out the wheel marked "resources". Or as one commentator observed wryly: "Nobody expected a Rolls-Royce, but it looks as though we'll end up with a Reliant Robin!" The government's self-congratulation on its community care resource allocation in chapter eight simply doesn't ring true and should be set against what is happening in the acute sector of the NHS.

Care management should ensure a much clearer and faster route to assessment, and resource identification and procurement. Some voluntary societies have, however, already expressed reservations that "meeting long-term needs with a series of short-term contracts could result in a very disjointed and inconsistent experience for service-uses" (Roger Singleton, director of Barnardo's at the "Brave new world?" conference, 19 January,

1990). In the field of mental health, Professor Rolf Olsen has voiced uneasiness that "we may develop a superb system for purchasing from empty shelves". With any sea change, such as social care is experiencing at present, the likelihood of its success will depend on whether that change is "carried out in deference to . . . the traditions of the people or . . . to abstract principles, and arbitrary and general doctrines", as Disraeli remarked in *Sybil.*

As we do not know the future we can only judge its possible outcomes by a study of the past. What we do know from the past is that people with learning difficulties have until now been as hidden from history as from the rest of life, what history they do have is not so much theirs as the history of others either acting on their behalf, or against them (Ryan and Thomas, 1987). Both public and private sector provision, followed slavishly, have failed in the past. Perhaps the "age of the consumer" will fare them better, but if it is to do so then there will have to be a genuine listening to the individual, support from society and an overall commitment from government. As Sir Roy Griffiths pointed out in his report, there is a feeling that "community care is a poor relation; everybody's distant relative but nobody's baby" — there is a need to adopt it, and quickly!

P Abbott & B Sapsford (1987), *Community Care for Mentally Handicapped Children,* Open University Press

A Alaszewski, 'From villains to victims' in A Leighton ed. (1988), *Mental Handicap in the Community,* Woodhead Faulkner

Audit Commission (November 1987), *Community Care: Developing Services for People with a Mental Handicap,* Occasional Paper No.4, HMSO

Audit Commission (1986), *Making a Reality of Community Care,* HMSO

Audit Commission (October 1989), *Developing Community Care for Adults with a Mental Handicap,* Occasional Paper No 9, HMSO

M Bayley (1989), *Welfare — A Moral Issue?* Diocese of Sheffield Social Responsibilities Committee, chapter II

M Bulmer, (1987), *The Social Basis of Community Care,* Hyman

Paul Cambridge & Martin Knapp ed (1988), *Demonstrating Successful Care in the Community,* Personal Social Services Research Unit/University of Kent

M Dear & C Wolch (1987), *Landscapes of Despair: From Deinstitutionalisation to Homelessness,* Polity Press

P Dickens & P Gilbert (1979), *The State and the Housing Question,* University of Sussex

J Dunne (1989), "A radical philosophy for mental handicap services", in P McGenley ed., *Research and Practice in the Service of People with Learning Difficulties,* Galway

P Gilbert (1985), *Mental Handicap: A Practical Guide for Social*

Workers, Community Care/Reed Business Publishing
R Griffiths (1988), *Community Care: Agenda for Action*, HMSO
C Hallas *et al* (1982), *The Car and Training of the Mentally Handicapped*, Wright, chapter 1
C Hill (1989), *John Bunyan and His Church*, Oxford University Press
House of Commons Social Services Committee (1985), *Community Care: With Special Reference to Adult Mentally Ill and Mentally Handicapped People*, HMSO
K Jones (1975), *Opening the Door*, Routledge & Kegan Paul
K Jones (1988), *Experience in Mental Health*, Sage
K Jones, J Brown and J Bradshaw (1978), *Issues in Social Policy*, Routledge & Kegan Paul
C S Lewis (1945), *That Hideous Strength*, The Bodley Head
N Malin ed. (1987), *Reassessing Community Care*, Croom Helm
Office of Health Economics/MENCAP (1978), *Mental Handicap: The Way Forward*
W Parry-Jones (1972), *The Trade in Lunacy*, Routledge & Kegan Paul
T Philpot ed. (1989), *The Residential Opportunity?: The Wagner Report and After, Community Care*/Reed Business Publishing
D J Rothman (1971), *The Discovery of the Asylum*, Boston
D J Rothman (1980), *Conscience and Convenience: The Asylum and its Alternatives in Progressive America*, Boston
H Reid & A Wiseman (1986), *When the Talking has to Stop*, MIND
J Ryan & F Thomas (1987), *The Politics of Mental Handicap*, Free Association Books
R Snaith (1989), *Neighbourhood Care and Social Policy*, HMSO
B Stratford (1989), *Down's Syndrome: Past Present and Future*, Penguin
J Taylor (1986), *Mental Handicap: Partnership in the Community?*, Mencap/Office of Health Economics
R H Tawney (1922), *Religion and the Rise of Capitalism*, Penguin
R Titmuss (1968), *Commitment to Welfare*, Allen and Unwin
B Tonkin (1987) "Voices in the wilderness", *Community Care* 15 January
W Wolfensberger (1975), *The Origin of Nature of Institutional Models*, Human Policy Press

2

Closing the institutions

"You want your freedom, don't you. It's a free country, I ken, but you're not getting your freedom . . . The people outside . . . can go where they like. They don't have people telling them where to go . . . "
Hospital resident quoted in M. Cattermole (1988)

"Any fool can close a long-stay hospital: it takes more time and trouble to do it properly and compassionately."
House of Commons Select Committee (1985)

"Enabling people to live as independently as possible in the community is at the heart of community care."
Caring for People (1989)

"Seriously folks, the only way to really know when a villa is due for closure is when you see the painters on the horizon or the planning officer hiding in the bushes."
Leybourne Grange Hospital, *Staff Bulletin* (1990)

In a short story entitled "SQ", the science fiction writer, Ursula le Guin, depicted a world state where everybody had to take an annual SQ (sanity quotient) test (*The Compass Rose*, Panther, 1984). Those who failed were placed in humane asylums, and increasingly these turned into self-sufficient reservations with their own factories, power plants, schools, and so on. Eventually the chief psychologist himself is committed and his secretary runs the world government!

The growth of the mental handicap and psychiatric hospitals in America and the United Kingdom had some of this remorseless logic. The march towards the asylum, as we saw in chapter 1, had its origin both in economic and attitudinal factors. The institutions were designed to be therapeutic, and to protect both society and the handicapped or the insane person from each other. In the end, as Wolfensberger shows, they developed a momentum of their own (see Figure 2.3.1).

Most of us know individuals who have spent many years in the hospital system and yet now live very successful and satisfying lives in community settings. Harry Daneman, who one of the authors knew in London, spent many years in one of the large outer London hospitals yet often held down a full-time job outside in the community. He now lives in a group home and, though a pensioner, is still to be seen painting his house — or other people's. The question has been and still is — why were such people kept apart from life "outside"?

Figure 2.3.1: *Graphic summary of the evolution of institutional rationales and practices*

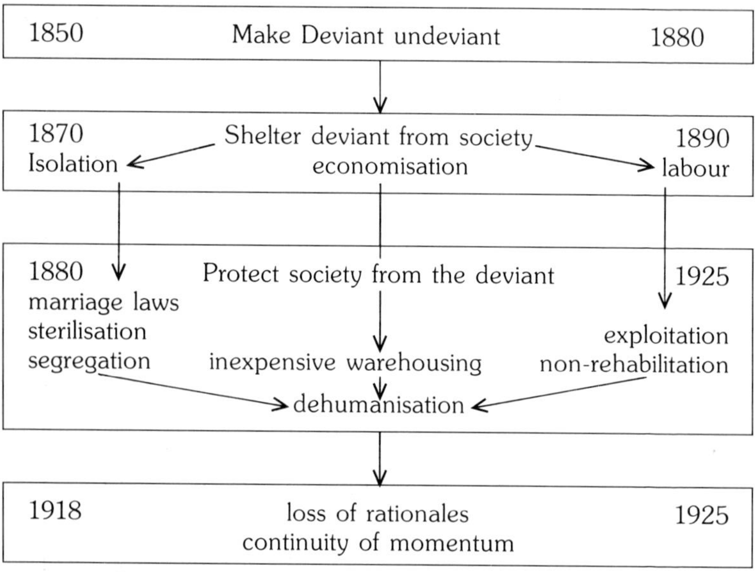

(From W Wolfensberger, 1975)

Many of the old long-stay hospitals are closing or have already closed (see Table 2.1.1). In some regional health authorities, such as North Western and Wessex, bed numbers have halved over the past ten years. Many of the smaller hospitals have closed altogether, while a number of the mammoth institutions have seen large reductions: for example, St. Lawrences (South West Thames RHA) from 1,350 residents in 1978 to 792 in 1986; Calderstones (North Western RHA) from 1,050 in 1983 to 595 in 1989, and Coldeast (Wessex RHA) from 533 in 1978 to 310 in 1988.

Closure programmes have often depended on the motivation and energy of particular politicians or officers, which has meant an uneven progress across the country. North Western Region has a firm policy of community-based provision, backed up by a model district service; a regional development team, a training team and a financial strategy (*Community Care*, 27 October 1988). South East Thames region hasa had a long-term strategy with a coordinated approach, regional training programmes for staff (the "Bringing People Back Home" material and so on); and a special development team to cater for people posing special challenges.

At the same time there have been doubts about the wisdom of closures raised by RESCARE, on one pole of the debate, as to what they see as "an abdication of responsibility by the State", as Richard Jackson said at a conference in 1987. At the other pole the Campaign for Mentally Handicapped People has pointed out that, in a study of 414 people leaving long-stay hospitals most transferred to other hospitals in transinstitutionalisation rather than deinstitutionalisation, to use the jargon. The latest statistics from

Figure 2.3.2: *Admissions to mental handicap hospitals and units in England 1976-1986*

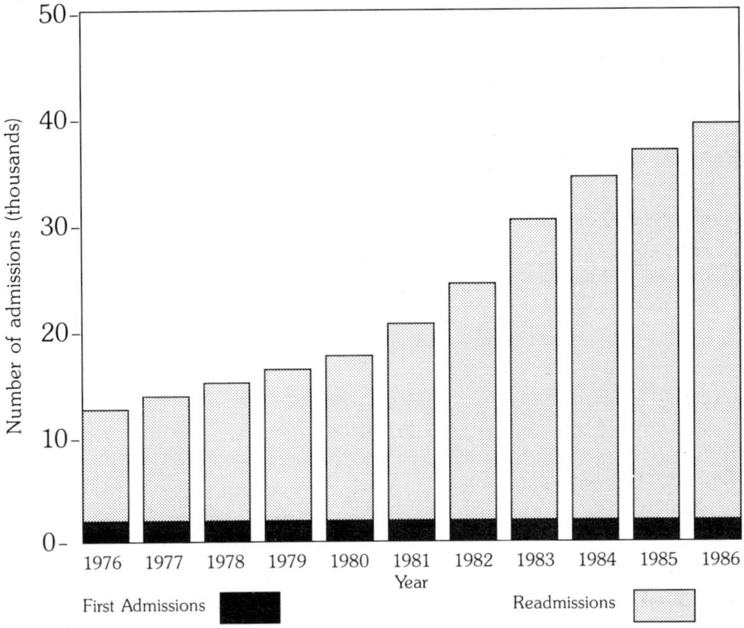

(From DHSS, March 1988)

the department (DHSS, 1988) show a steep *rise* in admissions to long-stay hospitals for short term care. The number of people admitted for the first time in 1986 was 1800, 300 more than in 1985 and the highest annual number in the decade (see figure 2.3.2). No reason is given for this disturbing trend but it is probably due to dowry monies being used to finance solely those individuals discharged from hospital with little or no resource for assessment or short-term care being set up for those already living in the community (see chapter 1).

Despite the poverty of human relationships in the long-stay hospitals described by Goffman, Coser, Morris and others (see Jones, 1975, pp 117/118 and Morris, 1969, chapter 13), there is a tendency now to see the hospitals through rose-tinted spectacles just as they are disappearing. Compare for example the words of junior health minister Roger Freeman on 6 February 1990 to Enoch Powell's in 1961. When the latter asked his audience: "Do not for a moment underestimate their (the Victorian Asylums') power of resistance to our assault." "Our Victorian forefathers were excellent builders. They built hospitals to last, and it seems to be to be economic nonsense to demolish a soundly constructed building simply because it looks shabby".

Table 2.1.1: *Moving out of hospital*

		Individuals	(% of total)
NHS hospital		282	68
NHS hostel or community unit		72	17
Local authority hostel		12	3
Staffed housing:-			
Local authority	4		
Private	12	16	3.75
Unstaffed housing:-			
Vol. org.	5		
NHS	1	6	1.5
Returned to family		4	1
Fostered		1	.25
Old people's home		4	1
Council housing		2	.5
(Died during the year)		15	3.5
		414	99.5

(From A. Wertheimer, 1986)

But in some ways the hospitals are no longer the issue. "Change", as Disraeli remarked "is constant" in a "progressive country", and services have to adapt to consumer demand. The local authority or private home may be more institutionalised than a hospital ward and the small satellite unit less attentive to individual needs than the 150 place social education centre. As the experienced nursing manager, Tom McClean, points out (McClean, 1988), some of the worst scandals in the 1960s and 1970s occurred in the smaller hospitals. The changes required by evolving philosophies and consumer demand throw up challenges to staff on the ground. Many projects in which residents and staff have moved from larger to smaller units have noted a similar finding to Paul Chamberlain's. He writes: "But as other properties were opening, so the level of support decreased. Staff in the house began to feel isolated. Most had worked in institutional settings, and began to speak fondly of the camaraderie which existed in such places" (Chamberlain, chapter 8 in G Horobin and D May, *Living with Mental Handicap*, Jessica Kingsley, 1988).

This chapter looks at two practical examples of service which have undergone dramatic change. But it also raises the issue (examined again in chapter 14) that change is constant and we cannot afford to become institutionalised in our attitudes and methods. When the *Observer* newspaper exposed the barbaric conditions on the Greek island of Leros (16 September 1989), we were scandalised, but conditions not too dissimilar to those have been documented in offical enquiries in Britain. The Mental Welfare Commission for Scotland's report on Lennox Castle Hospital (February 1989) condemned conditions there as "appalling", but the Scottish Office's response was to pour £4.5m into making physical improvements to a grossly outmoded facility (leading article, *Social Work Today*, 23 February 1989). Why is Scotland still holding back on community care? Why are some authorities in England developing staffed housing schemes while others are still building 25-bedded hostels and social education centres? Why is it only in Wales (as shown clearly in the 1989 White Paper) that the government are backing community care to the hilt?

Most consumers (see, for example, *Community Care*, 1988) wish to move to more valued settings. Booth and Simons (1990) found that the majority in their study welcomed a move from hospital to hostel, but "having found their feet in the community, many movers were now looking forward to branching out on their own". Institutionalisation is in many ways an attitude of mind. Often staff members have transformed drab settings by imaginative personal touches. The people they have worked with have appreciated that, as one ex-hospital resident remarked to Peter Gilbert on his return to his former "home" to visit friends: "There are some good people here, good staff, but you should bomb this place!"

Darenth Park Hospital

Background

Darenth Park Hospital was in many ways unique. It was one of the oldest institutions in England, and also the first major hospital to close when it was replaced by alternative services in 1988. The hospital, with a catchment area that included five London boroughs and part of Kent, was situated two miles from the centre of Dartford and established in 1878 as a training school for some 500 children. Ten years later its original role had extended to the admission of adults with the population reaching 1,000. Early in this century it became an industrial training colony, and in time housed over 2,000 patients. Further changes in name and emphasis followed throughout the years up to 1936 when it became Darenth Park Hospital, being taken over by the NHS in 1948.

Factors promoting change

The origins of the plans for the closure of Darenth Park began in the mid-1970s when a cement company approached the regional health authority with the view to purchasing the hospital as it was situated on chalk stratum, and was also conveniently located to a nearby processing plant. In view of the concerns about improving services the regional health authority saw the sale of the hospital as an attractive proposition as it would provide the capital required to replace the increasingly outdated service being offered by the hospital.

The decision on the sale of the site went to a public enquiry in 1978, but in the meantime representatives of the health authority and social services department involved had formed a working party (The Darenth Park Steering Group), to oversee the closure programme, which would need to work with haste if it was to meet the deadline of 1985 set for the vacation of the hospital site. In 1979 the public enquiry turned down the application to extract chalk from the site. Nevertheless the steering group decided to carry on with the closure plans as a commitment had by then been built up to develop alternative services.

Providing alternative services

With a deadline of April 1987 as the date for closure, the team planning the closure of the hospital and the movement of patients to alternative services were dependent on health districts providing accommodation, particularly with the withdrawal of social services department representatives from the steering group, over differences concerning the transfer of funds for residents moving from health to social services accommodation. In their account of the history of the closure of Darenth Park Korman and Glennerster (1990) describe the response of the districts to the resettlement of residents of Darenth Park. Early plans included the use of converted hospitals or purpose built large-scale accommodation. This thinking was quickly changed by the work of Mansell and his colleagues (1988) who convinced managers that ordinary housing was not only preferable to the institutional alternatives planned, but offered a more rapid response to the accommodation needs of residents, rather than waiting for specially planning buildings that would not meet the short closure time the Steering Group had set itself. The successful promotion of staffed housing as a cornerstone of the alternative services provided for Darenth Park residents, eventually resulted in districts working with housing associations, and later consortia of agencies, including social services departments, in the provision of accommodation. Although there was some slippage on the original date for closure, the hospital saw the last residents leave on the 12 August 1988.

What helped change happen?

Korman and Glennerster (1990) state that at the time of their interim research report on the closure of the hospital in 1984 they had private doubts about whether it would close at all. But the hospital did close, and they list a large number of reasons why this closure plan was successful. In addition they also suggest some important requirements that need to be built into service changes in the future. Some of the factors that operated across both region and district health authorities will be of particular interest to managers working in services where similar, if smaller scale changes are taking place:

- ☐ a clear statement of the timescale for change, with participants required to adhere to this as far as possible, as part of a continuous pressure to succeed. This was seen as the strong incentive needed to urgently develop new services and force the issue on to planning and budgetary agendas.
- ☐ strong leadership, and importantly continuity of leadership, with a group of senior staff meeting regularly to maintain the impetus of the project.
- ☐ a shared philosophy based on normalisation and ordinary living, that provided a rationale for the alternative provision which was eventually accepted by districts as appropriate for people with learning difficulties.
- ☐ professional support, through the provision of training and consultancy, for staff who were building the new service, including providing a specific service for staff working with people with challenging behaviour, in order that these users were not rejected by the new service.
- ☐ involvement of agencies and individuals who had a valuable contribution to make to the development of the new service, including consulting with people with a learning difficulty from the outset.
- ☐ employing a core of senior staff who eventually manage the new services, but initially will be involved in planning and monitoring the implementation of the plan. The range of decisions that need to be made while developing new services highlights the need for senior staff to be in post early in the life of a project. The employment of these senior staff for two years or more while services are developing means extra costs have to be carried, if a high quality service is to result.
- ☐ offering staff an opportunity to play a role in the new service, including orientation to new service philosophies.
- ☐ staffing the service with people who have the right balance of age and experience, with a commitment to providing continuous training in order that staff develop appropriate skills, teamwork and high morale.
- ☐ services tailored to the needs, hopes and wishes of users, starting with accommodation. Korman and Glennerster (1990) recognised that this was only the beginning of providing appropriate services. The need for an integrated lifestyle, with friendships, social activities and meaningful occupation would

be required in the future.

- ☐ recognition on the part of senior managers, health authority members and councillors that developing new services inevitably means experimentation. As a result mistakes may be made, for example, where staff underestimate the needs of users, and services have to be modified that can result in additional costs.

Early lessons from the closure of Darenth Park

Although the plan to close Darenth Park and provide alternative accommodation was successful, Glennerster and Korman (1990) have documented some of the issues that arise from such a major service change.

Alternative residential accommodation, particularly in the early phase of movement of residents, was other hospitals, hostels and private homes, as new accommodation planned by health authorities had not been built. In the second phase from 1986 until the hospital closed in 1988, residents were able to move to small staffed houses. The shift to using ordinary housing offered many advantages both to residents, in terms of more appropriate accommodation, and to the health service, in avoiding planning permission problems associated with large-scale facilities, and reducing expenditure through social security benefits payments to residents, and grants paid to housing associations.

The opportunities available to residents moving out of Darenth Park were dependent upon the district to which they returned. Some areas were able to offer a wide range of accommodation, while others offered limited choice. Although alternative residential accommodation of varying quality was provided for all residents, opportunities for day activities have been more difficult to arrange, with work training and employment the least developed of all day activities.

In spite of residents moving to community settings, integration has been slower. The need to develop links with community facilities is highly dependent on staff, both in terms of knowledge of local facilities and skills in helping build links. Here Glennerster and Korman point out that many of the staff in new services are young and not well integrated with local communities themselves, and therefore have few local contacts to share with users. Other concerns were about the lack of staff who needed to help build community links, and absence of community facilities that people could use. Occasional intolerance on the part of the public and professionals towards people living in the new services are also voiced as an area of concern. The need to promote social activities and the encouragement of friendships with people who are not part of the service, was seen as a high priority alongside the development of personal and self-help skills.

A further area of concern was the need to develop new ways of managing a community-based service, that enabled the service to support staff working in dispersed housing throughout the community. Staff can become isolated working in such dispersed settings, and structures need to be built that enable them to meet together for mutual support, to learn from each other in order to find new ways of helping users, and to maintain the quality of the new service through access to practice by service managers. Finally, Glennerster and Korman describe how health authorities came to develop relationships with other service providers, particularly housing associations, that enabled residents to take advantage of social security benefits, which helped fund the change to a community-based service. It is in the area of costs that some of the most difficult future questions rest. The move from hospital to alternative services brings with it substantially increased costs, as services that were once provided on site become an extra cost, no matter how limited in quality. Costs of the new service are on average half as much again as the hospital, with social security benefits playing such a significant role in enabling health authorities to fund these service changes. Glennerster and Korman raise the question about how much the White Paper changes, with the government concern to control social security spending, will undermine similar hospital closures in the future, or force the clock back, with a return to large scale institutional services.

The Forest Hospital

Background

March 1990 marked the end of a particular chapter in the history of mental handicap services in Britain. That month the Forest Hospital, Horsham, West Sussex, closed, an establishment which had as its roots the birth of the institutional movement in the mid-nineteenth century. The Forest was for many years an annexe to the Royal Earlswood Hospital, Redhill, Surrey, which began its life in 1847 as the innovative and educational Highgate Asylum but had become by the 1960s a monolithic institution of several thousand beds.

The Forest itself was set up in 1812 as the Horsham Workhouse, well away from the main town as it was then constituted. It stood near to the future site of the railway station — a common occurrence for workhouses and asylums as both they and the railways were regarded as noisy and a general nuisance by the townspeople! In 1860 the impressive Victorian frontage was added adjoining the road. The Poor Law under which the Forest was built only came to an end in the 1930s, and two hospital workers in the early 1980s were children of the former workhouse superintendent!

During the Second World War wards were erected on a temporary basis for Canadian service personnel. Perhaps no-one would be surprised to learn that these temporary buildings soon became a permanent fixture.

In 1974 the health service reorganisation placed the Forest firmly in the West Sussex Area Health Authority and most links were severed with the Royal Earlswood.

In a further reorganisation in 1982 district health authorities were formed and the new chairman of Mid Downs DHA, Martyn Long, decided that there had to be a new ethos of care for people with learning difficulties currently resident in the Forest (M. Long, 1988).

Conditions of care

The Forest in the 1970s and early 1980s had both some of the benefits one might expect in a small unit and also a number of the problems identified by Tom McClean (McClean, 1988). Although situated within an expanded Horsham town and near to neighbourhood facilities the Forest had, like many long-stay hospitals, become isolated if not geographically but "from the mainstream of both medical and educational advances" (P. Morris, 1969).

Care was often provided in 60 place, single-sex wards with the recreational areas having bare wooden or lino-covered floors, a few chairs and a boxed-in TV set in one corner. A number of nursing staff had battled against the odds to bring touches of homeliness to a stark setting. The conversion of an old sluice room into a kitchen on one ward made an enormous difference to residents who had been used to food appearing, as if by magic, from hospital kitchens.

During the mid-70s two "Crossman units" were set up in other parts of West Sussex. These smaller units, put up nationally as a response by Labour Social Services Secretary, Richard Crossman, to the inquiry at Ely Hospital, were newly built and better resourced than the old institutions. Ironically, however, many professionals and parents found the new units very "clinical" and less "homely" than the wards of the old workhouse, where staff had used energy and imagination to reshape the environment.

Move towards closure

In 1983 the chairman of the health authority set up a district health authority members working party with officer support. The chairman himself had been shocked by the conditions in the hospital and put his weight behind the report's recommendation to close the Forest by March 1990.

Figure 2.3.3: *Length of stay in the Forest Hospital*

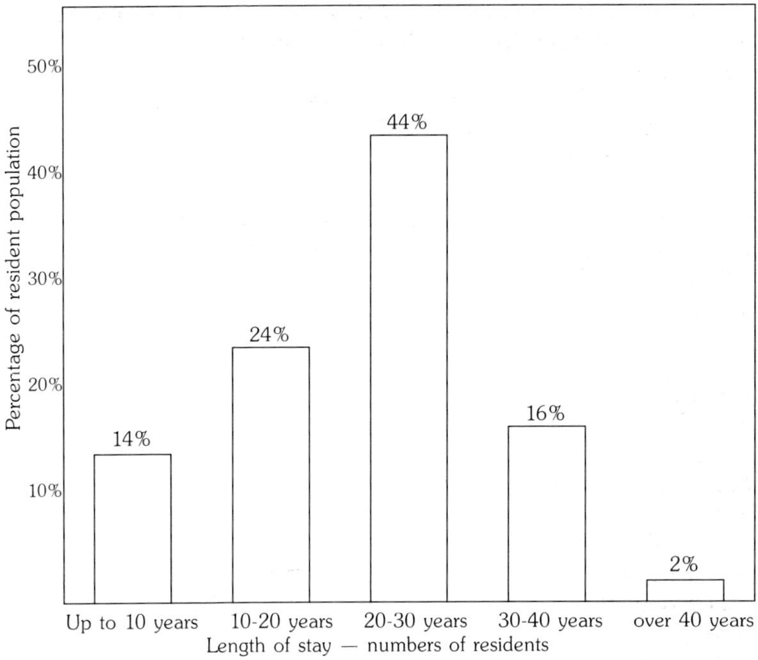

There was, as might be expected, considerable opposition to the idea of relocating services away from the hospital site from within the establishment, but changes within the management team included a new consultant, and an agreement with the social services department and the two neighbouring health authorities enabled a definite plan to be established (*The Way Ahead: Strategic Proposal 1985-1995,* Mid Downs DHA).

The social work role in assessment

Multi-disciplinary assessments, involving individual residents and their carers was an essential part of the process. The social worker role (see Gilbert, 1987) was to look at each individual in terms of his or her relationships with other residents, staff, voluntary visitors and community groups; the dependence on the setting itself (for example, in the case of an elderly person or one with sensory disabilities); the relationship with parents and relatives, or community groups; the wishes and anxieties of the relatives which may be complex and ambivalent; the wishes of the resident, their need for choice and their general social needs.

The assessment operation was complicated because of the Forest's former role as an annexe to the Royal Earlswood. Residents had come to this small hospital from all over the country because of the Earlswood's reputation. In fact 76 per cent of the

Forest's residents came from outside the district health authority area and 36 per cent from outside the county of West Sussex. Of 193 adult residents in 1985 45 originated from Mid Downs, with a further 77 from the two other West Sussex health districts; 27 residents came from 13 different London boroughs; and 44 people had come to Forest from 12 counties, as far apart as Yorkshire and Somerset.

Some moves had taken place because of family moves, others were victims of the notorious "swop" system between consultants. Arnold Baker had no personal details on his file except his date of birth, religion and dates of moves from institution to institution across the country. Barry Jones had a reputation for "deviousness", but a tendency to canniness was entirely understandable when staff read his history: his childhood spent in and out of care and his adulthood in a number of long-stay hospitals.

The first task of the social workers was to consider the residents they had worked with for some years as people facing a major life crisis. Many had no known history, but if they had then they needed it recorded, and for those who did not have a written history, social work staff wanted to ensure that their memories of their current life were preserved in story and photographs. However inadequate the hospital seemed to staff as a "home", it certainly was perceived as such by most of its residents.

A major exercise in life stories then took place, first with relatives, partly as a way of eliciting their views on the development plans. In many cases the story that they had to tell was a harrowing one. Many parents had been advised by powerful figures, doctors, other parents, and so on to put their child away and forget about them; this had led to repression and guilt. As another parent said in similar circumstances, "It was like a criminal conspiracy, and we could not even talk about the crime" (*The Visit*, BBC Film).

Others had gradually found the old hospital system too much to cope with; illnesses such as cancer and depression, and family breakdown were frequent occurrences; and there were the brothers and sisters whose parents had never talked about the handicapped child and who, in their turn, had hidden the secret from their children.

Many parents found it a cathartic experience to talk to someone at last; others were angry at being contacted after such a long time; some wanted to get involved in decision-making; others again began visiting after a gap of many years. For the residents choice was a major issue — how do you elicit a genuine choice after many years of hospitalisation? Fortunately, local community facilities were generous in their time in offering visits and social activities to give people a wider perspective.

Factors promoting change

☐ A DHA chairman, Martyn Long, who had a personal and

professional commitment to produce a new model of services; a powerful position in the county council; links with national bodies; and the personality to ensure change was achieved.

- Coterminous boundaries between the social services department and the three district health authorities.
- The small scale of the hospital and its valuable land site.
- An accent on communication with relatives and staff.
- The presence of a social work team with both a hospital and community focus which enabled social services' resources to be utilised in preparation for community living and good links to be maintained between the SSD and the DHA.

Paradoxical factors

- Conflicting views about the new model of service to be adopted. A strong lobby for a safe solution outweighing any idea of going for ordinary housing.
- Four local MENCAP branches within the health district with widely differing views.
- A very strong parental lobby for a "village community" on the hospital site.
- The depression which descends on staff during a time of change even when they approve of the new model of service.

Perhaps the most inspiring thing about being involved in a large-scale service relocation is how service users themselves rise to the challenge. A social worker undertaking assessments to enable long-stay hospital residents to move to community settings found the following in an old psychologist's report: "I asked 'James' what he would get if he added five apples to six apples, and he said, 'I prefer oranges'. I then asked him to subtract three eggs from ten and he replied 'I like mine scrambled'. Sadly 'James' will clearly not have the intellectual capacity to cope with community living" (quoted in Gilbert, 1987). Fortunately for "James" this pessimistic prediction has proved unfounded.

The future pattern of care

Because of conflicting views both within and outside the Forest, it was not easy for the planners within the DHA or SSD to settle on a new model of care. Some urged the need for ordinary houses but anxiety among some parent bodies and staff groups led to the main service model being the 25-bedded unit, though the Crawley unit is ingenious in the way it blends in with ordinary housing on a new estate. With the Forest being a prime town site in an expanding commuter zone, the land was sold to a developer prior to the relocation of the service and thus "capital-rich" the district was able to build its own units and finance a capital "dowry" for those residents to be cared for by the SSD. For ordinary housing schemes to have been set up there would have had to be backing from the South West Thames Regional Health Authority, but up until the appointment of its new chairman, Mrs Julia (now Baroness) Cumberledge, in 1988, the authority had been content to let each district seek its own salvation.

The change goes on

In the introduction to this chapter it was stated that many hospitals are moving towards closure. Where closure has taken place, for example in the two hospitals described in this chapter, this has not been achieved easily. Closure has occured at a time of changes in national policy; also changes in organisational structures and the presence of severe funding restrictions. As closures have gathered pace, parental concern and staff resistance have also played their part in reducing the speed of change towards the creation of better services.

As we have seen in the accounts of the closure of Darenth Park and Forest Hospitals, the services that have succeeded them still have many challenges to overcome in providing a genuinely high quality lifestyle for the previous residents of these two hospitals. Korman and Glennerster (1990) go so far as to warn that the facilities which have replaced Darenth Park have hardly started with the task of sustaining quality provision. This remark, based on a discussion about the difficulties of developing services underpinned by normalisation, suggests that the risks of recreating the institution exist in all services, whether they are found in large hospitals or small community-based services. It suggests also that for whatever reason they have been unable to maintain a high quality service, or may be designed in such a way as to perpetuate the problems experienced in the old service.

The particular problems that Korman and Glennerster refer to, concern the way that services must continually adapt according to the needs of users, if they are to avoid repeating the mistakes of the past. Some services, which have replaced hospitals, risk creating new institutions by their size and structure, and will be under pressure to adopt more appropriate facilities in order to avoid the problems that beset the services they superceded.

So change goes on. Not just the major change involved in closing hospitals, but the continuing smaller-scale change where services are required to adapt to new ideas and expectations about what constitutes the ideal model at a particular point in the history of provision. Senior managers need to start from an awareness and understanding of the way in which services enable people with learning difficulties to achieve a high quality lifestyle through their presence and participation in natural communities. If this is to happen we will witness a continuing process of change with today's preferred services changing to meet the new expectations of tomorrow.

Community Care (1988) "Leaving long-stay hospitals", INSIDE Supplement, 27 October.

Martin Cattermole *et al*, "Life in a mental handicap hospital: The view from the inside", *Mental Handicap*, December 1988.

DHSS, *Mental Handicap Hospitals and Units in England*, DHSS Statistical Bulletin, 2 March 1988.

P. Gilbert, "Part of a team", *Community Care*, 15 October 1987.

P. Gilbert, "Strangers in a strange land", *Community Care*, 22 October 1987.

House of Commons Select Committee on Social Services (1985), *Community Care*, HMSO.

K. Jones (1975), *Opening the Door*, Routledge & Kegan Paul.

N. Korman and H Glennerster (1985), *Closing a Hospital: The Darenth Park Project*, Bedford Square Press.

N. Korman and M Glennerster (1990), *Hospital Closure*, Open University Press.

H. Glennerster and N. Korman, "Success costs money", *Community Care*, 26 April 1990.

H. Glennerster and N. Korman, "Normalisation is not easy", *Community Care*, 3 May 1990.

M. Long, "Delivering a balanced service", *Community Care*, 28 January 1988.

Tom McClean, "Closing the hospitals and changing provision", in A Leighton ed. (1988), *Mental Handicap in the Community*, Woodhead Faulkner.

J. Mansell (1988), *Staffed Housing for People with Mental Handicaps: Achieving Widespread Dissemination*, South East Thames Regional Health Authority.

P. Morris (1969), *Put Away*, Routledge & Kegan Paul, 1969.

S. Sharkey and S. Barna eds (1990), *Community Care: People Leaving Long-Stay Hospitals*, Routledge.

V. Shennan (1983), *A Home of their Own*, Souvenir Press.

D. Sines ed (1988), *Towards Integration: Comprehensive Services for People with Mental Handicaps*, Lippincott.

A. Wertheimer (1986), *Images of Possibility*, CMH.

A. Wertheimer (1986), *Hospital Closures in the Eighties*, CMH.

L. Wing (1989), *Hospital Closure and the Resettlement of Residents*, Gower.

W. Wolfensberger (1975), *The Origin and Nature of our Institutional Models*, Human Policy Press.

T. Booth, K. Simons & W. Booth (1990), *Outward Bound*, Open University Press.

Consumer's View: Locked away
David Barron

In March 1939, I was taken, at the age of 14, from my foster mother to the mid-Yorkshire Institution at Whixley, near York. I was collected by two men and we were all met by the superintendent and the matron. I was instructed to wait until they had finished talking. As the men left, they said: "Goodbye, lad. We hope you'll soon settle in."

I was marched from the room and into a large dining hall. It was massive. I had never seen so many people sat at tables. A patient told me that the hall held 485 people. I asked him lots of questions. Suddenly, he frightened me almost to death. He sent a pot of tea flying, fell from the chair and lay foaming at the mouth. Someone yelled "Tom's having a fit," and an attendant came over.

I left the table to chat to other patients and was immediately told to sit down until the necessary permission was granted after the saying of grace. I was taken down a long corridor to the ward. The attendant pulled out a big bunch of keys fastened to his pocket on a long chain. Eventually he found the right one, we entered and he locked the door behind us. The ward seemed like a prison. He took me through to the locked bathroom.

Bathing completed, he took me back to the ward. I sat on a chair and talked to some other patients. I was wasting my time. I couldn't get through to them. Looking around, I saw that the windows were barred. The whole place shone with cleanliness. At 6.30 pm we were given our suppers, a pot of cocoa each. At 6.50 pm we were told to go upstairs to the bedrooms and get undressed. I was shown my bedroom and given a nightshirt to wear. The attendant locked me into the bedroom. I crawled into bed and cried my eyes out.

I learned later, I was in the punishment ward. It was an institutional ruling that you spent the first few months there. You weren't allowed to speak to other patients; all possessions were taken away; we were on half rations; a discipline of hard physical labour like scrubbing concrete with a brick and half a bucket of cold water.

After a few months, I was transferred to Ward Two. One night, I was woken up with a start. A hand had grabbed my bed clothes at the bottom. All the bed-clothes were pulled expertly away from me. It was the superintendent.

"Come on now, son," he said, "Get them off."

Playing dumb I just lay there.

"You know what I mean — those socks."

I took them off.

"Right, son. Don't let me catch you with your socks on in bed again or you'll know what to expect." He meant shunting back to the punishment ward.

On Friday, when I went up for my meagre pay, I had another shock.

"I have stopped your money for a fortnight," he informed me. All for wearing a pair of socks in bed!

Another trick was the rubbish hunt. They were really trying to find out how much money we had. We had to turn our pockets out and if you had anything, particularly money, you shouldn't have had, there were severe punishments. Some got money by selling breadcrusts. We were all hungry. One patient sold two crusts for a halfpenny. I only got a halfpenny a week and so was soon in debt. Kitchen workers could easily smuggle bread and cake out to exchange for money or cigarettes.

The paying-out ceremony was a grand occasion. We all trooped into the main hall. Anyone seen talking could say goodbye to their pay.

"You were talking just now."

"Yes sir."

"Right. Your money is stopped for a fortnight. Off you go and sit down."

"But . . . "

"Take him to the punishment ward for answering back."

Some months further on I got my first taste of freedom. One Sunday morning, I went to see outside the grounds for the first time since admission. At 9.30 am prompt we left our wards to go round to the main drive where we lined up in twos for inspection. This proved a long process. There were nearly 450 patients and some had their shoes on the wrong feet. Some had no ties or had tied them incorrectly. Others, like myself, had failed to comb their hair or clean their shoes.

After an age, we marched off. I called it the "Whixley crawl" or the chain gang. It was an ordeal we should never have had to undergo. The superintendent deliberately made us a spectacle for all the surrounding villages to see. I suppose it was OK for the lower-graded patients who had no way of knowing they were the laughing stock. But we could sense the public's ridicule. The attendants shouted at us like a herd of cattle. It was a two hour walk. I made it for 18 years until I could have walked it blindfold.

After my first week in Ward Two, I was assigned to the sewing room. There were eight of us darning socks and sewing buttons on shirts under the supervision of a female instructor — Miss Hawkins. I could never do anything right for her. She had me spending more time dunce-like, standing in the corner, than sewing.

One day, Miss Hawkins told me to clean the windows. I climbed up a step ladder and felt faint.

"Why haven't you cleaned the windows?" she snapped when I returned.

"I don't feel well."

"Rubbish. You're just putting on an act to get out of the job. Get on with it or else."

Back on the high ladder again, I felt faint and passed out. I came round and saw Miss Hawkins standing over me.

In the line for my pay on Friday, the superintendent said, "Your pay is stopped for a fortnight. You know why that is?"

"No sir."

"For not doing what you were told and cleaning the windows as instructed."

Besides having non-qualified attendants, there were also tradesmen in four different trades — tailor's, the mat shop, the occupational therapy room and the cobbler's shop. The tailor's shop made everything in the suit line from new suits for patients to those specially for the staff. The mat shop made everything from carpets to rugs to big heavy doormats. They were practically all epileptics in the OT room. They made baskets, tablemats, hand sewn goods. This was run by a fully qualified male nurse, Mr Tynegate, who was a perfect gentleman.

For four years, I worked in the cobbler's shop. I felt no longer a patient working among the boots and shoes. I felt as if I was working outside. The cobbler, Mr Webster, was a good man. However well we were treated here, we had to remember we were patients when we returned to the ward in the evenings. He taught me all about repairing shoes. With his passionate temper and ripe language, he was full of respect and kindness. When Mr Webster died suddenly, the cobbler's shop was taken over by a private firm.

After this I was transferred to Ward Four. This was the pre-discharge ward. I was allocated to work with Mr Tynegate in OT who had 40 patients under him, mostly epileptics. My task was to put out the various jobs for patients — painting, drawing, sewing and basket work. Eventually I became an assistant instructor, learning a lot on the medical side, coming to know and understand the patients in the same way that a parent understands his children.

When certain patients were about to have a fit, they seemed to gain the strength of a horse and took off their boots to throw at the staff. It was all Mr Tynegate and I could do to see they came to no harm. We inserted a special medical implement in their mouths to stop them biting their tongues.

We had to guard against patients who had fits without warning. They often became violent. Some people got injured as they fell. It used to break my heart but Mr Tynegate gave me a piece of sound advice.

"You mustn't let your emotions get the better of you, David. They need a bit of understanding."

Rumours were going around about lots of patients being sent out to hostels in Tadcaster, Bubwith and further afield. It spread like wildfire when tons of suitcases were delivered and every other day, patients were sent for by the tailor and measured out for new suits.

A good 12 months rolled by and I had just returned from a walk. Mr Tynegate called out: "The tailor wants you, David." I was to be fitted for a discharge suit.

A few days later, my suitcases were put in the back of the superintendent's car and I was taken to Bubwith Hostel near York. After a few months there, I went under licence to Leeds to live with Mrs Shaw. I found her harsh but got most of my company through the Salvation Army.

One day, when I came in from work, Mrs Shaw was waiting for me. "Don't go to work in the morning, David, someone is coming to see you."

At 10.30 am the following day, I sat in her front room when in came Messrs Perry and Hoyle, the same two men who had taken me to Whixley Institution nearly 20 years before.

"Hello," said Mr Hoyle with forced cheerfulness, and turning to Mrs Shaw, "you are sure you won't change your mind?"

"No," she cried out harshly, "he's a bloody menace. Get him out of my house."

The fear of going back to the institution was too much for me. I bolted for it. I ran quickly down the back alleys to my friends in the Salvation Army — Mr and Mrs Sharpe.

Mrs Sharpe gasped "Why, David — you look as if you've seen a ghost." Breathlessly, I explained.

"I will arrange for you to go and stay with my sister who lives in Tingley — just near Wakefield."

I was on the run. The Yorkshire police would be out looking for me. After a cup of tea and a bite to eat, I caught the various buses to Tingley. I had to change buses bang opposite Dewsbury Road police station.

I had to explain to Mrs Furniss, Mrs Sharpe's sister, who was most welcoming. I knew that it was only a matter of time until the police caught up with me. At 6.20 pm on the Friday, the policeman's knock came.

"Come on David," he said, "I don't like having to do this but it's my job and you have to come with me."

I was kept overnight in Morley police station. I cried myself to sleep. In the morning, the superintendent called with an escort to take me back to Whixley Institution. I was taken out of the car and with sickening inevitability placed in Ward One.

Next Monday, I was completely taken by surprise when they

came for me. There, outside the Board Room, to my joy, was the Sharpe family. As I greeted them, the superintendent called me into the board room. I stood at one end of the long room so the committee could see me. The superintendent spoke.

"Well David, what have you done wrong to make Mrs Shaw have you brought back here?"

"Nothing Sir."

"Nothing, eh?"

"I couldn't put a razor blade down but what it took legs and walked."

The committee laughed and a few words were exchanged. The superintendent turned to me. "Alright. You can go and wait outside."

Mrs Sharpe and Mrs Furniss asked me how I had got on. "I don't know," I said.

Then they were called into the Board Room. They were a long time. Afterwards they told me about the questions. The committee wanted to know why they were offering me a home. Was it because of the money? "I told them," said Mrs Sharpe, "the money never entered my head. I had come to know you as one of the family. You spent most of the time with us when you weren't at work."

The superintendent came out. "David. You can go back with Mrs Furniss on licence and I will send her the necessary forms to fill in in due course," he said.

I left with the two ladies, in great joy, never to return.

Reprinted from Community Living *(July 1987) by permission of the editor.*

3

Care in the community or by the community?

"We are living at a time when the principle of looking after number one is widely proclaimed as a respectable principle of personal and public morality".
Mark Santer, Bishop of Birmingham

"No one would choose a life without friends, even if he could have all the other things in the world'".
Aristotle

When, in its 1985 Report, the House of Commons Select Committee on Social Services considered the subject of community care, it stated firmly: "The stage has now been reached when the rhetoric of community care has to be matched by action, and where the public are understandably anxious about the consequences." In fact, as the committee pointed out: "The phrase 'community care' means little in itself, it is a phrase used by some descriptively and others prescriptively: that is, by some as a shorthand way of describing specific services provided in certain ways and in certain places; by others as an ideal or principle in the light of which existing services are to be judged and new ones developed. It has in fact, come to have such general reference as to be virtually meaningless. It has become a slogan, with all the weakness that implies". (*Community Care: With Special Reference to Adult Mentally Ill and Mentally Handicapped People*, HMSO, 1985, paras. 26 and 8 respectively).

For the phrase "community care" to have any meaning the reality must consist of people with learning difficulties being part of the community, not just in it; working alongside local people and being supported by them, where that is necessary. It means engaging in reciprocal relationships, not just being recipients of paternalism — or maternalism — however benevolent.

Over the past 15 years many techniques have been devised to assess the ability levels of people with learning difficulties and to teach specific aptitudes and everyday living skills. Many parents will now say to a keyworker, that their Jenny, Nick or Amy are able to cook or go to the shop on their own, sew on a button or work a computer. Recent studies by Malin (1981) and Raynes *et al* (1987), have demonstrated the proficiency of many to cope in independent living situations, but also highlighted the difficulties encountered in being an integral member of the local community. For many their only "friend" is the social worker or community nurse. Dorothy Atkinson (1989) quotes a social worker talking about a married couple with learning difficulties living in their own home, and their relationship with their former workers: "They don't see them as social workers . . . they are friends, it's more of a friendship. They simply don't expect to be cut off".

People with learning difficulties in Atkinson's research group expressed similar sentiments. Laura, in a letter to her social worker, writes:

"Dear Friend,

"When are you coming back as I miss you quite a lot . . . hope to hear soon. Hope it won't be long before I see you.

"With Love, Laura".

Raynes *et al* quote (1987) the instance of Bill Harrison, who lives in his own home after a number of years in a long-stay hospital and hostel. As Mr Harrison himself says: "I clean every day when I come in from work, Mrs Keenan [social worker] sometimes helps sort out money . . . neighbours are not so bad, really, I only know two what's next door. Nobody comes to see me only Mrs Keenan . . . I go to me sister's on Sunday, she doesn't come here. I watch television mostly, sometimes reading. Get books from the library."

The social worker is aware of this dependence but our whole "care" system is geared to personal dependence rather than independence. Parents are naturally protective of their children (not just parents of children with learning difficulties as some texts suggest), and it is school and friends who gradually widen the individual's experiences. Most people with learning difficulties, however, still go to special schools which are often situated out of town. The special school has a wide catchment area so that it is unlikely any one child will have a friend in the immediate vicinity of their home (see P. Seed, 1988 and C. Cullen in Horobin & May, 1988). In one of the Scottish schools examined by Seed, a teacher described the work of the school, its parents and the Friends organisation as "fighting a way out of the ghetto of handicap into a world of genuine relations with ordinary children". Special schools, however, still tend towards a nurturing rather than a developing approach, while those children who are in ordinary schools do not always have the backup necessary for them to take full advantage of this integration. As Cullen points out: "Simply putting mentally handicapped children together with non-handicapped children, does not lead to the benefits we might anticipate. Special help is required and we are still some way from knowing exactly how to arrange that help".

The majority of young people with learning difficulties move from school to adult training centre or social education centre.

These organisations do splendid work, as do the special schools, but they are attempting to inculcate skills in an unrealistic setting and promote interaction with a public which has no natural contact with the centre. Living situations raise similar issues. Raynes, Sumpton and Flynn's comparative studies of homes for people with learning difficulties showed that, as one might expect, residents in long-stay hospitals had very little control over their own lives, but this lack of choice and personal autonomy was also mirrored in local authority hostels, the private and voluntary sector homes, and living with parents. In local authority hostels more involvement in everyday living was encouraged but it was clear to the researchers that "most of the residents we saw had no friends outside their residences". Living with parents usually meant a much greater sharing of "family tasks" but, as the authors point out: "Being physically within the neighbourhood did not seem to make going out more frequent for most of these adults than for those who lived in the hostel for example. Sixty three per cent did not get out in the evening during the week, and 53% did not get out at weekends. Contact with friends again appeared to be very limited . . . and for several, the integration extended to one's family, the ATC and the bus to get there and back."

Trying to make connections

Margaret Flynn's extensive studies of people in the north-west of England living in their own homes (Raynes *et al*, 1987 and Malin ed., 1987, chapter 13) have illuminated the struggle of people with learning difficulties to achieve and retain their own independence. Flynn has described movingly how many of her interviewees sat clutching their front-door keys as a symbol of their new-found independence, and despite the difficulties facing them the great majority would not wish to return to hospital or hostel (lecture at St George's Hospital Medical School, London, 1987). Some of the positive comments were: "I like being here best . . . it's alright here. I've got a key and I can see who's outside. My things are safe. I can keep them safe. I like it. I can see my friends when I want and I can do what I want when I'm here". And: "I always wanted a place of me own".

Dorothy Atkinson's study (Atkinson & Ward, 1988) of 50 people who left long-stay hospital and moved into varied domestic housing in Somerset, paints a similar picture — as one of them says of her neighbour: "Mrs Williams is nice, she talks to me in the garden. Marjorie, who lives on the other side, calls in every day for a chat".

Living in ordinary housing in ordinary streets increases the possibility of reciprocity. One in Flynn's study talked about having "very good neighbours". "If they want to use the phone, like Mrs Hall next door, she's a bit crippled and she can't go far, so we let her use the phone".

Living in a house of one's own, however, is not as Raynes *et al* point out "an easy option". Of the 88 people interviewed by Flynn (N. Malin ed. 1987, chapter 13), about 75 per cent were leading, what their keyworkers described as, a "successful life in the community". A number of the group, however, had problems with unfriendly neighbours or downright harrassment and victimisation; some were lonely; others had dropped out of SECs but had no visible alternative for occupation and companionship, although a few had made very good use of their increased freedom of action. Financial problems were a source of anxiety, with training in handling money being inadequate for the complexities of life outside of the institution, especially with the continual changes in DSS benefit claim rules. As Atkinson (1980) has written: "One problem is that, almost always these days, we discharge people into poverty, a subsistence level with few, if any, extras".

Not enough attention has been given to people's need for companionship, and for those of us who have worked in rehabilitation services for people moving out of the long-stay hospitals, one of the major criteria for success or failure is the preservation of friendship networks. For many people moving out of institutions their only friends are "those professional friends", the social worker or community nurse. Both individual and keyworker are in an ambiguous position if old friendships have not been maintained or new ones developed. The professional has personally invested a great deal in the success of the venture, but their professional goal is to set things going and then withdraw. Social work supervisors, using a task-centred approach, would expect them to start giving more attention to other clients. But as Atkinson (1989) and Flynn have pointed out, the keyworkers are well aware of the strength of these ties.

One of Dorothy Atkinson's discussion groups described a relationship which even transcended the death of the professional concerned: "Mrs Hart used to take us all out in the car, for rides to see different places. That was when I lived in the group. She died later, after I'd moved here on my own. I'm still a friend of her family though. I'm going to her daughter's wedding party on Saturday".

Research into counselling has shown that people, either in helping or helped situations respond to others who are young, attractive, have good eye-contact and are both good listeners and interesting conversationalists. Many people coming out of long-stay hospitals don't fit this description, and we professionals have often failed to build up the social skills necessary to enable people to succeed in becoming a real part of a community. This is not just true of hospitals, however, but in families, special schools and centres, we have maintained a paternalism that ensures that the majority of people with learning difficulties continue to look to professionals as a source of warmth, guidance and approval. Perhaps one of the great disservices we professionals have done for people with a learning difficulty is to ensure that they relate to paid staff rather than their peer group and other friends (see Gilbert, 1987).

Forms of integration

The word community, from the Latin *communitas,* — meaning "common" — means people living in one locality and/or having cultural, religious or other characteristics in common. As we have said, the precise definition of community in the sense of "care in the community", is often left unstated. The concept of community sometimes has a tendency to pitch camp in different locations like a travelling circus. In hospital reviews "community" can mean the local hostel, in hostel reviews "community" a group home or adult family placement, and so on.

Nirje (1969), one of the Swedish exponents of valued lifestyles, describes six types of integration:

Physical Integration — involving the sharing of normal physical settings.

Functional — allowing people with learning difficulties the opportunity to participate physically in normal experiences.

Social — involving social interaction and acceptance in routine settings, for example, shopping, pubs, neighbourhood activities etc.

Personal — that is, the development of significant personal relationships and the opportunity to maintain, respond and gain from these in the normal way.

Societal — involving people with learning difficulties in active participation in society in terms of self-determination, legal rights and opportunities, as a full citizen, to the same extent as the rest of the population.

Organisational — the use of systems, structures and services, designed for the general public, as opposed to specialist services administered separately.

Flynn's research into the lives of people in homes of their own, and research into integrated schooling, shows that physical and functional integration can stop short there unless positive action is taken. A study of residents at St Lawrence's Hospital, Caterham, found that of the 1,400 residents, 48 per cent had had no visitors for over 10 years. Of the 52 per cent remaining, 50 per cent had had no contact in the previous year, and the remainder had had contact of a varied kind (Dr Akuffo, lecturer at Leybourne Grange Hospital, July 1989). David Felce discovered that in institutions people wasted 96 per cent of their time. In local hospital units activity was more positive but there was still considerable lassitude.

In the small homes that were set up in the Wessex region, purposeful activity increased dramatically, partly because staff set out to undertake domestic activities *with* residents, rather than do things *for* them, and encouraged the making of outside friendships and contacts.

Felce and Toogood (1988) carefully describe the sensitive and individualised action taken by staff to assist their residents to play an active part in community life. The change in demeanour and appearance was so marked that it led to one passerby asking a member of staff accompanying one of the residents (Catherine) on a trip: "Where's the big girl who used to sit down in the street?"

Contact with residents' families increased from 11 contacts per year on average, to 42 per year, once the move had been made to the small homes. Community contacts increased dramatically from an average 10 events a year, to 250. Even then it is probably only when another resident, Shirley, gained a job in a local pub, that full integration, in Nirje's sense, took place: "She has achieved the status of an employee, paid at parity with other citizens who have no disabilities who undertake similar employment, but not only that, she is doing something which is entirely individual to her. Part of her life is arranged with just her in mind, and for her own benefit".

The BBC/MENCAP television series, *A Life of our Own*, stresses the importance of work and leisure in integration, and shows what can be achieved. Gary was enthusiastic about his job with Sainsbury's. His mother spoke of his increased independence and pride in his appearance. "He's one of the community now", she said, "he's a completely different person since he's working. He's more aware of things, and he'll go out to places on his own now which he never did before". Dorothy Atkinson (1989) has spent a considerable amount of time researching the leisure activities of people with learning difficulties. She found the leisure time of people discharged from large mental handicap hospitals into independent living situations was full, and allowed them to mix with a wide variety of people. She did, however, find a number of disturbing trends:

'Giving up pursuits' through a lack of money, ill-health or interest waning over time, either on the part of the individual or the group.

'Getting stuck' — people having talent but lacking the confidence to take their interests and hobbies into local community groups.

'Being fixed in sex-role activities', with the men getting involved in outdoor activities, while the women were actively encouraged in domestic pursuits.

'Getting fixed in handicap roles' — attending special clubs and classes and, therefore, being out in the community but not a part of it.

Many people with learning difficulties seemed to get stuck into the status of an on-looker rather than a participant and it often took active but sensitive intervention from a local or professional friend to break the cycle.

Figure 3.3.1 *Positive and negative cycles*

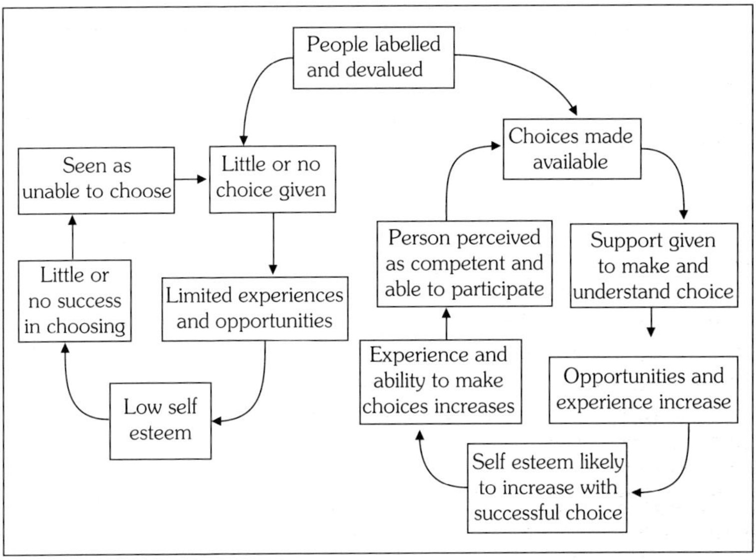

(From work by Nan Carle and David Brandon)

Community, what community?

"There is no such thing as society. There are individual men and women and there are families"
Margaret Thatcher

"The truly religious man looks after his own soul and other people's bodies. The hypocrite looks after his own body and other people's souls".
Rabbi Lionel Blue

In Brighton in 1952, a reporter from a local paper penned this description of a council housing estate: "I walked last week through Moulsecoomb . . . I found a world of climb and turn, of starched white collars and oil-stained overalls in fairly equal proportions — a world of happy children running home from school. It is at once a place of noise and quiet. And its streets and houses — council grey and tudor half timbered, spell the word 'home' to a community that is as united as any tiny hamlet planted deep in a forest" (quoted in P. Dickens and P. Gilbert, 1979).

The sentiment may be hopelessly idealistic but it does speak to us of a British society which had been united in a war, that had meant a fight for both national survival, and indeed, for certain fundamental principles. Britain was led by politicians from both main parties, who thought it best to retain "the family silver" and move forwards toward a better quality of life for all citizens.

The sense of community is a strong myth within Britain, a myth which Banton *et al (The Politics of Mental Health*, MacMillan, 1985), have described as the "fantasy of the 'remembered community'". Four main features characterise it: it is small, and separable from other communities; everyone understands the experiences of everyone else; each shares responsibility for each other's lives; and each participates in a common, unifying cause.

Although the ideal may never have existed in its entirety, many people experienced a common sense of identity and purpose as in the East End neighbourhoods described in Wilmott and Young's famous studies. One of Aneurin Bevan's fundamental beliefs about a social housing policy was that whereas the 1920s had provided "castrated communities", with private enterprise providing for one income group, and local authorities for another, it was "essential" he felt "for the full life of the citizen, to see the living tapestry of the mixed community".

This living tapestry is not how Britons see themselves now. In an ICM poll in the autumn of 1989, nearly three-quarters of the electorate saw Britain as an unjust society, with one law for the rich and another for the poor. Fifty per cent of all voters, and a high proportion of Conservative voters, thought better services and high taxes were preferable to lower taxes and worse services. In the 1980s we have seen a return to the concept of the "rich man in his castle" (detached house with burglar alarm), and the poor man at his gate (in a cardboard box by the litter bins). Even one former Tory Cabinet Minister, John Nott, described the 1980s as an era of "public squalour and private affluence" (BBC2, *Newsnight*), echoing J. K. Galbraith's famous aphorism about social extremes in the United States of America. As needs increase the needy turn more to private charities, while government withdraws its support. But *Charity Trends* (1989) shows private companies and individuals lagging well behind the American levels of charitable donations, which is the example Britain is supposed to emulate.

Although "Victorian values" are held up as a shining example, it is worth noting that many Conservative politicians in the Victorian era, and indeed up until the late 1970s, recognised that the evils engendered by societal neglect as graphically described by Dickens in *Dombey and Son* threatened not only the poor but the rich as well: "Those who study the physical sciences, and bring them to bear upon the health of Man, tell us that if the noxious particles that rise from vitiated air were palpable to the sight we should see them lowering in a dense black cloud above such haunts, and rolling slowly on to corrupt the better portions of a town. But if the moral pestilence that rises with them, and in the eternal laws of outraged Nature is inseparable from them, could be made discernible too, how terrible the revelation . . . then should we stand appalled to know, that where we generate disease to strike our children down and entail itself on unborn generations, there also we breed, by the same certain progress, infancy that knows no innocence, youth without modesty or change, maturity that is mature in nothing but in suffering and guilt, blasted old age that is a scandal on the form we bear."

Conservative municipal politicians, such as Chamberlain in Birmingham, saw the public control of utilities as essential in promoting social harmony and reasonable standards of life for all citizens.

Although the standard of living has risen for many, the sense of division within society has risen also. Monetary success has become the main criterion for measuring individual worth, while individuals themselves have become evermore isolated from their fellows. The Archbishop of Canterbury in his now notorious interview with the *Director* (October 1989), spoke of the temptation for the successful to "regard their success as a sort of blessing or reward for rightiousness. This can lead to judgements being made about the unsuccessful . . . which are both uncharitable and untrue". Or as the BBC journalist, Brian Redhead, put it, Thatcherism is "suburban prejudice made flesh". The growth of home ownership is cited as a major social advance, and yet rising interest rates have turned many people's dreams into a nightmare. When social ownership was a reality earlier in the century rent rises would produce a sense of solidarity across a wide range of citizens, and considerable mutual assistance (see P. Dickens and P. Gilbert, *op cit*).

The East Germans and Czechs gathered in their hundreds of thousands to force their monopoly governments to stand aside and introduce democracy. The irony is that our many years of freedom — now increasingly oligarchic not democratic — could almost certainly not produce the unity through peaceable strength that the more socially conscious East Europeans have used so effectively. The British protest against injustice tends to be the letter from the individual bunker of "Disgusted of Tunbridge Wells" or the street riot where protest ends in looting by people who, as Conor Cruise O'Brien pointed out, are only taking the "everyman for himself" idea to its logical conclusion. They are indeed *Homo Thatcheriens*.

Professor Howard Newby, chairman of the Economic and Social Research Council, pointed out that the value system of the New Right "appeals to self-interest, and works against the grain of any sense of community. People only come together out of

Income

The 1988 budget made an explicit statement that the present government wished to see the rich getting richer. With the ending of all higher income tax rates above 40 per cent, £6 billion was lost to the Treasury, much of it given to the top one per cent of society, who already had incomes of between £100,000 and £2.5 billion per annum — apparently as an incentive to them to be more productive! At present the richest one per cent of the population own 21 per cent of the wealth, the richest 10 per cent own 52 per cent and the poorer 50 per cent only seven per cent.

Policies since 1979 have seen a relative and absolute increase in poverty for those on benefits. In 1979 the government cut the benefit link with earnings so that they now go up by the increase in prices. The end result is that people who are on benefits fall behind the increase in prosperity of those in work. When the second report of the comprehensive survey by the Office of Population Census and Surveys was published in the autumn of 1988, it indicated that two-thirds of Britain's 6.2 million disabled adults, found themselves in financial difficulties or just managing to cope after stringent economies. People with disabilities have to spend a significant amount of their income each week because of their disability (See J. Martin and A. White, *OPCS Surveys of Disabilities in Great Britain: Report two: The Financial Circumstances of Disabled Adults Living in Private Households,* HMSO, 1988). These findings reinforced those of Judith Buckle in 1984 (*Mental Handicap Costs More,* Disablement Income Group).

It must be stated that all figures should be treated with some caution as this government has been more prone than previous ones, to both change the basis on which statistical information is collated, and to change the rules around the claiming of benefits. The Institute for Fiscal Studies, in its report *Counting People with Low Incomes,* pointed out that the government had removed more than a million people from the poorest group in the population by changing how the figures were calculated. The new method for identifying living standards shows that 4.35 million people are on half average incomes or less. The institute's calculations, based on the methods used by the government until 1988, show the number to be 5.5 million.

Housing

Housing is supposed to be one of the government successes of recent years. Owner-occupation has risen from four million in 1951 to 14 million in 1986. More than 63 per cent of households own or are buying their own, and four in five of these are houses rather than flats (*Britain — An Official Handbook,* HMSO, 1988).

Since 1975, however, there has been a steady decline in council house building from 130,000 in that year, to less than 30,000 in 1987. The private-rented sector, which has been shrinking since the turn of the century, has also continued its fall, though this sector may receive incentives to develop in the latest government Housing Acts. At the same time there has been a concurrent rise in homelessness: 53,000 in 1978 to 113,000 in 1987. The figure now (1990) is estimated to be approximately 150,000. In London the local authorities completed 25,000 homes a year in the mid-1970s, but in 1988 produced only 1,391. The pressures on family life and the attraction of the capital has meant an estimated more than 30,000 people sleeping rough in central London with a high proportion being young blacks. Housing charities in London speak of street gangs that are beginning to assume the menacing complexion of those found in Latin-American cities.

Shelter (*A Bad Start in Life — Children, Health and Housing*, Shelter Publications, 1989) postulates that two million homes suffer severe dampness that may cause respiratory problems in children, and that "throughout Britain, childhood can mean growing up in conditions with which Victorian health inspectors would be at home".

The slow-down and effective halt in council house building has been disastrous for people with disabilities. Many people with a mental illness have not been rehoused from psychiatric hospitals, but have been left to wander the streets of London or seaside towns. In fact, it was partly the scandal of the growing "Cardboard City" next to the Houses of Parliament, which led to a move towards a more paternalistic care strategy for people with a mental illness, in the 1989 White Paper, *Caring for People: Community Care in the Next Decade and Beyond.* For people with a learning difficulty moving into independent living situations many schemes have been held up because of the lack of housing, or at least suitable housing. One of Margaret Flynn's criticisms is that many of the people she interviewed in the north-west were living in sub-standard accommodation which nobody else wanted. Some schemes have taken the risk of holding out for accommodation of a good standard. There is in fact, money available for public housing: £8 billion of capital receipts have been accumulated by local authorities from council house sales. Unfortunately 75 per cent have been targetted, at the insistance of the past Secretary of State for the Environment, Nicholas Ridley, for the repayment of debt rather than new building, exemplifying Mr Ridley's often proclaimed belief that "the proper role of government is nothing". The latest Housing Acts offer little hope for improvement, as the 1989 Housing Act is more concerned with the repair of a deteriorating housing stock, than providing special needs housing. Even in the private sector the new group of home owners are under pressure, with the cost of the average mortgage having risen by £2,000 a year between autumn 1988 and autumn 1989.

The revised edition of the National Federation of Housing Association/MIND handbook on housing, states: "The outcome for special needs housing is not altogether clear, although the government has promised to give 'special consideration' to this part of the housing market". The handbook itself is titled, *Housing: The Foundation of Community Care* — how high a priority the government gives this is yet to be seen.

Employment – Disability and race

The features of employment have become increasingly difficult to scan in recent years, partly because the government has changed the method of calculating the statistics over the past ten years, also because a number of people with disabilities do not care to register as such because of the stigma, and a large percentage of young people from ethnic minorities are kept in government training schemes so that the statistics are kept favourable.

As the unemployment rate rose during the mid-1980s, racial minorities were hardest hit. By the Spring of 1985 the unemployment rate for black men had more than trebled, and was almost twice that for white men. Black women had a 19 per cent unemployment rate, compared with 20 per cent for white women; and for blacks within the 16-24 age band, there was a 33 per cent rate, compared with 16 per cent for young whites. Some sections of the black community were even harder hit, with 48 per cent of economically active 16-25 year olds amongst the Pakistani and Bangladeshi communities being unemployed, and the disparities were far greater within the inner cities (Walker & Walker, 1987). Bayley points out that while at the end of July 1988, the national unemployment rate was 8.2 per cent, in Sheffield the figure was 13 per cent, and this average figure for the city hid marked disparities between 5.8 per cent in a reaonably prosperous area, and 27.5 per cent in an inner-city ward (Bayley, 1989).

For people with learning difficulties the dramatic rise in unemployment from about a million in the late 1970s, to three million in the mid 1980s was a disaster. Coupled to this, changes in employment law to protect the employee, meant that many employers were not prepared to take the risk of taking on somebody who might be prone to long-term sickness. Many people with learning difficulties lost their employment in the mid 1980s, and a number of successful enclave schemes were scrapped by over-anxious employers. Now, even in areas of low unemployment, agencies such as MENCAP's Pathway, Shaw Trust and The Disablement Advisory Service, are having to work hard to persuade employers to take on people with disabilities.

Public attitudes

The historian, Lawrence Stone, once remarked about the sixteenth century wars of religion, that "religious tolerance would probably only come about through public indifference". Writers such as Bulmer, have focused on the lacuna in community care caused by dangerous assumptions being made about the strength of informal care networks, assumptions which lie at the heart of the policies themselves (Bulmer, 1987). Yet many people would say that there is an increasing acceptance of people with learning difficulties, as individuals and small groups are seen out and about in ordinary settings, and as representatives make appearances in soap operas (the ultimate acceptance?).

Sheila Manning's research in Lincolnshire (Malin, 1987), found that:

- Many people had a sympathetic view of people with learning difficulties, with a surprising high number (44.1 per cent) indicating that they had seen some form of written material. The term "mental" in mental handicap was seen as increasing stigma and causing confusion with mental illness.
- In terms of living situations, 24.5 per cent mentioned the "family home" but with support and alternatives if the family couldn't cope. Opinions as to integration were divided, some saying that people should be "surrounded by everyday life and be a part of it", others that "it was not right to foist them on a generally uncaring public".
- Respondents did not expect families to shoulder the whole burden, and 64 per cent believe that professional people should take responsibility, with the government having a clear duty not to opt-out.
- 76.5 per cent had no reservations about living next door to someone with a learning difficulty. But there was a marked change in attitudes when the question was about living next door to an institution for 150 people — then feelings of fear and anxiety were aroused.
- Seventy per cent would help neighbours, *if asked,* while a lower number, 40 per cent would feel able to *volunteer* help.

MENCAP's national survey in 1987/8 (Leighton ed, 1988), mirrors a number of Manning's findings, picking up a considerable confusion between mental handicap and mental illness, but also discovering that "those who have personal contact with people with a mental handicap, are generally much more knowledgeable and positive about their needs". There was strong feeling about the need for supervision in the community, and a lack of confidence in people's ability to make meaningful contact. Leighton identified four main cluster groupings: avoiders; protectors; naive acceptors; and confident acceptors.

Witherspoon's small study (1988) of people who had moved

from a residential training unit into small group homes in a South London borough, took a number of negative hypotheses, and the author was pleasantly surprised by her findings. The staff had not sought permission from neighbours for the move (and in fact Manning's study indicates that many people do not expect to be consulted), but had made contact during the moving-in phase with the result that there was considerable interaction between the neighbours. Whereas Manning's hypothetical question about visiting had elicited a willingness to visit, but not invite back, Witherspoon found a reciprocal visiting pattern; a considerable use of community facilities; people in the neighbourhood were mainly friendly; and new friendships were forged through the use of local facilities.

It is often put forward that rural communities would be more accepting than urban ones. When Janice Sinson looked at a rural and an urban community in Yorkshire however, she discovered that whereas 24 per cent of townspeople had a negative image of people with Down's Syndrome, 54 per cent of people in rural areas held a negative attitude (J. Sinson, *Attitudes to Down's Syndrome*, Mental Health Foundation, 1986). This is in line with Bulmer's review of American research, which shows that urban dwellers have just as many friends as those living in rural areas, and seem to be able to form friendships quicker, and Seltzer and Seltzer's opinion that negative attitudes are more probable in stable neighbourhoods than transient ones (quoted in Witherspoon, 1988). NIMBY (Not in My Back Yard) attitudes, are more likely in well-to-do-neighbourhoods, but Flynn's research points to the risk of vandalism and victimisation in decaying areas where a scapegoat is required.

Who cares?

"This city has 10 million souls — some living in mansions, some living in holes,
But there's no place for us my dear. There's no place for us".
W. H. Auden.

Most young people share their leisure time with a friend or a group on a regular basis. Many people with learning difficulties have to rely on parents, as table 3.1.1 shows, and therefore have a very restricted lifestyle.

Research from the NIMROD project in Wales shows a more encouraging picture, especially in areas, such as the Rhondda Valley where there is considerable community solidarity. The NIMROD experience of placing people with learning difficulties in ordinary housing won considerable "negative acceptance" within local communities, in that people were tolerated, but still there were a number of barriers to positive acceptance, that is, becoming a real part of the local neighbourhood. Some of the barriers identified were:

- The difficulties in communication or lack of interactive skills in the individuals themselves.
- The effects of institutionalisation.
- The lack of a focus for relationships to be fostered, e.g. employment.
- Community attitudes and lack of confidence.
- The availability of staff or volunteers to initiate relationships.
- Staff can get in the way — undermining the status of the individual.

Table 3.1.1: *Companions of adults with a learning difficulty*

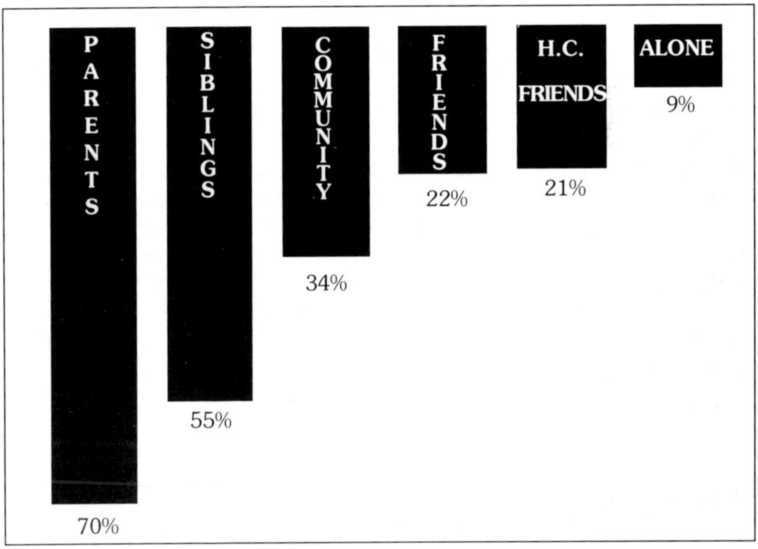

(McConkey and McCormack, 1983)

Roy McConkey's research in Dublin (McConkey, 1987) demonstrates that it is possible to predict who in the local community might be interested in creating a relationship with a disabled person. McConkey's view is that people with learning difficulties are their own best ambassadors, as the most likely to get involved are those who have had past contact with someone with a disability and are confident in their ability to make relationships.

Witherspoon (1988) found the respondents in her survey were generally positive in sharing community facilities with people with learning difficulties, and interested in learning more about them. An overwhelming majority felt that longstay hospital care was inappropriate and that people should live in ordinary housing.

Building positive networks

"Care out of the community need not concern itself with the community from which it is removing the client. Even care in the community need not concern itself overmuch with what the community is or the way it functions. But care by the community demands understanding of what it is, sympathy with the way it works and insight into the way the community can help". Michael Bayley's perceptive analysis of community care in Sheffield (1973) is even more relevant now with a greatly increased number of people with learning difficulties living in the community, but not always part of it. Service planning needs now to focus on the five accomplishments set out by O'Brien and Lyle (*Framework for Accomplishment,* 1987): community presence; community participation; promoting choice and protecting rights; improving competencies and acquiring skills; and enhancing status and self-respect.

Community workers can usefully carry out the networking analysis undertaken by Seed (1988) to ascertain the contacts individuals and families actually have, and then build on to these natural care networks.

Increased real integration has to take place at a number of levels:

Passive integration

- ☐ *Integration through community presence* while as Nirje says, "isolation and segregation nourish public ignorance and prejudice", an increased community presence over the past 20 years appears to have increased public tolerance and understanding, if not to any great extent, actual involvement.
- ☐ *Macro-public education pogrammes* through media coverage and charity advertising has often tended to promote an "object of pity" image, series such as *A Life of our Own,* and the appearance of, for example, a child with Down's Syndrome in the *Crossroads* serial, help promote a positive image of achievement. The achievements of individuals like Cathy Hebden (See J. Hebden, *She'll Never Do Anything, Dear,* Souvenir Press, 1985) need to be given the same prominence as fund-raising events, and McConkey's work encourages specific programmes targetted at groups, for example, local churches.

Active integration

- ☐ *Community living and integration* Both a philosophy of human dignity and practical experience counsels against asking permission of existing residents in a locality where an independent living scheme is being set up. Sensitive work once individuals or a group arrive in a neighbourhood is far more effective. When local people perceive people with learning difficulties as people first, then prejudice tends to fall away.

- *Micro-education programmes* Targetting specific groups in particular neighbourhoods would seem to be a way forward indicated by the available research.

  North America is considerably in advance of the UK in this sphere. Agencies like the Office of Community Education in New Jersey, have designed programmes aimed at various age groups in different settings, utilising a variety of mediums. For example, "kids on the block", an interactive puppet show for 8 year olds has had considerable success in this country, as well as with a probably more spontaneous audience the other side of the Atlantic. Britain is beginning to follow this lead and a *Community Care* Enterprise Award winner in 1988 was the NCH Options Project in Cardiff comprehensive schools. (see Bartlett, 1989). GPs and churches (see Gilbert, 1988) are important groups to involve in a community education strategy. Steve Dowson has suggested that five factors need to be considered in building up a public education strategy (from the CMH conference, "Changing attitudes", 22 September 1989): sensible time targets; a specific target group; adapting the message to the audience; choosing the best medium; and setting an effective style ("Don't become enveloped in the bad news").
- *Leisure* Edgerton remarked in his often quoted study *The Cloak of Competence* (California 1967) that ". . . the use of leisure time indicates better than anything else the richness or impoverishment of their lives". Walsh's study (1986) hinged on the need to think further than bricks and mortar when building a new service and projects such as the MENCAP IMSC "Bridge-In" scheme in London fulfills this kind of integrative function.
- *Further and adult education* Extended education in its broader sense is an ideal opportunity both for integration, making friendships and developing competencies. Many schemes started off like the Islington Adult Education Link Scheme (see Shearer, 1986, chapter 7, and Richardson and Ritchie, 1989, chapter 3) as a special project and have now been taken on by local authorities as a mainstream service.
- *Befrienders schemes* These can begin as schemes explicitly designed to foster one-to-one relationships, or may start off as a respite care programme for carers, which grow into more reciprocal friendships. McConkey's survey indicated a desire on the part of potential volunteers for "support and back-up from professionals", and an evaluation of schemes points to a need for good co-ordination and a counselling component for befrienders as well as users.
- *Legal* Some Scandinavian countries believe that legislation is the best method of making a clear statement of values.

Increasing competence

Relationships are interactive and based on a satisfaction of mutual needs. People with learning difficulties need to acquire interactional skills if they are to survive and flourish in an ordinary life situation. As Becker pointed out in his *The Denial of Death,* a person's self-worth is constituted symbolically. Most people with learning difficulties, however, are less able to conceptualise and are therefore more dependent on concrete relationships (J. Dunne, 1989).

The crucial role here is that of families (or staff where people do not have a family) whether they have a "she prefers to be with me, she really does" attitude, or one that says he needs "a place that's his . . . where he's socially accepted" (quoted in Richardson and Ritchie).

Government action

In one of the most influential studies of the theory and practice of community care, Martin Bulmer has described the concept as being particularly prone to "vagueness, confusion and misconceptions. At the heart there is a vacuum" (Bulmer, 1987). He describes current government policy as "minimalist" with as much responsibility as possible placed on families.

Central funding of public education, integration and carer support projects would be an option, like those care in the community projects monitored by the Personal Social Services Research Unit (see chapter 1).

Towards a more caring community?

"The history of mental handicap demonstrates how easily the best-intentioned reform can turn to repression, especially in conditions of economic stringency and hardening social attitudes, such as those we are witnessing now."
Joanna Ryan and Frank Thomas, *The Politics of Mental Handicap.*

"No, England's not a bad country. It's just a mean, cold, ugly, divided, tired, clapped-out, post-imperial, post-industrial slag-heap, covered in polystyrene hamburger cartons. It's not a bad country at all, I love it".
Margaret Drabble, *A Natural Curiosity*

The treatment of vulnerable people has always been based both on the economic ability (or perceived ability) of a society to care for those who are not themselves economically independent, and also how the particular group of people are regarded by their fellows.

Societies have reacted very differently to apparently abnormal behaviour. Corporatist social organisms might be expected to react more favourably than individualistic ones, but the Bejing psychiatrist, Professor Jian Zuo-ning has stated clearly that prejudice against people suffering from mental illness in China is deep-rooted and discriminatory (see K. Jones, *Experience in Mental Health: Community Care and Social Policy,* Sage, 1988). Jean Vanier, the founder of L'Arche, believes that a community's development, and indeed the human race's survival, is translucently tied to the discovery of knowledge as to how to transform aggression into co-operation and the perception of difference as a value not a threat (J. Vanier, *The Challenge of L'Arche,* Winston, 1981). Public policy and public education cannot be translated into care and collaboration unless society itself acknowledges values which hold these as life-giving and life-enhancing. The support for relief agencies in Ethiopia and Romania seems to speak of a public concern, but the zenophobia about admitting Hong Kong residents betrays a darker side.

The 1980s have been the age of a reborn justification by wealth and rampant individualism. The trouble with this ideology, as the late Victorian reformers discovered, is that in a shared world the neglect of one part of the body politic grievously affects the whole. As one modern commentator has put it: "Unless [people] act as a community, no amount of private affluence will compensate for the general public squalor. And unless they recognise that money is not everything, nothing of real value can ever be defended. When people can be bought and sold as commodities, where money is the bottom line, the casualties are first people of quality and then the quality of everything. For the world to be pleasantly habitable it needs people who have no price, who believe that there are things beyond price, and to do much without hope of reward. It needs people who have ideals and will not sell them for 30 nor 30 million pieces of silver" (Harriott, 1989).

D. Atkinson (1980) "Moving out of mental handicap hospitals," APEX, volume 8, No.3.

D. Atkinson (1989), *Someone To Turn To,* British Institute for Mental Handicap.

D. Atkinson and L. Ward (1988), Talking Points Number 3, *A Part of the Community: Social Integration and Neighbourhood Networks,* CMH.

N. Bartlett (1989), "First Steps forward", *Community Care,* 25 May.

M. Bayley (1989), *Welfare — A Moral Issue?,* Diocese of Sheffield Social Responsibility.

M. Bayley (1973), *Mental Handicap and Community Care,* Routledge and Kegan Paul.

H. Brown and H. Smith, "Whose 'ordinary life' is it anyway?", *Disability, Handicap Society,* Vol 4, No 2, 1989.

M. Bulmer (1987), *The Social Basis of Community Care,* Unwin.

P. Dickens & P. Gilbert (1979), *The State of the Housing Question*, University of Sussex.
J. Dunne, "A radical philosophy for mental handicap services", in P. McGinley ed. (1989), *Research and Practice in the Service of People with Learning Difficulties*, Brothers of Charity/Dublin.
D. Felce and S. Toogood (1988), *Close to Home*, British Institute of Mental Handicap.
P. Gilbert, "Strangers in a strange land", *Community Care*, 22 June 1987.
P. Gilbert *et al* (1988), *We are one People*, Diocese of Arundel and Brighton.
John F. X. Harriott, "The trouble with materialism", *The Tablet*, 9 September 1989.
G. Horobin and D. May ed (1988), *Living with Mental Handicap: Transitions in the Lives of People with Mental Handicap*, Jessica Kingsley Press, chapters by Chris Cullen and Philip Seed.
B. Jordan (1976), *Freedom and the Welfare State*, Routledge and Kegan Paul.
Kings Fund (1988), *Ties and Connections: An Ordinary Community Life for People with Learning Difficulties*, Kings Fund.
A. Leighton ed. (1988), *Mental Handicap in the Community*, Woodhead Faulkner.
N. Malin ed. (1987), *Reassessing Community Care*, Croom Helm.
R. McConkey (1987), *Who Cares? Community Involvement with Handicapped People*, Souvenir Press.
R. McConkey and B. McCormack (1983) *Breaking Barriers: Educating People about Disability*, Souvenir Press.
B. Nirje (1969), "The normalisation principle and its human management implications", in R. Krugel & A. Shearer eds., *Changing Patterns in Residential Services for the Mentally Retarded*, Washington DC.
Office of Population Censuses and Surveys, 6 reports from the OPCS on surveys of *Aspects of Disabilities in Great Britain*, September 1988 to July 1989.
T. Philpot ed. (1984), *Group Care Practice: The Challenge of the Next Decade, Community Care.*
N. V. Raynes *et al* (1987), *Homes for Mentally Handicapped People*, Tavistock.
J. Renshaw *et al* (1988), *Care in the Community: The First Steps*, PSSRU/University of Kent, Gower Publishing.
P. Seed (1988), *Children with Profound Handicaps*, Falmer Press.
A. Shearer (1986), *Building Community*, Kings Fund/Campaign for Mentally Handicapped People.
D. Sines ed. (1988), *Towards Integration: Comprehensive Services for People with Mental Handicaps*, Harper and Row.
D. Towell ed. (1988), *An Ordinary Life in Practice*, Kings Fund, especially chapters 2, 5 and 7.
A. Walker and C. Walker ed. (1987), *The Growing Divide: A*

Social Audit, 1979-1987, Child Poverty Action Group.
J. Walsh (1986), *Let's Make Friends,* Souvenir Press.
D. Wilkin (1979), *Caring for the Mentally Handicapped Child,* Croom Helm.
P. Willis and C. Kiernan (1984), *A New Way Evaluated: Adult Education Integration, MENCAP/Thomas Coram.*
C. Witherspoon (1988), *Community Care and Individuals with Mental Handicap,* unpublished MSW Thesis, University of Sussex.

VIDEOS

A Life of our Own, BBC/MENCAP, 1989.
Open University (1986), *Patterns for Living,* Sections 2 and 3.
NB: *Patterns for Living* is an entire course, not just published material.

with mental handicaps, which I love doing. I have now reached a stage at which I can read anything printed or typed.

My constant companion for two and a half years was a budgie, Peter, who survived a broken leg and was a non-stop chatterbox. I spent hours teaching him to talk. Unfortunately he escaped and I now have a grey cockatiel.

My life has now gone round in full circle. I have been adopted by a family in Leeds — Bob and Lesley Priestley and their children Kenneth and Elizabeth and have changed my name by deed-poll to Priestley. All being well, I shall return to Leeds to live with them in the near future.

Reprinted from Community Living *(October, 1987) with permission of the editor.*

4

Supporting a valued lifestyle for service users

". . . There's a beautiful world out there and we want to be part of it . . . "
Quoted in Ann Shearer (1986)

"Anyway, after a while, I got a new flat in a nice area. I have been here nine months and I'm very happy. I got promotion at the dockyard. I now work in the store and I enjoy my job. I also made a lot of friends at my workplace and I play pool with some of them. I also go to Country and Western concerts.
"I'm totally independent and I'm enjoying myself. All I need now is a girlfriend."
Quoted in D. Atkinson and F. Williams (1990)

Traditionally people with a learning difficulty have experienced restricted lifestyles. These have offered little in the way of choice, with few opportunities to make personal decisions about everyday domestic activities, or major decisions about home, work and personal relationships. This lack of power over decisions has resulted in people living lives that are limited in experience and opportunity. This can lead to institutional behaviour, and a restricted lifestyle that has little to do with a person's learning difficulty, but mainly the result of service systems that have systematically, often in the name of caring, ignored the needs of users, to the extent that they are unable to undertake everyday tasks that most of us take for granted.

Socially valued lifestyles

Although there are many descriptions of what it means to live a socially valued life, in the context of services for people with learning difficulties, the Kings Fund Centre's document *An Ordinary Life* (1980) has much to commend it for brevity and clarity. It states: "Our goal is to see mentally handicapped people in the mainstream of life, living in ordinary houses, in ordinary streets, with the same range of choices as any other citizen, and mixing as equals with others, and mostly not handicapped members of their own community."

This aspiration of an "ordinary life" symbolised the guiding philosophy of the movement towards community-based services, which are now increasingly accepted as the pattern for provision.

It provides a valuable starting point for the manager who wishes to develop a service that enables users to live their lives in a manner that is as close as possible to that of any other citizen, irrespective of their degree of disability.

Moving a stage further in the attempt to define a valued lifestyle, Williams and Tyne (1988) have identified some characteristics of a lifestyle that everyone is likely to value:

- having easy physical access to a wide range of people and places;
- not living in close proximity to large numbers of people who are likely to be seen as "odd";
- having a good reputation;
- having lots of opportunity to meet people;
- being treated as an adult, with corresponding freedoms and responsibilities;
- not being made to seem "odd" or negatively different;
- having intensive help to overcome any disabilities or disadvantages;
- comfortable settings to live or work in;
- being treated as an individual;
- being respected and treated well;
- being served by organisations and programmes that have the structures and supports to enable all these things to happen and be maintained.

They see this list as a useful starting point for identifying good practice in the application of these values. When managing services they also offer an important basis for examining what happens to users of services, and how much we are able to develop service structures and processes that provide the crucial opportunities to support valued lifestyles.

Wolfensberger (1983) in his description of social role valorisation has stated that the primary goal of services "is to create, support and defend valued social roles for people who are at risk of social devaluation". O'Brien (1987) has developed a practical approach that enables Wolfensberger's statement to be used with his description of the "five essential accomplishments". These accomplishments can be used as a basis for questioning the service provided and begin to introduce activities that will give users an increasingly wider range of opportunities in their lives. The accomplishsments are:

Community presence where service users are physically present in their local community. This would include non-segregated settings, such as home, work, education and leisure. In other words all those ordinary places that constitute community life.

Choice is concerned with extending the service users' opportunities to make decisions about everyday activities, such as what to eat and what to wear, and major decisions such as where to live, who to live with and where to work.

Competence is about the opportunity to learn and use new skills with whatever level of assistance is required. This would particularly focus on the supports people require in order to increase their competencies in personally and socially important areas of their lives.

Respect is concerned with users having a valued place among a network of people and roles in the community. This is particularly important in reversing the perception of people with learning difficulties as second class citizens, with the devaluing consequences that stem from such perceptions.

Participation is important for people with learning difficulties who may need help and encouragement to meet non-handicapped people in their day-to-day lives. Particular assistance could be provided to enable service users to form relationships and become part of a growing network of people, including those who are not involved in the service.

Case example

Quarry Hill Centre is a day centre that has been redeveloping its service following the appointment of a new manager in 1987. Since then a number of changes have been gradually introduced that reflect a growing awareness of the need to provide valued daytime activities for service users. Initially, a series of workshops for staff were organised that explored ideas of valued social roles for people attending the centre. The five essential accomplishments were adopted as a framework for developing the service, followed by the introduction of activities in the day-to-day work of the centre that reflected the outcomes described by the accomplishments.

This centre, although outwardly still presenting a traditional service, has now begun to change quite radically the opportunities offered to users. The application of the five accomplishments is used to illustrate what can be achieved when a manager and staff have a clear operational framework for enabling people to establish a valued lifestyle.

Community presence is demonstrated by the opportunities offered to users who are provided with a timetable that encompass periods in the centre, along with periods spent in ordinary community settings, including work experience, use of leisure facilities, shops and public transport. A steadily increasing number of users have now left the centre and have moved into ordinary jobs. Others spend a great part of the week outside the centre, for example learning domestic skills in their own homes.

Choice has been tackled at many levels, but two particular areas are worthy of mention. Individual planning has been introduced with the emphasis placed on listening to users' views and respecting their wishes, and making a genuine attempt to incorporate their wishes into the subsequent plans. Second, for people who have never been asked their opinion about the most insignificant aspects of daily life, this has required slow and painstaking work, starting with simple choices about food and drink, and later as confidence grows extending this to more substantial areas related to choice in daily activities.

Competence has been increased by expanding the range of activities available to users, including valued activities in the community. Traditional light assembly work and time filling routines have been largely abandoned and replaced by activities that relate to needs identified in individual plans. Activities include job skills, social skills, basic DIY and leisure skills. As far as is practical these activities are located in the community rather than the day centre, in order that the skills are learnt in real life settings where they are most relevant to users' needs.

Respect with its emphasis on being seen and valued as an individual started in the day centre. Staff were encouraged to examine their own attitudes towards users, with emphasis placed on acting respectfully when interacting with users. Taken a stage further, effort has been placed on users becoming involved in community activities that enable them to be perceived by members of the community as valued individuals, through involvement in work, leisure and shopping like other people in the community.

Participation in a network of people, including friendships and relationships, has been facilitated by a number of the other accomplishments. Some users have friendships with other people attending the service, others have formed friendships for the first time with people they have met through their jobs. For example, one previous user of the service has struck up a friendship with a fellow worker he met in his new job in a supermarket. The opportunity to develop a friendship at work was something he had never achieved during many years' attendance at the day centre.

This example from practice suggests some of the ways a traditional centre has been able to change its service and improve the lifestyle of users by identifying a range of valued options for people using the service, and focussing on individual needs, through the individual planning system, with its stress on listening to the person and their hopes and wishes.

The role of staff in supporting valued lifestyles

Staff have a critical role to play in supporting service users establish a valued lifestyle. A number of studies (Flynn, 1989, Evans *et al, 1985,* and Atkinson, 1988) of people who have moved into the community from hospitals point to the importance of staff in enabling people to adapt successfully to more independent living. The quality of the environment, particularly ordinary housing, offers greater opportunity for domestic control and access to the community, and is a highly significant factor in terms of improvement in lifestyle. Nevertheless, the role of staff should not be underestimated. Staff who can positively assist users adapt to, and participate in ordinary community activities, are providing one of the most important functions in supporting valued lifestyles.

To undertake this work Atkinson (1988) sees staff needing to develop positive relationships with service users, treat them with respect, value them as individuals, and enable them to express their views and opinions about their current and future lives. Evans *et al* (1985) point to the constant need for staff to offer opportunities and encouragement to users so that their repertoire of activities can be expanded and they can become increasingly discriminating in what they do. Here Evans and colleagues mention the importance of staff helping initiate contacts and supporting the development of relationships with non-handicapped people. Although a move to the community increases the likelihood of such relationships, the commitment of staff is needed to increase the potential for this to happen.

Staff needs in supporting valued lifestyles

If staff play an important part in supporting users to achieve a valued lifestyle, then in turn they need support. A number of key factors have been identified in meeting the needs of staff and have been described by Chamberlain (1988).

- staff training is central to any attempt to develop high quality services that offer users the potential for a valued lifestyle. Emphasis needs to be placed on training in values, attitudes and skills as these are important areas that influence how staff perceive and respond to users as individuals, and in turn what users experience.
- staffing levels should be sufficient to enable staff to respond to the needs of users. Unless there are adequate staff it will be difficult to design programmes for users that respond sensitively to their individual requirements.
- staffing structures need to be designed and organised in ways that enable staff to practise the skills they have acquired during training, and be rewarded for doing so. To train staff then not provide opportunities for practice is a waste of both human and technical resources that are increasingly difficult and costly to replace.
- staff need guidance and support from their line manager if they are to be clear about the objectives to be achieved, components of good practice, and outcomes expected for users. Regular supervision that focusses on the development of the

worker, in the context of improving the quality of service provided to users should be the goal of the manager. Where staff are working in dispersed housing, managers need to establish support systems that avoid the risk of isolation and deterioration in the quality of the service, that is a particular risk in these services.

- staff and managers need the stimulus and reflection on their practice that can be provided by a system of monitoring and evaluation, particularly when this is conducted by people external to the service. The use of the values-based approach found in the PASS instrument (Wolfensberger and Glenn, 1975) offers an opportunity to evaluate the progress of a service, in creating and supporting socially valued lifestyles. The individual planning systems now being used extensively (Chamberlain, 1985) also offer staff an opportunity to monitor and evaluate their service. A further approach to evaluating service effectiveness is to actively seek the views of service users. The greater the level of user involvement in the planning and monitoring of service, the greater the likelihood that alternative perspectives on the service will be identified.

Summary

If we are to enable people with learning difficullties to achieve valued lifestyles, then services need to provide opportunities for users and the staff who support them, with the resources to translate good intentions into practice. First, this requires a thorough understanding of the risks to service users of social devaluation, and the critical importance of socially valued roles. Second, staff need a framework such as the "five accomplishments" to guide their practice. Third, staff need support if they are to strive creatively to facilitate users' integration and valued place in the community, with a service system that recognises the demands such work places on individual staff by providing them with the skills and resources to achieve this fundamental service goal.

D. Atkinson and F. Williams (1990), "*Know Me As I Am": An Anthology of Prose, Poetry and Art by People with Learning Difficulties,* Hodder and Stoughton.

D. Atkinson, "Moving from hospital to the community", *Mental Handicap,* Vol 16, March 1988.

P. Chamberlain *et al* (1985) *Life Planning Manual,* BABP.

P. Chamberlain (1988), "Moving into ordinary houses supported by staff — key factors for success", in G. Horobin and D. May (eds) *Living with Mental Handicap: Transitions in the Lives of People with Mental Handicaps,* Jessica Kingsley.

G. Evans *et al* (1985), *A New Style of Life: The Impact of People Moving into an Ordinary House on the Lives of People with a*

Mental Handicap, Research Report No.17, Mental Handicap in Wales — Applied Research Unit.
M. Flynn (1989), *Independent Living for Adults with Mental Handicap: A Place of My Own,* Cassell.
King's Fund (1980), *An Ordinary Life: Comprehensive Locally Based Residential Services for Mentally Handicapped People,* Project Paper 24.
J. O'Brien (1987), "A guide to life-style planning", in B. Wilcox and T. Bellamy, *A Comprehensive Guide to The Activities Catalog,* Paul Brookes.
A. Shearer (1986), *Building Community,* King's Fund and CMH.
P. Williams and A. Tyne (1988), "Exploring values as a basis for service development", in D. Towell (ed) *An Ordinary Life in Practice,* King's Fund.
W. Wolfensberger, "Social role of valorisation: A proposed new term for the principle of normalization", *Mental Retardation,* Vol 21, No.6, December 1983.
W. Wolfensberger and G. Glenn (1975), *PASS-Programme Analysis of Service Systems* (3rd edition) National Institute on Mental Retardation.

Consumer's View: 'People I could talk to'

Brian Johnson

Brian Johnson is in his forties and has experienced many changes, resulting largely from our changing approach to people with a learning difficulty. He has lived in various hospitals, a social services hostel and is now with a small group of other people with disabilities living in a private home. He talks about some of his life experiences, his feelings and his hopes.

I've been in hospital for about 19 years. As a little boy I went to a London hospital, Fountain Hospital and all the staff looked after me there. Then I left that hospital and they put me in another hospital and then I went to Hastings. I know all the staff there. They all missed me. I left there and went to the Forest Hospital in 1962, that was a Friday, January 26. I remember that year. After that I went to Hobbs Field Hostel

A lot of people have left the Forest now. After a bit I wanted to leave Hobbs Field, go to somewhere smaller, with people I could talk to. I wanted to go to Lyn's home but I was nervous, but it's no good being nervous. And then I went to Lyn. That's the last time I moved.

It's alright at Lyn's. Nice, smart home and all that. Everything's all upside down but we're making it all warm now, got the boiler now, keep ourselves warm in the winter. This year the kitchen's going to be done nice, take the wall down and make it look bigger, larger to put all our stuff in. Got to keep everything tidy, make sure the plates are clean. And the garden, doing all the weeds and take all the leaves and everything up.

There's six of us there, and Lyn and Dennis. It's like a home, like a family. I don't know how long I'm going to be with Lyn. I don't want to go anywhere else. The best of the lot is Lyn's.

I've always worked, always done work. In the Forest I did needlework and basketwork and I used to do carpet work. I used to get money for that. At the moment I'm thinking of something else. I'd like — it'll take a long time — to work in a shop in the town — clothes and all that. It'll take me a long time to get it worked out. I like working five days a week; Saturday and Sunday I stay indoors.

In the summer time I have a holiday, when the warm weather comes. I went on holiday this year to Jersey, stayed in a caravan, near a big windmill. There's lots of people there, nice there. Nice and warm. Lovely.

I look after myself very well, have a bath in the morning, wash, get my own clothes. I make my own tea or coffee. I am a man. Some people say I'm a baby. I'm not, I'm a man.

I'm having a good time and everything. I'm very happy.

Reprinted from Coping with Mental Handicap *by P. Gilbert & J. Hollingdale, West Sussex County Council, 1984.*

PART II
Managing services

"The deepest wisdom consists of doing the next thing you have to do, to do it as well as you can and to find joy in doing it."
Meister Eckhart (1260-1327)

"Nothing could be more radical in the public sector than to spell out responsibilities, insist on performance and accountability and to evidence that action is being taken; and even more radical, to match policy with appropriate resources and agreed timescales."
Sir Roy Griffiths, *Community Care: Agenda for Action*

"Leaders should be a sign of contradiction."
Pope John Paul II

5

Manager or leader?

"Management is out of date now, we're talking about leadership. We have too much management in this country and not enough leadership."
Walter Goldsmith, chairman of Food for Britain

'"I'm Prime Minister now . . . I am going to rule the country". "What are you going to do for us first?"
"Do for you?" repeated William indignantly. "I'm not going to do anything for you. I'm going to RULE!"'
Richmal Crompton, *William, Prime Minister*

"Women have always had to be strategic"
Beatrix Campbell, BBC2 *Arena*

In the 1970s social services departments had a number of people with the title of "leader", usually in charge of "teams". Whether they led and others followed and whether the people they were designated to lead had the cohesion of a team, orientated to undertake a specific task, or rather individuals following their own instincts, is a matter for conjecture. Those posts now, however, have, in the main, been redesignated as "managers", to show that greater control and more effective direction of human and material resources is required in social services departments in this decade. In the National Health Service it is quite hard to find someone who is not designated as a manager of some description or other! In the London Borough of Merton in 1989, the local health authority were starting to call their charge nurses "homes managers" and their nursing officers "direct service managers".

Is this a change to fashionable jargon or does it reflect a genuine devolution of power and responsibility to those who are closest to clients and those staff working directly with them? Certainly the changes in job terminology spell a move away from professional titles, such as "nursing officer", to ones which correlate more to the deployment of resources. These changes may be entirely positive but we have to be aware that it is a change affecting not only welfare agencies but industry as well.

John Adair (1983), points out that in the early stages of a manager's career he or she tends to rely on specialist/professional skills and it is only later on that he or she is concerned with more general management attributes. Now, partly in an attempt to make everybody using material and personal resources aware of the cost of those resources, staff at a relatively junior level are becoming involved in allocating and auditing money for specific programmes. Following the White Paper on the National Health Service, *Working for Patients* (February 1989), GP's were engaged in a debate as to whether their clinical judgement would be warped by having to meet treatment for patients within a fixed budget or whether conversely it would make them more thoughtful over, for example, drug prescriptions.

Care managers in pilot community care schemes in Gateshead and Kent have found that devolved budgets and responsibilities have enabled them to provide a better service to their clients and also derive more autonomy and personal satisfaction through empowerment. As David Challis, assistant director of the Personal Social Services Research Unit, said: "Most of the staff have said they don't want to go back to straight social work where they don't have control and have to give their managers a hard time to get resources" (*Community Care,* 13 July 1989).

Is there a dichotomy between "leadership" and "management"? Field Marshall Bill Slim, one of the most inspiring generals of World War II, used to say that to him leadership was about people while management was to do with money and materials. Slim had to deal with both, taking over the British Army in Burma (the "forgotten Army" as it was popularly called) under fierce attacks from the Japanese in 1942, and leading them during a long and traumatic retreat and then in an equally arduous but ultimately victorious campaign.

"Management", writes John Harvey-Jones, the man who revivified ICI, "is about people and manufacturing is about harnessing, motivating and leading people" (Harvey-Jones, 1988). The bureaucratisation of both industry and local government in the 1970s stressed the value of systems to the detriment of people, perhaps because many were under the delusion that the introduction of computers would absolve them from the need to plan on a human scale or communicate with staff. This led to organisations producing "matrix" systems, which were impossible to understand and slow to respond to the needs of consumers, staff, or the aims of the organisation. One book on people as the first resource in organisations states that: "It is almost as though there has been a rediscovery of the importance of leadership" (Fowler, 1988). The writer, with extensive experience in industry and local government, draws the conclusion from the failure of the more mechanistic management techniques of the 1960s and 1970s that "the management of people is a central function for all managers — not a peripheral activity which is subordinate to the technical or professional content of a particular service, or a specialist activity which can be left to personnel officers". However good the plans are, they will not be effective if the workforce is demotivated, suspicious, lacking the necessary expertise or out of tune or unaware of the organisation's aims and values.

Getting behind the word

The word "manage" comes from two words: the Latin noun *manus* — hand — and its derivative, the Italian verb *maneggiare* —to handle or train. It epitomises control but also a "hands on" coaching to increase skills and produce from something or someone with raw talent a controlled source of power and skill. "Lead" on the other hand is derived from the Old English *laedan*, related to *lithan* — to travel — and gives a more progressive feel of movement than "manage". The *Oxford Dictionary* defines "lead" as "to show the way to (an individual or a group) by going with or ahead: to guide; to guide, control and direct; to direct the course of; to give an example for others to follow".

"Leadership" has, then, quite simply a more dynamic ethos than "management", with leadership's connotation of adventure, exploration and pilgrimage. But the two go hand in hand; even an intuitive leader such as Alexander the Great built his spectacular marches and victories, as modern research shows, on effective, logistical planning (J. Keegan, 1987). The complex modern world of business and welfare provision requires proper controls, safeguards and standards to avoid the confusion Carol Satyamurti (1981) found in some social services departments immediately afte the 1971 Seebohn reorganisation, where meetings of senior managers were held on an *ad hoc* basis; the setting of priorities was left to basic grade workers; there was distrust not only between managers and other staff but between different branches of the Service; and organisational requirements were ignored or overlooked.

Conversely the more complex the environment and the larger the organisation the more essential it becomes to have leadership at every level. To create a sense of mission, hold and transmit values, communicate, motivate and quite simply get things done. Tom Peters, one of the gurus of management in the United States, put his gut feelings on the line in a co-authored book with Nancy Austin: *A Passion for Excellence: The Leadership Difference* (Collins, 1985). A gut feeling about the need for a new style of management, based on experience of a large number of successful and unsuccessful organisations: ". . . for the last 25 years we have carried around with us the image of *manager* as cop, referee, devil's advocate, dispassionate analyst, professional, decision-maker, naysayer, pronouncer. The alternative we now propose is *leader* (not manager) as cheer-leader, enthusiast, nurturer of champions, hero finder, wanderer, dramatist, coach, facilitator, builder".

This is a model which relates back to our earliest traditions of leadership, as a reading of Greek literature and the Anglo-Saxon heroic poems will demonstrate. Management/leadership is not merely a matter of donning a particular shade of suit and holding a filofax but more like stiffening the sinews and summoning up the blood!

Manager or practitioner — Two sides of the same coin?

"Some withdraw themselves from works of mercy" wrote the philosopher Thomas Aquinas "*Lest* they be involved in other people's misery". Many practitioners feel precisely that this is what managers do — that they have withdrawn themselves from the fray for reasons of ambition or squeamishness. The Wagner report (HMSO, 1988), however, makes clear that "expert management is essential for staff to be able to give of their best and to be able to ensure that high quality services are achieved" (chapter 7).

The apparent dichotomy between management and practice transmits itself in a lack of trust both ways, and yet surely they are two sides of the same coin, with some complementary and some congruent skills, making practice and management attributes transferable from one sphere to another. The manager must be adept at active listening so that he or she can understand and evaluate a situation before planning and acting. The practitioner who cannot organise himself or herself and his or her immediate environment will be of little help to the client who wishes to gain or regain control of his or her own life. The successful practitioner, nurse, social worker, residential or day care officer, therapist etc., will look, listen, plan, act, evaluate and plan again. So will the successful manager. The practitioner will be sensitive to the wishes of the consumer and so will be the manager if he or she is going to provide a service which is consistent with its own objectives. Some would say that the practitioner is too subjective in situations to achieve effective results. The advent of care management will mean practitioners having responsibility to translate their skill diagnoses into effective outcomes for clients within an efficient budgetary parameter.

Ken Young, former chief executive of the Spastics Society, perceives the dichotomy between practitioner and manager as one that is often artificially constructed. "Social workers" states Young, "have to take very tough decisions . . . All of this is a strong school for decision making. Social worker skills are eminently transferable to a management environment" (Fielding, 1989).

The effective social or health service practitioner will move from positive listening to positive action. Gerard Egan (1986) writes: "Helpers are seen as competent because they are active, because they listen intently . . . talk intelligently . . . are understanding, genuine and respectful". In all this Egan argues that "helpers must be able to *deliver*".

Many managers of residential establishments, as Chris Payne of NISW points out (Payne, 1988), tend to either cling to practice through guilt or an inability to delegate, or to shut themselves off from practice and become desk bound: "It is a sad fact that there are many residential "managers" who interpret their role either in terms of "doing" all the things for which their staff are paid to do or who become administrators pure and simple. Instead of which they should be building on their knowledge and understanding of practice to take a more rounded and prospective view of the services being offered; to initiate sensitive programmes of, for example, staff recruitment and selection, development, supervision, training and stress management; to create a sound "foreign policy" for their establishment; and most importantly to offer skilled professional leadership to staff. But they will be unable to do any of these things competently unless they can trust in the abilities of their staff to 'manage', and staff have similar confidence in them. Such reciprocal trust does not come about if managers and practitioners operate from completely different assumptions".

Managers should use their organisational skills to create the space to get alongside staff and coach them in the art of good practice. To do this they will need practice credibility but also the ability to stand back and evaluate the interactions of staff and clients and staff with staff, so as to monitor standards.

Clearly the practitioner turned manager will need to take on new skills (see chapter 6), such as:

- ○ The ability to lead diverse groups of people.
- ○ Managing money and 'bricks and mortar'.
- ○ Getting the best out of information technology.
- ○ Operating quality.
- ○ Planning for operational effectiveness and change.

These skills are what some call the "outer game of management". In many ways, however, it is the "inner game" that counts. As one woman entrepreneur was quoted as saying: "In recruiting we look for attitude . . . I couldn't care less about their skills because they can always improve them" (quoted in R. Goffee and R. Scase, 1985).

Management in social services and the NHS has tended to lurch from a need to be liked to an attitude where humanity is seen as weakness. In fact, as Flamholtz and Randle (1989) point out, neither of these extemes makes for successful management in an increasingly complex world. The Greek Xenophon believed that there was small risk of a leader being "regarded with contempt . . . if, whatever he may have to preach, he shows himself best able to perform". The general manager in a large organisation, however, has to co-ordinate a range of professional experts and to plot a way ahead for the unit as a whole. Flamholtz and Randle set out three key requirements for playing the inner game of management successfully:

- ○ Being able to manage your own self-esteem so that you derive satisfaction from the things managers are supposed to do, that is enabling rather than doing.

○ Being able to manage your need for direct control over people and results.

○ Being able to manage your need to be liked so that it does not interfere with performing the managerial role.

In a consultative document drawn up by the South East Thames Regional Health Authority (*A Review of Policy for People with Learning Difficulties*, February 1989) the region took the step, seldom taken unfortunately, of seeking and recording the views of consumers, parents, paid carers and managers. The views of the staff were not flattering to their managers but give clear pointers as to how things could be improved:

● Carers saw better managers as essential in enabling them to give of their best. They needed close guidance and support in their work especially when it became necessary to take risks in order to develop their clients. Such support was rarely forthcoming so carers chose safe options for their clients who then faced limited opportunities, under-stimulation and delayed personal development.

● Some managers were characterised as being inaccessible, ignorant of good modern practice, unfamiliar with clients and their needs, and more interested in the organisation above them. Some were unaware, dishonest and lacking in humility.

● They did not set standards of what was acceptable and did not monitor performance. This was because they were poorly trained or had unrealistic workloads or a combination of the two.

● Paid carers received little praise for their efforts and were not taken seriously by their managers.

● This lack of direction and of explicit standards of performance were symptomatic of poor communication, up and down the organisation and between the organisation and its consumers.

Both clients and staff needed honest and open feedback from staff and managers so they knew how well they were doing. Staff wanted to have team meetings, be listened to and involved in planning. They wanted to know what happened to suggestions they had made. They wanted their managers to use their wider perspective to alert them to good practice and to keep them well informed.

● The demands of their work required considerable and wide-ranging skills. This in turn required improved, more relevant and ongoing training. The training needs of staff needed to be identified by managers as part of regular performance appraisals.

Conclusion

In an increasingly complex and fast-changing welfare system the cool-headed control of “the manager” is required to assess situations and plan appropriate action. The same circumstances also call for “the leader” to evoke a sense of purpose, and motivate people towards the goal of better services for people with learning difficulties.

Practitioners must be challenged to become more purposeful. Practice knowledge and skill are needed if management is not to lose touch with the aim of providing a valued service; otherwise it could become like the Mock Turtle's "branches of Arithmetic — Ambition, Distraction, Uglification and Derision"!

J. Adair (1983), *Effective Leadership,* Pan.

S. Etherington, "Managing at the sharp end", Three articles in *Insight,* in July 1989.

G. Egan (1986), *The Skilled Helper,* Brookes/Cole.

E. Flamholtz and Y. Randle (1989), *The Inner Game of Management,* Hutchinson.

A. Fowler (1988), *Human Resource Management in Local Government,* Longmans.

R. Goffee and R. Scase (1985), *Women in Charge: The Experiences of Female Entrepreneurs,* Allen and Unwin.

J. Harvey-Jones (1988), *Making It Happen: Reflections on Leadership,* Collins.

J. Keegan (1987), *The Mask of Command,* Jonathan Cape.

N. Fielding (1989), "Hard head takes charge of a charity's soft heads", *Sunday Times,* 9 July.

NISW (1988), *Residential Care: A Positive Choice* (The Wagner report), Volume I, HMSO.

C. Payne, "When management skills are part of basic practice", *Social Work Today,* 23 June 1988.

C. Satyamurti (1981), *Occupational Survival: The Case of the Local Authority Social Worker,* Blackwell.

6

Leading from the front

"He [Alexander] showed much concern about the wounded, visiting each, examining their wounds, asking how they were received, and encouraging each to recount and even boast of his exploits."
Arrian on Alexander the Great.

"Leadership is a priceless gift which you earn from the people who work with you and you have constantly to earn that right."
John Harvey-Jones, former chairman of ICI.

"What used to bore me when I worked at the advertising agency, was these regular management meetings. Instead of thinking of how to get more clients and more business, the men would always be talking about their cars and getting a space in the garage. Men are motivated by those sorts of things, and women are not."
Jean Wadlow, managing director of Wadlow Grosvenor International, quoted in *Women Mean Business*.

"He [the abbot] must know what a difficult and demanding burden he has undertaken: directing souls and serving a variety of temperaments, coaxing, reproving and encouraging them as appropriate. He must so accommodate and adapt himself to each one's character and intelligence, that he will not only keep the flock entrusted to his care from dwindling, but will rejoice in the increase of a good flock."
The Rule of St Benedict, A.D.550.

"In enterprise of martial kind
When there was any fighting
He led his regiment from behind
He found it less exciting".
The Duke of Plaza-Toro, in Gilbert & Sullivan's *The Gondoliers*.

As we said in the introduction to this book, it is not easy to write about leadership in social care settings. This is partly because many of the professions making up the pattern of services are relatively new, and second, for the precise reasons that they are professions. The professional is an individual relating to a code of ethics and accountable primarily to him or herself. Nursing has always been medically orientated until recent times, while social work has often been the port of call for doctors *manqué;* clinical psychologists are now in positions where once only doctors dared to tread, and social care workers in day and residential settings, have conversely had a hard battle to gain any professional recognition at all — despite doing the bulk of the work!

Management, therefore, is still a comparatively new genre, where services for people with difficulties are concerned. Team building is often ignored or done as a "one-off" and then no more; communication systems are embryonic; staff development in some of the old hospitals is still, as we still remember it, the senior nurse bellowing down the corridor! Social services departments are less than 20 years old and too callow to have produced many acknowledged heroes or heroines — though the media have created a few villains. The fledgling departments have been through a number of organisational metamorphoses from functional to geographic to patch or specialist. They have witnessed a huge growth in staff but an even bigger increase in legislative duties, consumer expectations and public pressure. The first generation of directors had to transform itself from primarily professionals, turned small-scale, professionally-orientated administrators into general managers overnight. The county mental welfare officer or children's officer who became a director of social services in 1971 had to make a hyper-leap, even more complex than the manager of a local retail chain being transported to be a director of Marks & Spencer. In the health service, too, the traditional administrator has given way to the manager, though ironically general management in the Griffiths' mode has opened up senior posts to doctors and nurses as well as the specially trained administrators and the new intake from commerce and industry. The difference in orientation between "administrator" and "manager" is considerable, though often glossed over, and is neatly illustrated in Table 6.1.1.

In the 1980s a new breed of social services directors came onto the scene with more explicit views on management. Some of the more radical moves towards patch and other systems took place at this time, and a more abrasive style was adopted at all levels. Partly this was an acknowledgement of a lack of direction exposed by the child abuse inquiries, partly it was a reflection of a national leadership style, almost a *zeitgeist,* which eschewed consensus and opted for a clear action path at the risk of turning some complex issues into a black and white focus. Again the perspective of time needs to be added before it can be identified whether the benefits of such a change were transitory or long term, and indeed whether a period of conflict was needed before a transmuted consensus could be restored.

Andy Main, a former director of social services, St Helens Council, commented on the appointment of a former BASW colleague, Tim Brown, as the new director of St Helens: "Maybe Tim and I did not agree. I was a consensus man and he would see an objective and go for it" (*Social Work Today* 27 April 1986).

This is the change in attitude in a nutshell.

Table 6.1.1: *The different characteristics of administration and management*

	Administration	*Management*
Objectives	Stated in general terms and reviewed or changed infrequently	Stated as broad strategic aims supported by more detailed short-term goals and targets reviewed
Success criteria	Mistake avoiding. Performance rarely measurable	Success seeking. Performance mostly measurable
Resource use	Secondary task	Primary task
Decision-making	Has to make few decisions but affecting many and can take time over it	Has to make many decisions affecting few and has to make them quickly
Structure	Roles defined in terms of areas of responsibility. Long hierarchies; limited delegation	Shorter hierarchies; maximum delegation
Roles	Arbitration	Protagonist
Attitudes	Passive: work-load determined outside the system. Best people used to solve problems	Active: seeking to influence the environment. Best people used to find and exploit opportunities
	Time — insensitive	Time — sensitive
	Risk avoiding	Risk accepting but minimising it
	Emphasis on procedure	Emphasis on results
	Doing things rightly	Doing the right things
	Conformity	Local experiments: need for conformity to be proved
	Uniformity	Independence

(From Rees, 1984)

Attracted by the mirage of increased responsibilities and creating a new Jerusalem of Seebohm's reciprocal services, directors of social services in the 70s and 80s took on an increased burden of care for people with long term chronic needs which the NHS was only too glad to shed in its pursuit of its own technological nirvana of high-tech acute services.

Senior managers are a vital part of the jigsaw because it is they who lay down the standards and procedures to be followed within any organisation, and perhaps more importantly they set the tone. Leadership, however, is not their sole prerogative — far from it. People with learning difficulties are often hidden from history, as Ryan and Thomas (1987) have so perceptively written (see chapter 1) and so are many of their co-workers and carers. The management of circumstances and the leadership of people takes place at all levels and many situations. The person with a learning difficulty who forms a local branch of People First or who states his or her mind in a packed conference hall; the small staffed house which is well integrated in its local community; the employment officer persuading firms of the benefits of taking on his clients; the parent managing the complex daily needs of a sick and disabled child with calmness and humour — all these are as much examples of leadership as a well-run department with thousands of employees and multi-million pound budget. As George Eliot wrote in her preface to *Middlemarch,* "many have been born who found for themselves no epic life wherein there was a constant unfolding of far-resonant action". Many people contain "spiritual grandeur ill-matched with the meanness of opportunity". The leader needs must bring to fruition the spiritual grandeur of those they lead and attempt to manage the environment so as to release potential of those in their charge.

As Peters and Waterman (1982) made clear one of the prime functions of management is to "give attention to the care, feeding and unshackling of the average man". All of us have a role in showing leadership and taking responsibility in both day-to-day decisions and planning ahead; and the thrust of much of the management texts coming out of America (e.g. Peters and Waterman, 1982 and Peters and Austin, 1985) is that every individual in an organisation should be a hero or heroine. When one reads Peter and Austin's chapter on leadership in a *Passion for Excellence,* one feels sure that Alexander the Great must have been on a Tom Peter's management study course! In the quotation from Arrian, at the beginning of the chapter, Alexander is giving his personal attention to each individual and making each one a hero. As Robert Waterman (1988) pointed out, "attention is all there is".

Because social care is a stripling in the scheme of things we have looked at leadership in other fields: the family, military service, business and the Church. It may seem strange, for example, to quote the Rule of St Benedict on the abbot (or leader) of a monastery. What does a monk born in the sixth century have to teach us? The fact is that the Benedictines developed successful communities of creative individuals up to and including the present day; adapting to a changing world but retaining their essential ethic and ethos. Benedict's warning that "by rubbing too hard to remove the rust he may break the vessel" is a timely reminder to those of us who like things done as soon as we thought of them — or before!

The interest in heroes is maintained by the "indispensability of leadership in all social life and in every major form of social organisation". This was written by Sidney Hook in *The Hero in History,* just after Europe had suffered a surfeit of "heroics" from Hitler and Mussolini. Hook (1955) extols leadership and warns of the twin dangers of selfish heroics and fatalistic determinism.

Theories and people

Although systematic writing about management issues is a

relatively recent phenomenon, practical management must have been in evidence from earliest recorded times — the Sumarians founded their archives at Uruk in circa 3000 BC; Egyptian pharaohs of the Third Dynasty started to build pyramids in 2600 BC; and the Yin dynasty developed complex political and social entities in the China of the 17th Century BC.

Philosophy followed hard on practical events. The codes of behaviour cultivated by Confucius in the fourth century BC held a prime influence in Chinese life at least until the Communist revolution, if not beyond. The Greeks and Romans expounded ideas on what made effective administration and put the concepts into action. The Renaissance philosopher and politician, Thomas More, in his *Utopia* argued that "the welfare of a state depends entirely on the quality of its administrators", while the much misunderstood Machiavelli was mainly concerned with encouraging effective organisation in divided city states surrounded by predatory foes.

Recent commentators such as David Clutterbuck and Stuart Crainer (1990) portray thought patterns about management going back for centuries and have resurrected some much neglected sages, such as Mary Parker Follett (1868-1933), whose early practice in social welfare and an ability to relate individual human experiences to general principles led her to articulate a humane management approach which was in sharp contrast to some of the more mechanistic ideology of her day, and remarkably consistent with modern thinking. Her remark that "what we want is co-ordination *from the bottom up* and all along the line" (our emphasis) is a potent marker for the way that today's outfits view planning and marketing. There are a number of ways of grouping management theorists but one possible method is as follows:

☐ **Scientific management** Often described as "the father of scientific management", Frederick W Taylor (1856-1917) was an engineer and inventor who had a genius for analysing individual tasks and used this not only to drive himself (he was a tennis champion as well as a businessman) but to set standards for industrial processes. Taylor saw people's motivation as based on material rewards.

☐ **The classical approach** It was Max Weber (1864-1920) who looked at how organisations developed from "charismatic", with the founder-leader at the helm, to "traditional", which emphasises custom and practice, and onto "rational-legal" with its finely honed framework of functions and procedures. Sometimes referred to as the creator of "bureaucracy" as a concept, Weber viewed it, at least at first, as a way of operating on a fair and rational basis without being prey to the whims of one person. As Charles Handy has observed, the rational-legal configuration, or what Handy terms the "role" or "Apollo" culture, "is excellent if it can be assumed that tomorrow will be like yesterday" (Handy, 1978). Unfortunately this is a world in which tomorrow is hardly ever like the day before.

French mining engineer Henri Fayol (1841-1925) formulated the simple, but often forgotten axiom that there should be unity of purpose at all levels within the organisation. Each part of the corporate entity must have a programme of action; a structure chart so that everybody knows his or her place in the scheme of things; clear communication; and universal control based on accessible information.

☐ **Systems theory** The systems and organisation theorists moved forward from the classical approach. Thinkers such as Luther Gullick built on Fayol's work and defined management tasks as planning, organising, directing, staffing, co-ordinating, reporting and budgeting. The British researcher, Joan Woodward (1916-71), argued that there is no best option for all organisations but that it all depends on the context. Clutterbuck and Crainer assert that the giants of systems theory are Peter F. Drucker (b.1910), who coined "management by objectives", which harnessed together the goals of the organisation with the developmental needs of the manager, and Henry Mintzberg (b.1939) who identified five different forms of structure.

Britain's main contributor to this school is Charles Handy (b.1932) whose famous *Understanding Organisations* (Penguin 1976) is a starting place for many. His later works, such as *The Age of Unreason* (Hutchinson, 1989), consider the type of entity required when the pace of change becomes furious.

☐ **The human relations approach** The Hawthorne research project based in Chicago in the 1920s and 30s was led for much of the project's life by Elton Mayo (1880-1949). The Hawthorne experiments demonstrated people's motivation by social needs in strong contrast to Frederick Taylor's' materialistic creed. Strengthened by observations of individuals and groups under war conditions the behavioural scientists explored the concept of motivation, which we look at in more detail later in this chapter.

Robert Blake and Jane Mouton considered various management styles combining different weightings of concentration on the task and concern for the workers. Douglas McGregor (1906-64) formulated "Theory X" and "Theory Y" with their contrasting views of human drives. Abraham Maslow (1908-70) is famous for his "hierarchy of needs", while Frederick Herzberg (b.1923) went further than both with his definition of "satisfiers" or "motivation factors", and "dissatisfiers" or "hygiene factors". Chris Argyris (b.1923) writes about the "psychological energy" in each individual and urges managers to look towards helping each employee become as involved as possible and work towards self-fulfilment as a means to achieving organisational goals.

☐ **Value-based approaches** Of course, every organisation has values, however obscure or covert, but in recent years a growing number of bodies have held up "excellence" or "quality" as the value underpinning all their operations and corporate life. As recent commentators have observed, when a firm says it has a quality system it may mean simply an inspection process. Many organisations, however, have worked through inspection, quality control and quality assurance, and "the most progressive companies are now working towards total quality management" (B G Dale and J J Plunkett, 1990).

W Edwards Deming (b.1901) and J M Juran (b.1904) are two of the most impotant proponents of quality management, with many local initiatives now in progress (see Richie and Ash, 1990).

The best known exponents of a culture of excellence are obviously Tom Peters (b.1942), Robert Waterman (b.1936) and Rosabeth Moss Kanter (b.1943). Although some of the *In Search of Excellence* companies have hit difficulties since the book's publication in 1982 and Peters is sounding somewhat pessimistic these days, many of the maxims of him and his fellows have a timeless ring of truth about them. Many social care agencies would do well to note when Peters and Austin urge that "neither superior customer service nor constant innovation — the two sustaining edges of excellence — is built upon genius in the executive suite . . . Both are built, instead, on a bedrock of listening, trust and respect for the dignity and the creative potential of each person in the organisation."

☐ **A renaissance in leadership** Warren Bennis and Burt Nanus (1985) quote a message in the *Wall Street Journal:* "People don't want to be managed. They want to be led". It is the lack of innovation and dynamism in the managerial approach which has led to this renaissance in leadership studies. John Adair, Warren Bennis and John Kotter are some of the most quoted exponents of leadership as a concept, with Kotter recently arguing that while "the real challenge is to combine strong leadership and strong management and use each to balance the other", only leadership can cope effectively with change and move groups of people into the new directions they need to take (J. Kotter, 1990).

A good deal of research is now going into how differing theories and national cultures affect leadership practice (for example, P. Smith and M. Peterson, 1988), and Robert Kelly has asserted that too much attention is paid to leadership and not enough to how we all work as "followers" — as most of us have "follower" as well as leader roles ("In praise of followers", *Harvard Business Review,* November/December 1988).

Of course most of these theories overlap and many of the thinkers on management could be placed in a number of theoretical contexts. Most have something significant to offer but it is foolish to go overboard on any one theory (for example, McGregor's "X" and "Y" factors) without considering the situation at hand. It is also important to note that most hypotheses are a rediscovery of old truths with something added. Many nations, groups and companies have worked exceedingly well before the late 20th century! As one historian has observed about ancient Athens (Forest, 1986): "It is not the least of Athenian achievements that she contrived to diminish or delete the distinctions across the country while building up the city as the acknowledged capital, preserving at once local pride, national identity and individual dignity".

The singer or the song?

If it is true that we are betrayed by our virtues, as Graham Greene opined, then it is also true that in certain situations vices will become meritorious. Writing in 1928 about Winston Churchill, A P Nicholson in his *The Real Men in Public life,* said of Churchill: "The wise direction of men or events is not within his compass." The historian, Robert Blake, has pointed out that Churchill's weaknesses in peacetime as a minister of state — "simplistic views", "single-mindedness verging on fanaticism", "fascination with decisive action and a temperament for being a chief rather than a colleague" — were all positive virtues when his "immense energy" was put towards winning the war (*The Conservative Party from Peel to Churchill,* Eyre and Spottiswode, 1972).

So it is the leader who brings forth the right vision for the time rather than dreaming mere dreams who is likely to be effective. But is it the time that calls forth the leader or the leader who kick-starts events? This may well depend on whether the individual is an "eventual person", inspired by changes to mould them to a compelling purpose, or an "event-making person", seizing the diffuse material of time and creating a direction of their own making.

We aren't just talking about Winston Churchill here. By creating changes in our own attitudes and working practices, at whatever level we are, we can all manage ourselves, our use of time, our presentation, our practice, in such a way to make ourselves more purposeful and achieving. As Field Marshall Bill Slim once said: "There is nobody who cannot vastly improve his powers of leadership by a little thought and practice". Churchill was only able to take advantage of the change in world events through the rigorous work schedule he had put himself through during the wilderness years.

The deputy of a social education centre, a staffed housing scheme or a hospital ward, may either be devastated when their long-serving boss retires, or alternatively be able to lead the staff group into either new directions or positive consolidation. The deputy who has schooled himself to be more personally effective (see, for example, John Adair, *Effective Time Management*, Pan 1988), and alert to current thinking will be an asset to their team, the deputy who hasn't will not.

At this point we need to emphasise again two points we have already made. One is that parents of people with learning difficulties are often an extremely potent role model for us. When Joan Hebden's daughter, Cathy, was born with Downs' Syndrome "the so called experts seemed to concentrate solely on the difficulties to parents, pointing out what the child could not, and never would do" (Hebden, 1985). Cathy's innate determination and that of her parents, coupled with her mother's careful planning and persistence resulted in Cathy leading a very rich life and gaining a Duke of Edinburgh's Gold Award.

Our second point is that professional skills and managerial skills are not necessarily exclusive. The disorganised professional is unlikely to be more than marginally helpful to his or her clients, the soulless manager may be effective in the short term but alienate those around him.

As the individual moves away from direct practice, however, professional knowledge is less important than the ability to get a team of people together who can work on a project without getting in each other's way, and distil other people's ideas rather than their own. Commercial history is full of brilliant technicians who became abysmal managers. At some stage in a career people have to ask themselves where their strengths are and what path they want to follow. So often in social care only the management path has been rewarding both financially and in terms of status. The new career grades introduced by some authorities, in social work and national grades for nurses are a recognition of the divisiveness of this.

Four theories

"The manager is wrapped in a rich and seamless garment under the name of management, which has become a pervasive religion of our time, but management like the emperor's clothes, does not exist".
Robert Heller (1972)

For someone who is atheistical about management Robert Heller has written a lot of books on it! The truth behind the words, is simply that effective management means keeping some simple rules constantly in mind. The main questions must be: Why are we here? What are we meant to be doing? and How are we going to achieve what we set out to do?

These are not ontological questions, but designed to keep us all on a course which is continually orientated to the customers we serve, the aims and philosophy of the service, and the staff who ensure service delivery. When people become "patients" when they enter an institutional setting a peculiar transformation takes place. F. F. Jacques (1983) offers an example:

"I'm brought into this hospital real sick and someone asks me a whole string of dumb questions. I tell them I feel I'm going to faint and they say: 'I have to ask you a few more questions or else we can't admit you'. I faint and fall to the floor. I come too, and someone's saying, 'you can't lie here!' My wife starts to help me up. The voice says: '*you* can't lift him!'

"They take my clothes away . . . I put on this gown split down the back. It doesn't have buttons, and they make you wear it backwards. My backside's always hanging out, or I'm clutching at my gown with my only arm. See, the other one has an IV in it and I have to push that pole along every time I get up to go to the bathroom or brush my teeth . . . "

That hospital had clearly forgotten that care of patients is to do with far more than technological medicine, and that the preservation of individuality and dignity is vital to us all. Peters and Austin (1985) stress the simple virtues of attention, common courtesy, ownership, innovation and keeping close to the consumer.

Management also can be described in straightforward terms as "getting work done through others" (Rees, 1984), and as far back as 1908, the Frenchman Henri Fayol listed the functions that managers perform as planning, setting objectives, forecasting, analysing problems and making decisions — functions which would remain essentially unchanged to the present day.

Theories of leadership have revolved around four main concepts.

Personal traits

"Mad — possessed — perhaps she was. A demoniac frenzy had seized upon her . . . For years she was in hourly expectation of death. But she would not rest . . . there was the work to be done".
Lytton Strachey on Florence Nightingale in *Eminent Victorians*

"I am resolute, you are stubborn, he is bloody-minded"
Anon

The idea that leaders are born rather than made is a persistent one encouraged by the hagiography of heroes on which we were nurtured at school. All the heroes and heroines we heard of seemed, like Greek godesses, to have stepped, fully prepared for the fray, direct from the brow of Zeus! Yet we have all worked, not only with leaders who immediately impressed us with their personality, but also those who got the job done by quietly setting goals, careful briefings and consistent supervision. In the case of the "personality"leader, there are many different ways that this is demonstrated: by a quiet intensity, extrovert ebulliance, a razor sharp intelligence or irresistible energy. Churchill was an exhuberant inspirer, while his intelligence chief, William Stephenson, was known as the "quiet Canadian". Despite Stephenson's extraordinary talents over a number of disparate fields of work, his was a quiet and unobtrusive personality.

Even with the universally regarded leader the qualities may not have been apparent at an early age. The Duke of Wellington's biographer describes him as "lonely and withdrawn" as a boy. Sir Jonah Barrington declared acidly that he had known Wellington at all stages of his career: "In the first stage . . . I was his equal, in the last nobody is" (quoted in E. Longford, Wellington, *The Years of the Sword*, Weidenfield, 1969). The transformation from the withdrawn boy to the hawkeyed, resolute and decisive "Iron Duke" is dramatic. Wellington had innate talents such as the way his mind could consider a complex task "and suddenly a whole train of reasoning comes before you like a flash of light — you see it all", but much of his success appears to have come from a basic determination and singlemindedness.

Rosemary Stewart (1985) quotes two studies of leadership qualities: Edwards and Townsend of British managers of successful businesses and Argyris on American executives. The first list is as follows:

- Strength and willingness to work hard, immensely hard in some cases.
- Perseverance and determination.
- A taste and flair for commerce and an understanding of the market place.
- Audacity — a willingness to take risks that are sometimes large gambles.
- Ability to inspire enthusiasm in those whose co-operation and assistance are essential.
- Toughness, amounting in some to ruthlessness.

The American list is somewhat different:

- Exhibit a high tolerance of frustration.
- Encourage full participation and are able to permit people to discuss and pull apart their decisions without feeling that their personal work is threatened.
- Continually question themselves, but without being constantly hyper-critical of their own integrity.
- Understand the "laws of competitive warfare" and do not feel threatened by them.
- Express hostility tactfully.
- Accept victory with controlled emotions, and conversely are not shattered by defeat.

- ○ Understand the necessity for limits and are able to say "no".
- ○ Identify themselves with groups, thereby gaining a sense of security and stability.
- ○ set goals realistically.

The lists have common attributes but with different emphases. The first stresses primarily competitive traits, whereas the second demonstrates more social characteristics laced with competitiveness. Part of the difference as Stewart points out is due to the first list being compiled by economists and the second by a psychologist.

It is significant that the Rule of St Benedict, to which we have already alluded, has a chapter entitled "The qualities of the abbot". But the chapter never mentions any specific qualities at all; rather it is a series of injunctions to remember what the task is and how to fulfil it, for example, "the abbot must always remember what he is and to what he is called" (chapter 2).

Arthur Young (1986) advises any manager to know himself or herself and his or her strengths and weaknesses, and then "ensure your weaknesses are covered . . . delegate . . . learn to improve". The problem is that many managers don't evaluate themselves and therefore allow their strengths to become weaknesses or fail to recognise their own faults in others. A popular and amusing instance of this is James Herriot's portrayal of veterinary boss Seigfried Farnon in *All Creatures Great and Small,* who is always pontificating about a course of action and then does the opposite with a sanguine air of saintliness! Self-awareness is a vital quality because, as Aristotle said, we only learn from our mistakes not our successes. We might think that military personnel would tend to be rather unaware of their weaknesses, and that social services and health care managers would have gained self-awareness in their training. Experience does not teach that this is so. An interesting example from the services is that of Admiral Halsey, the fiery and combative American admiral, who being taken ill before the vital battle of Midway in the Second World War, recommended to his boss, Admiral Nimitz that his successor should be the methodical and quiet tactician, Raymond Spruance. Halsey was able to correctly perceive Spruance's talent, despite the fact that he was the complete opposite of Halsey in character and did not have the detailed knowledge of aircraft carrier tactics that Halsey had. In the event Halsey's judgement proved correct and the Japanese advance in the Pacific was halted.

We can consider a number of qualities (which J. Adair, 1983, has written about), where drawbacks may turn strengths into disadvantages. To take just three, first, efficiency may be useful especially in a task area, as measured by a constant comparison of work done with its cost in energy, time and money. This is relevant to team work and self-management as well. But efficiency is not useful when carried to extremes, ignoring the human factor. Then it can become an end in itself, divorced from effectiveness.

With another quality, intelligence, it is useful when offering the ability to assess people and the organisation and to see what challenges may be ahead. It is not useful when it leads to arrogance and an attitude which says: "Only I can do this job properly." In this case a centralising of decision-making may result which again leads to a loss of self-confidence among subordinates.

Last, communication is useful in getting across the plan and building the team. It is not useful when telling staff too much too early which may be merely a means of passing on the manager's own anxiety.

If everything is so situational are there any essential qualities? Winston Churchill used to say that courage was the essential quality "because it was the quality that guaranteed all others". When Carlo de Benedetti turned round the Olivetti Company from slump to renewed growth, he said looking back that he had given "a little *courage* to the company". From that courage came a sense of belief, purpose and then renewed energy and enterprise.

Integrity, which evokes trust from those depending on the leader, and those with whom he is negotiating at his own level or above him, is a character quality rarely absent from great leaders. Harold Macmillan once remarked that the problem with the man who trusts nobody is that he "is apt to be the kind of man that nobody trusts".

It would be nice to think that humour was an essential trait, even though Margaret Thatcher is recognised as not having a great deal of it. While humour may not be needed in a Prime Minister, for anyone in middle management it can lighten both their day (and night!) and those who work for them. Our best teachers in this respect are parents and carers and people with learning difficulties themselves. Their humour, often in adverse circumstances, is a constant inspiration.

Style

"Different strokes for different folks"
Blanchard, Zigarmi and Zigarmi, *Leadership and the One Minute Manager*

In the best-selling American book, *The One Minute Manager,* Blanchard and Johnson allude to the fact that "it was as though most managers in the world were primarily interested in results *or* in people . . . the young man thought each of these managers — the 'tough autocrat' and the 'nice democrat' were only partially effective. It's like being half a manager, . . . "'Effective managers' he thought, managed themselves and the people they work with so that both the organisation and the people profit from their presence."

When research was carried out by Lewin in the 1930s, into leadership in a boys' club, he identified three styles: autocratic, democratic, and laissez-faire. The autocrat was found to be effective in getting the work done, but if the leader wasn't there a "when the cat's away . . . " attitude developed. Lenin had to be autocratic to achieve results quickly in the Russian Revolution in 1917. When he died Stalin drew the reins of power in tighter and choice at the ballot box in The Soviet Union only returned in 1989. The stagnation of the Soviet economy is a good illustration of the stutifying effect of autocracy. Mikhail Gorbachev's *perestroika* was a bold attempt at political empowerment.

Democratic leadership was popular with the consumers of leadership and proved reasonably effective. It can, however, degenerate into a state of laissez-faire which is ineffective and unpopular with the workforce who want to achieve something and perceive only a rudderless drift onto a series of lee shores.

Social services departments have reacted strongly against a *laissez-faire* image and some have adopted a more autocratic style. This too can be ineffective if extended over a long period or used on a well-motivated workforce, thus infantisising them. One manager we know recalls joining a group of well-motivated middle managers who had recently come into a reorganised department. Attending a seminar on the ethos of the organisation they were expecting an inspirational speech and were disappointed when the senior manager uttered a long string of threats as to what would happen should they make any mistakes. There is plenty of evidence to suggest that fear has only a limited influence and is not productive of a healthy and achieving organisation in the long term. Fear is not only demotivating but induces a sense that the organisation lacks confidence in itself and its people; in the end it can become a self-fulfilling prophecy as only inferior people submit to bullying. John Harvey-Jones (1985), former head of ICI, takes a very different tack when he writes "everything I have learnt teaches me that it is only when you work with rather then against people that achievement and lasting success is possible".

Blanchard, Zigarmi and Zigarmi set out four styles which give room for individual staff and groups to develop:

○ *Directing* The leader provides specific instructions and closely supervises task accomplishment.

○ *Coaching* The leader continues to direct and closely supervise task accomplishment, but also explains decisions, solicits suggestions, and supports progress.

○ *Supporting* The leader facilitates and supports subordinates' efforts toward task accomplishment and shares responsibility for decision-making with them.

○ *Delegating* The leader turns over responsibility for decision-making and problem-solving to subordinates.

The debate over style brings us back to one of our original premises — that the competent and effective professional should be able to develop into an effective manager because they will be able to organise themselves and the environment to set and achieve realistic goals. The social worker who sees his or her client needs rehousing, doesn't indulge in family therapy. The nurse will undertake skills and circumstances assessment before teaching someone with elastic-sided shoes to tie their shoelaces! The occupational therapist does not put in a lift before seeing if the consumer can be helped to recover mobility. In the same way, managers cramp themselves and indeed their organisation, if they cannot vary their style in an eclectic manner to meet the needs of their staff at any one time depending on external pressures and the competence and commitment of the individuals. As such the autocratic or in Blanchard's terms "the directing" style becomes something that is not fixed but only used with new staff who lack knowledge, with competent but uncommitted staff who need a push, or in a 'change state' when the organisation needs to react quickly.

Situational

"Management and industrial leadership is an art, not a science. Each of us approaches the problem from a different background and each of us is dealing with a different situation, and a different culture, and from a different starting point."
John Harvey-Jones

"There are many ways to get where you're going, but I wouldn't start from here."
Irish proverb

The situational theory states that there are four variables: the leader; the lead; the task; and the context. Leaders and leadership styles are very dependent on how these four interact.

Rosemary Stewart (1985) quoting Robert Tannenbaum and Warren H. Schmidt's famous article "How to choose a leadership pattern", (*Harvard Business Review,* Vol.36, No.2, 1958) sets out the various characteristics which need to be acknowledged in deciding how to manage.

The manager's characteristics

- Value system.
- Confidence in his or her subordinates.
- Own leadership inclinations, e.g. whether he or she is more comfortable being a member of a team or being highly directive.
- Feelings of security in an uncertain situation, hence his or her ability to delegate.

The characteristics of the subordinates

- The strength of their need for independence.
- The readiness to assume responsibility for decision-making
- Their tolerance for ambiguity, for example, some subordinates have a preference for clear-cut directives, others prefer more freedom of action.
- The interest in the problem and their views on its importance.
- Their degree of understanding of, and identification with, the goals of the organisation.
- Their knowledge and experience.
- Whether they have learnt to expect a share in decision-making.

The characteristics of the situation

- The type of organisation, including the kind of behaviour that is customary, political constraints, freedom over the use of budgets etc.
- Group effectiveness.
- The nature of the problem.
- The amount of time available to achieve the task.

Tannenbaum and Schmidt (1958) conclude that successful leaders are those who are both keenly aware of the factors that are relevant to their behaviour at a particular time and who are also able to act appropriately. This is consistent with the "one minute manager" texts of 30 years later which also stress "different strokes for different folks". Unless the right components of purposeful action are brought together the result will be frustration, aimless activity or an addiction to the status quo.

Type

"A lot of people would probably say that in business you have to be ruthless. I would disagree. 'Ruthless' infers (sic) that you would do whatever it takes regardless of the cost and consequences for yourself or anybody else. I prefer to say: "I will succeed regardless of the many setbacks"."
Maureen Foers, entrepreneur

A colleague told Peter Gilbert that when she was a team leader for a London borough she could never work out why her team, which had so many excellent ideas, never seemed to achieve much. Later that year the social services department had assessed all field work staff using the Belbin system (see chapter 7), and the team was found to contain a high proportion of "plants" — people with creative ideas — but nobody was good at translating the ideas into goals and outcomes.

There are various theories of type, for example, the philosopher Carl Jung identified four main psychological types, who may well be complementary in a group and necessary for a group to function creatively — thinker, sensor, intuitor and feeler.

Michael Maccoby (1981) identified four character types having studied a number of successful managers in the American setting. As with Jung's findings most managers were not purely one type, but, in effect, one psychological characteristic was dominant. Macoby's four types are:

The craftsman who is painstakingly devoted to excellence in the product but tends to be weak at identifying external pressures and likely events, and neglectful in building a team to carry out the task.

The jungle fighter, often fuelled by a sense of righteousness and rectitude, the jungle fighter views life as the survival of the fittest in which winners destroy losers. This type can be protective towards those he or she sees as their "family" and is correspondingly ruthless to outsiders. But the aggression can also be turned against "members of the family" so that a shrinking number of people are seen as loyal, and those that are left are often weak-minded and dependent.

The company man who is an institutionally minded figure akin to Belbin's chairman. The company man will work on maintaining a corporate image but can become fearful and indecisive under the pressure of change.

The gamesman thrives on the new and can energise those around him. Greedy for fame the gamesman often over-reaches himself and ends up by being interviewed by Roger Cook or Esther Rantzen!

As we can see all four types have in them the seeds of their own failure. If we accept that people with the energy to take a lead are going to have some lack of balance to their personalities inherent in that very inner drive to achieve, then it demonstrates the need of organisations to ensure some balance of personalities and talents, and also a very clear corporate vision to maintain a sense of direction. The wise director may well pick out a manager to head a task force to sort out a crisis or set up a service. The very aptitude of that person to "sort" out a mess may militate against them setting a steady course over a period of years, so again the director moves in a different character, perhaps more of a "company man", in Maccoby's terms, to preside following the transitional stage.

Action-centred leadership

"The business that is not being purposefully led in a clear direction, which is understood by its people, is not going to survive, and all of history shows that that is the case".
John Harvey-Jones

The problems associated with reliance on personalities led the British Army in the 1960s to bring in John Adair, who formulated his concept of action-centred leadership based on the situational leadership theories of Blanchard and Hersey in America.

While social services has often concentrated more on the need of staff groups or on a vague consumerism, successful businesses and some branches of the services have tended to specify goals and harness corporate policy, the team, and individuals towards meeting those goals. We have always found the simple picture of the interlocking circles an extremely useful image to keep in mind as a plan proceeds. If the interface between the circles becomes distorted then the leader knows he or she must realign and bring the mission back on course.

Figure 6.3.1: *Leadership circles*

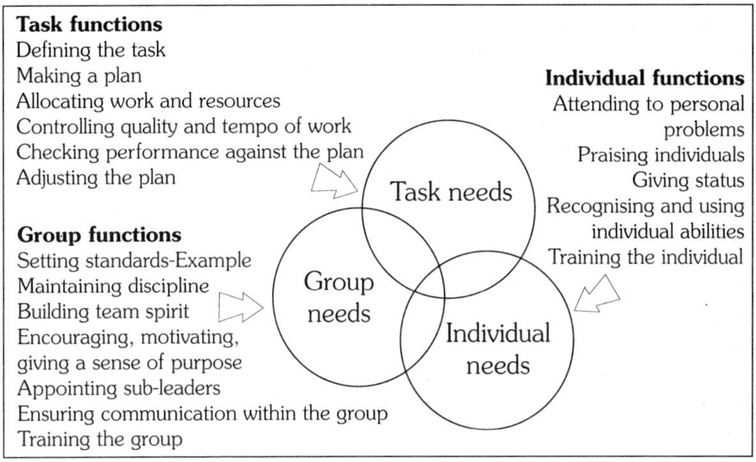

(From J. Adair, 1983)

The leader bucks responsibility for keeping the three circles in the correct alignment at his or her peril. Douglas McGregor, the writer on management and motivation, admitted that when he took up an executive position in an academic institution he tried to avoid the problems of being "the boss". In the end, however, he admitted: "I could not have been more wrong . . . I finally began to realise that a leader cannot avoid the exercise of authority any more than he can avoid responsibility for what happens in his organisation. In fact, it is a major function of the top executive to take on his own shoulders the responsibility for resolving the uncertainties that are always involved in important decisions. Moreover, since no important decision ever pleases everyone in the organisation, he must also absorb the displeasure and sometimes severe hostility of those who would have taken a different course" (quoted in W. G. Bennis and E. H. Schein, eds, *Essays of Douglas McGregor*, MIT Press, 1966).

Before proceeding with the task the manager will need to assess the organisation he or she works in, in terms of the three circles, and take management action to bring shape to it so that it creates a vehicle for action. A colleague of ours moved to a department which had reorganised into specialist sectors and she found a structure designed for an effective deployment of resources and speedy communication, as field, residential and day care services were all within the same group of services orientated towards the needs of people with learning difficulties and their families. Despite the fact that there were some excellent resources and staff there was also the "tribal warfare" referred by to Adair above, between different establishments and also a lack of co-ordination between different branches of the service. Although the geographical area covered by the department was only a few square miles in all many of the staff, serving the same client group, had never visited each others' establishments and there was considerable rivalry and distrust.

The response to this challenge was to:

○ Bring the managers of each establishment together for a regular meeting which had the clear functions of briefing; focusing on common issues to plan the way forward; and assessing applicants for admission to any of the units, so as to produce the best individual package for the consumer.

After about a year the 'tribal warfare' had reduced sufficiently that health service personnel could also join the meeting, and this helped to get over the worst obstacles in a split service.

○ Induction for staff was given a higher priority, so as to ensure that new staff saw themselves as part of a departmental-wide service, rather than just members of their immediate staff team.

○ "Tribal warfare" was outlawed and challenged every time it erupted.

○ Goals were set which orientated people towards tasks set rather than inessentials, and in-house training introduced which brought different groups together to focus on common issues.

Sterile dissention is often in evidence between fieldwork and establishments or between hostels and social education centres. Managers need to accept that co-operation and co-ordination are not empty words but vital to the consumers and the service, *and* necessary to our positive value in the eyes of other agencies.

The functions of leadership

The precise functions of the leader inevitably vary depending where he or she is in the organisation. The leader at any level can and should follow these basic steps if they wish to make progress with task, group and individuals in harmony. The middle manager, or officer-in-charge of an establishment, may not have much control over the department's vision — the department may not have one! They can, however, develop their own vision and this needs to be transmitted in the setting of objectives. As one of the most recent text books on developing comprehensive community-based services puts it: "Leadership is about gaining and maintaining support for the implementation of this vision. Looking 'upwards' and 'outwards' it is about building an authoritative mandate for change" (Towell, 1988).

The word "mandate" is vital here in that leadership is based on the delegated and consensus elements of authority (from the Latin *mandare* to command; *manus* a hand; plus *dare* to give). The manager who loses sight of the task is in danger of presiding over a cosy chat club; one who is authoritarian and neglects to build the team may gain short-term successes but will find the team fragmenting and "watching their backs"; while the manager who neglects the individual dimension may well find flaws developing in his team as the work progresses.

Defining and setting the task

"I keep six honest serving men
(They taught me all I know)
Their names are *What* and *Why* and *When*
and *How* and *Where* and *Who*"
Rudyard Kipling

The manager will set the general aim and break it down into objectives which should be specific, clear, understandable, obtainable and measurable. The correct task setting is necessary for the whole process to develop. "Nothing is more demoralising," write Peters and Austin (1985), "and ultimately useless than an unachievable vision."

Goal setting and planning should occur at each level of the organisation. It will vary according to the control the staff member has, but must dovetail in with the process going on throughout the whole organisation. For instance a manager of an SEC may have an action plan which may require him or her, amongst other things, to start up a self-advocacy scheme within the centre; and convert one activity room into a training kitchen. If the department as a whole, or at least the immediate service, is not in tune with consumer involvement then the local advocacy scheme may inform the rest of the organisation or risk being like the seed falling on infertile soil and be slowly strangled. If the SEC is setting up a training kitchen when domestic training is being targetted towards being carried out in people's homes then the plan is an expensive waste of time. Planning should fit, like the cogwheels of a clock mechanism between strategic, local and individual plans.

Planning

"When trouble is sensed well in advance it can easily be remedied; if you wait for it to show itself any medicine will be too late because the disease will have become incurable. As the doctors say of a wasting disease, to start with it is easy to cure but difficult to diagnose; after a time, unless it has been diagnosed and treated at the outset, it becomes easy to diagnose but difficult to cure" Niccolo Macchiavelli, *The Prince,* 1514)

"General Dalrymple has no plan, or even an idea of a plan, nor do I believe he knows the meaning of the word plan".
The Duke of Wellington

In the planning stage the broad goals are translated into stages with timescales and options. The overall aim, often now called a "mission statement", may be as all-embracing as the most famous split-infinitive of modern times: "Its continuing mission to seek out new civilisations, to boldly go where no man has gone before".

Planning should hone this down to make it specific depending on the nature of the goals which might be to do with strategic planning (long term, for the whole organisation); project planning (medium term, for example, the setting up of a day opportunities programme); and task planning (short term for individuals and teams).

At a time when social care agencies and even individual units are being urged to operate in a business-like way it is unwise to make too rigid a distinction between the three processes above. Each unit in the world after the NHS and Community Care Act will need to plan strategically and adopt both internal and external appraisals, or what is commonly called SWOT: Strengths — Weaknesses — Opportunities — Threats (see Young, 1986 and Drucker, 1964).

A facility looking for success in the new competitive climate will have to weigh up:

○ *Internal — Strengths and weaknesses*

People — leadership potential, attitude and aptitude.
Product — what is the service being offered and do consumers want it?
Organisation — willingness to allow autonomy; formal and informal relationships.
Information — how good are human and Information Systems/ Information Technology and communications?
Finance — adequacy of budget, income generation etc.
Knowledge — of the market, the competition and wider opportunities.
Reputation — credibility with customers.

○ *External — Opportunities and threats*

Legislation — what are the limits of what we can do?
Society — political and social realities.
Market — consumer demand, changes in perception and thinking, gaps in the market.
Competition — from and with the independent sector
and, how to protect itself to attract customers' co-operation.

In planning it is vital to consider, consult and then commit to a particular line of action. The time taken during the consideration and consultation stages will probably depend on the nature of decisions to be taken.

Sir John Harvey-Jones (1988) has pointed out that while the Japanese take some time to make a decision because of "the thoroughness of the involvement of people at every level of the organisation in the decision", when the "action stage comes they move like greased lightning". The Japanese management strategist, Kenichi Ohmae (1983) is critical of the monumental and inflexible corporate planning of both the former socialist Eastern Europe and capitalist USA and stresses that Japanese business strength lies in "understanding what is really happening in the outside world among customers and competitors" and keeping constantly in mind that "the workers know the business best and that innovation and improvement *must* come from the 'genba' (where the action is)". As the planning stage progresses a critical path analysis may be helpful, as a task of any complexity will depend upon the actions of others and will therefore need to be coordinated to ensure the continuation of the central thrust of the plan.

Organising

"Women seek to interpose the values of networking and peer group support into the cold, clinical 'scientific' model of male management styles."
Jean Lockley and Judy Fawcett (1989)

To succeed, the plan must have a vehicle which can move it forward without stalling or diving headlong off the road. The good manager will set the right people in the right place, give them the information they need and then sit on his hands! Leaders have to accept responsibility for their subordinates' actions but this often means that they get the itch to interfere at every opportunity.

As Robert Heller (1972) wrote, there is a manager somewhere who is in touch with reality, in that he knows what the consumer really wants. The longer the leading reins between that manager and the people in the penthouse suite "the more the company becomes an expensive device for generating unused information". The answer then would seem to be to delegate as much authority as possible, but this delegation has to be a realistic one in terms of a clear policy guideline and sufficient resources. It is a fraud to push responsibility down to people who don't have the confidence, information or resources to make the strategic plan work. This is where clear expectations and a contract between senior and junior managers comes in so that the activity demanded, for example, recruiting 20 link families in a year, getting ten people from social education centre into work placements and so on, measures up with the manpower and finance necessary to achieve those objectives.

Briefing

The leader now needs to communicate the task to individuals and groups in such a way that each person knows what is expected, the importance of his or her contribution, and the timescale involved.

The presentation of information is vital and should be reinforced at several levels, both in terms of the overall vision and specific objectives. The manager needs to ask himself or herself: "How many of my day or residential care workers have read the department's strategic plan?" The answer is probably one or two in every hundred. "How many people in my briefing group got the message I wanted to impart?" Again, almost certainly none, so communication will have to be reinforced without making it overly complicated.

John Adair (1983) gives five major skills in briefing — preparing, clarifying, simplifying, vivifying and being yourself — and some simple things to think about. For example, with preparing, he says that one should give a beginning, middle and end of a talk; prepare good visual aids; and arrange the room in advance. For vivifying there should be a use of vivid language or methods, even gimmicks; enthusiasm and an aim to enthuse the group and the use of humour, if possible. The presenter should breathe deeply, eliminate nervous habits and bear himself or herself well.

A popular image in communication these days is the "cascade" whereby information is passed from the top down to all levels. The problem is that those at the lower levels may only get the dirty water! Jets of information have to be aimed at all levels of the fountain to keep it fresh and the receivers refreshed.

Text books give a number of communication systems, but the thoughtful manager has to construct her or his own diagram of the communication system and remodel it as appropriate. A service manager may draw a linear model and then think how to ensure that communication isn't only linear and that the vision of the service is reinterpreted and renewed. Balancing on the tightrope comes from not being so outgoing that you undermine your own managers by short-circuiting them, but at the same time keeping in touch with what is going on and staying alive to the day-to-day issues. Just as in casework you need to feel the pressure but not be overwhelmed by it. Managing By Wandering Around (MBWA), as defined by Peters and Austin (1985), keeps the leader and their vision in the staff's mind and staff in the leader's mind. "Remember", urges Robert Waterman (1988), "that listening is not a passive activity. It's work and it's central to renewal."

The manager will be thinking about the advantages of different types of communication and how they might be combined, for example, a meeting between individuals or a group should be followed up with a short note as to what was decided on and who will be carrying out the actions later. A meeting with a considerable amount of information would derive more impact from a visual presentation. The Open University's *Open Business School Handbook on Communication* gives a number of advantages of verbal and written communication.

There are advantages in talking with people rather than writing to them —

- ○ can seem more *natural,* less bureaucratic or formal.
- ○ can encourage people to feel that they have been *personally consulted.*
- ○ allows the sender to tailor his remarks to the responses of his receivers, and therefore get his message across more *effectively.*
- ○ lends itself to the expression of *feelings* as well as ideas.
- ○ enables the *sharing* and *comparing* of ideas and feelings.
- ○ enables participants to "read" one another's *non-verbal* communication.

On the other hand there are advantages of communicating in writing:

- ○ enables you to choose your words more *thoughtfully* and reshape your statement until you are quite satisfied with it.
- ○ allows you to express your own ideas and feelings without the social pressure of having to cope with immediate responses from other people.
- ○ provides *physical evidence* that you gave certain information/instruction/advice/opinions and so on, to particular people on a particular date.
- ○ provides a means of *checking* exactly what was said, which may become useful when memories have become dim.
- ○ You can circulate a number of people with a written memo more easily than you can get them together for a meeting. Such a circulation would be less expensive (for example in lost working time) than having a meeting.

Motivating

"Of special importance . . . is the people's attitude to what they do . . . within the framework of *peristroika.* People have begun to change . . . we are moving towards the power of the people, involving the working man in all the economic and social processes . . . so that he may feel again like a human being"
Mikhail Gorbachev in April 1989

"Where the bland are leading the bland . . . all the behavioural scientists will not improve performance."
Robert Heller

The Soviet economy was for many years built on the wearily cynical premise that "they pretend to pay me, I pretend to work". One reason for this lack of motivation to work with any enthusiasm was clearly that pay is poor. Further on from that was the additional disincentive that the economy was so sluggish that there were few goods to buy anyway. In addition was the attitude of management, who themselves were unmotivated and failed to encourage their workers. *Peristroika* aimed to give people both financial incentives and the wider human energiser of citizenship.

Maslow's famous hierarchy of human needs has five rungs. In ascending order they are physiological needs; safety and security needs; social needs; esteem or egotistic needs; and (at the top) self-actualisation needs.

The Soviet system met the first two or three of the steps in the pyramid and the Gorbachev revolution was an attempt to add in the top of the structure in order to enable and encourage Soviet workers to raise their eyes to a higher level. In this he would agree with somebody from a different political system, the former chairman of ICI, John Harvey-Jones (1988), when he said: "People are self motivated. They do their best work when they have come to believe, through their own processes, that what they are going to do is worthwhile. The free man is always better than the slave".

In sociological terms Harvey-Jones and Gorbachev are following "Theory Y" first set out by the American social scientist, Douglas McGregor (1960) in the 1960s. McGregor's theories X and Y are really a pessimistic/optimistic or "original sin"/perfectability dichotomy, that is depending on how we view human nature. In theory X people are seen as naturally lazy and needing a stick and carrot approach, in Theory Y workers are seen as basically self-motivated but needing a favourable environment in which to work (see Table 6.1.2).

In the 1980s the work of Peters and Waterman in *In Search of Excellence* and William Ouchi (*Theory Z: How American Business can Meet the Japanese Challenge*, Addison-Wessley, Boston, 1981) were instrumental in trying to puzzle out why Japanese companies were so much more successful than their British and American counterparts. Ouchi came up with Theory Z which relies less than McGregor's on human beings' basic nature, which after all is rather hard to alter. Most managers can't wait for genetic engineering!

The work of Frederick Herzberg (1960) is useful in pulling these theories together. When he interviewed workers in the United States his survey groups identified two sets of factors: hygiene or maintenance factors, which would cause dissatisfaction if they were absent, and motivators which gave a positive incentive. The hygiene or maintenance factors were company policy, administration, supervision, inter-personal relations, status, salary,

TABLE 6.1.2: *Theories on individual motivation*

Theory X	***Theory Y***	***Theory Z***
People dislike work and try to avoid it.	People see work as fulfilling part of their psychological need to find value and meaning.	People identify with a corporate vision, value system and presentation which is accurate and explicit.
People only work if you use a "stick and carrot" approach.	Most people can be motivated if given a realistic and noble goal to aim for.	Workers respond to clear and achievable organisational goals.
People avoid responsibility at all costs.	Self discipline is far more effective than that imposed from outside. People enjoy the challenge of responsibility if given guidance and support.	Teamwork and intensive socialisation have worked well for Japanese firms in Europe and the USA as well as Japan.
Money and fear make things happen!	The desire to realise our full potential is even more powerful.	Individualised performance related pay is a motivator. Each individual should feel a hero/heroine in trying to improve their own performance.
People are only creative when it's a case of trying to buck the system.	There is a great deal of untapped creativity waiting to be released.	Creativity exists but organisations have the responsibility to ensure that knowledge and skills are made available to workers so as to translate motivation into performance.

security and impact of the job on personal life. The motivators were achievement, recognition, responsibility, advancement, interesting work, and possibility of growth.

Clearly many of these interlock and it is the responsibility of managers to look at an individual and small-group method rather than the blanket approach that has proved so unsuccessful in the Soviet Union or the British car industry. There is often very little room for manoeuvre in the public sector which has relied overmuch in the past on "job satisfaction" in the same unthinking way that the Soviets relied on job security. There are other motivators that can be used, however, such as recognition, opportunities for personal growth and the building of effective teams which enjoy working and playing together. Staff need to know that the work they are doing day by day is having an effect and achieving results. The example of "Chris" in Blanchard and Lorber (1984) (page 77-88) is an instructive one.

Alan Fowler (1988) makes eight key points:

- How well people work is influenced as much by attitude and motivation as by competence.

- Motivation is affected by an amalgam of influences — personal, job-related, environmental and managerial.
- Managers need to understand each employee as a unique individual.
- Jobs need to be meaningful and interesting, and people need feedback on their performance.
- Work needs to be seen as partially a social process, and motivation is affected by group attitudes.
- In organisations general culture has a strong motivational influence.
- Motivation can be stimulated by effective systems of recognition and reward.
- Managerial leadership is vital: there is no one leadership style, but qualities such as consistency, commitment, fairness, decisiveness and communication are common factors.

And he stresses that "for managers, the requirement is to know each employee well and so understand the individual characteristics which are likely to influence each person's motivation".

Supporting

Staff need support and encouragement, especially in times of change and stress. The greatest support a manager can give is attention, a listening ear and an appreciation both of the individual as a person and of the job being done. Again, there is a link between the practitioner and manager: the day care worker aiding a client move from a social education centre into employment will need to spend more time in teaching new skills, encouraging and supporting. Likewise, if the SEC is going to change its function from one of occupation to more specialist skills teaching then that day care officer will need support from his line managers.

Supporting isn't only for individuals but for groups of staff as well. One way of doing this, which ties in with motivating, is through spreading news of staff and consumer success via a newsletter or newsheet. This:

- reinforces service values.
- celebrates success.
- briefs people in straightforward terms.
- introduces new staff to the team and *vice versa*.
- gives a sense of purpose.

Support is given primarily through supervision, which will be dealt with in chapter 8, but also by Management By Walking About. We hear a lot today about the three "E's" — Economy, Efficiency and Effectiveness. We need to spend more time adding a fourth — Enjoyment. "Make it fun to work in your agency", urges David Ogilvy, advertising entrepreneur, "when people aren't having any fun they don't produce good advertising. Encourage exuberance . . . what kind of paragons are the men and women who run successful agencies? My observation has been that they are enthusiasts".

Monitoring/controlling/evaluating

Quality control will be dealt with in chapter 17, but in straightforward terms monitoring is the overseeing of what's happening; controlling is to intervene in the process to correct the thrust of the action; and to evaluate is to compare the end result with the stated aims that you started with.

In the 1970s a great deal of social care was, literally, aimless. Later, aims and objectives were introduced, but evaluation of what is, in many ways, essentially a human process, seemed somehow inappropriate. In fact, however, parents, one of our main consumer groups, are having to monitor, control and evaluate all the time. As Linda Scotson wrote: "In the final analysis parents are obliged to be prosaic" (*The Other Child*, Collins, 1988). When Linda's son, Doran, was born, apparently with insurmountable disabilities, his mother refused to accept a bleak prognosis and opted for the Dolman Delacato system of stimulation. This put an enormous strain, not only on mother and son, but also on Doran's sister, Lily, and their neighbourhood support. Friends and relatives sometimes questioned whether the whole process was successful or even sane. Lily's godfather wrote a challenging letter: "I think you inhabit a world where there is little proportion . . . it cannot be right to spend such enormous amounts of time and energy on Doran. Your life and that of your daughter are, if anything, more important".

Linda Scotson's battle to help her son achieve his full potential without it being at the long-term expense of her daughter and herself are the subject of continual evaluation throughout the book.

In Margaret Flynn's research into independent living (see chapter in N. Malin, *Reassessing Community Care*, Croom Helm, 1987), many people with a learning difficulty evaluate the pleasure of leaving an institution and having their own front door key, against some of the disadvantages of vandalism and unfriendly neighbours. If our consumers can evaluate so can we, and we must. The evaluation of a project will either show a need to intervene to correct the performance, a revision of the aims, or a decision to continue the process unchanged. The third option should be a positive choice and not simply the result of drift.

Doing things differently

"I think because of the way women are brought up, they pay more attention to detail, they are more conscientious . . . and I've always found the major difference between men and women is that men

are brought up to think of their short-term ambitions whereas women are brought up to think of the good of the whole. Women put the company before themselves."
Carol Wilson, former head of A & R, Polydor Records.

The American researcher Carol Gilligan (*In a Different Voice*, Harvard University Press, 1982) believes that in a number of Western cultures women are culturally conditioned to operate within an "ethics of responsibility". They tend to see individuals as woven into a web of relationships that have both a history and an anticipated future. This web leads to a sense of responsibility for those in it and for each other (presentation by women managers to Kent SSD departmental management team, in December 1989). Men tend to act according to set principles and override situational factors. We make no excuse for stressing in the middle of this chapter a set of action-planning principles, which is balanced by the emphasis on networking by Alexis Waitman and Kathy Johnson (chapter 12). The sad fact is that too many managers still operate on a management style of pure "adhocery". One of us once worked with a senior manager who came to important and complex planning meetings with no notion of what he wanted to get out of them and it was no surprise that he tended to leave empty handed!

The really proficient leader needs to combine the formal mode of planning with a subtle attention to and exercise in informal meshing. At the same time as a number of "Women in management" courses have been set up, consultants like Michael Simmons have been developing a programme called "Creating a new men's leadership", assisting male managers to realise and release the attributes they and their organisations need to operate in a world which the experts reckon will change increasingly rapidly as time goes on (see C Handy, *The Age of Unreason*, Hutchinson, 1989).

Although some psychological and physiological research is indicating fundamental differences between the sexes (see A Moir and D Jessel, *Brainsex*, Michael Joseph, 1989) too much can be made of this. The "stiff-upper-lip Englishman" is mainly a Victorian creation, while historical study shows men in previous ages far more in touch with their emotions and more willing to embrace other cultures. An acceptance of "Victorian man" as the only model has led to many misunderstandings, not least to women attempting to assume exaggerated "male" characteristics in order to succeed, or surrendering the use of humour.

Faced with male opposition to her presence in the House of Commons in the 1930s, Nancy Astor tackled Winston Churchill. The latter told her: ". . . I find a woman's intrusion into the House of Commons as embarrassing as if she burst into my bathroom when I had nothing with which to defend myself, not even a sponge". Nancy hit back instantly with: "Winston, you're not handsome enough to have worries of that kind"!

To talk of masculine and feminine facets is too simplistic but a harnessing of all attributes is needed in order to progress the service and stay human.

Setting the style – Or doughnuts at dawn!

"The essence of leadership is, however, simply stated: it is the capacity to inspire men to give of their individual and corporate best in all circumstances, but especially when the odds against them are greatest".
Geoffrey Bennett, *Nelson the Commander*

"No man is a continent"
Arthur Daley

Peters and Austin (1985) quote the example of Sam Walton, head of the successful Wal-Mart Corporation, wandering down to share doughnuts at 2.00 am with his people at the distribution centres. "Have you shared doughnuts at the loading dock at 2.00 am?" ask the authors, "If the answer's no . . you're out of touch".

Leaders should set the style. If they don't, then their team, sector, division, home, centre, hospital, department is going to be colourless and joyless *or* somebody else is going to impose a style from outside, or perhaps a negative influence from within will set an anti-style. If the team has no *élan* don't blame the troops, see what the manager is doing or not doing.

If the manager regularly comes to work late and leaves early, then he can't complain if others follow his example. If he is one of Robert Heller's "18 hour menaces", then others in the organisation may also be working long, but not necessarily productive hours. The manager who draws all decisions to himself, makes eunuchs of those around him.

The Audit Commission (1986) highlighted the fact that progress had been made where there was local commitment, co-operation and leadership. Ann Shearer's excellent *Building community* (Kings Fund, 1986), demonstrates the same point in her description of community projects. Much of the ongoing success of such enterprises is due to patient support for and coaching of staff. One big question faced by dispersed operations, however, is what happens when managers aren't around? It is on the nightshift or in the "ordinary house", several miles away from the core support unit, that the failure of autocratic management is most clearly shown. Unless staff are commited to their job, their clients and their colleagues, then "the Friday car" mentality, which dogged the motor companies in the 1970s, rears its head.

When Peter Gilbert's mother was in the Royal Marsden Hospital, London, with cancer the night staff would converse or sit with patients in the small hours, when life is fearful of itself. When he met the director of nursing, it was evident that this value system of supporting patients when they were at their most vulnerable, gained backing from the very top. Contrast this with the comment by a manager in a residential unit on a form concerning training. When asked to fill in what imagination the staff member showed, the reply was: "Night staff don't need imagination"!

One way of doing a Sam Walton in social care is working a shift with staff. In the Forest Hospital community mental handicap team all the social workers did an occasional shift on the wards they served, and the special schools they worked in to. In the hospital, the practice of hands-on care created a bond of solidarity between social workers and ward nurses; aided our understanding of the abilities, needs and aspirations of our clients; built up trust; and gave social services a human face whilst breaking down élitist barriers. The middle managers should work shifts in their residential homes. If you and the care assistant are still coping with double incontinence at 2.00 am with a 7.00 am start to the day looming, then you know your staff levels or rotas are wrong! If you work with very severely multiply handicapped young people, as one of us did, then you will have to look to the regular staff for guidance on how to interact and help those clients. Vulnerability to those whom you manage is not a fault or a weakness, on the contrary, it is a strength, as these staff are the experts in the same way that parents are within their own home. Only the insecure personality expects themselves or other people to be omnicompetent. Working side by side with people may be the only way to get to know them. It requires some personal risk-taking and a lot of listening, but it works.

"Doughnuts at dawn" is a style which enables and forces managers to regard their staff as something more than pawns who live to work. It blends attributes which are often seen as opposites, but which need to be congruent. Vince Lombardi, a legendary sports coach in America, once said to the American management association, that "mental toughness is humility, simplicity, Spartanism. And one other love . . . Love is loyalty. Love is teamwork. Love respects the dignity of the individual. Heart-power is the strength of your corporation".

Every manager is a chief officer

"It was going to one of Rabbit's busy days. As soon as he woke up he felt important, as if everything depended upon him. It was just the day for organising something, or for writing a notice signed Rabbit, or for seeing what everybody else thought about it . . . it was a captainish sort of day, when everybody said, 'Yes, Rabbit', and 'No, Rabbit', and waited until he had told them."
A. A. Milne, *The House at Pooh Corner*

"Captainish" people in any branch of life are a pain, and this image of management is what turns so many people off the whole concept. As we have seen, however, you don't have to be captainish to get things done. In the same way it would be natural to shy away from the idea of following the model of a chief officer. But in fact chief officers and local government organisations have put a considerable amount of thought into how they should orientate themselves, and the organisational roles of the chief officer, as outlined by M. Clarke and J. Stewart (1988) are very much the kind of roles that the middle manager should adopt in order to effectively manage services:

The strategist who can stand apart from day-to-day pressures and anticipate changes ahead and how to meet them.

The tactician who harnesses resources to meet everyday commitments.

The reader continually assessing his or her team so as to assess its strengths and needs and correcting imbalances.

The teambuilder who ensures that the team is strong enough to meet the task and carry with it a wide group of individuals.

The builder of the culture who gives a system of values, using verbal and non-verbal ways to communicate it.

The leader, enabler and motivator giving a sense of purpose.

The communicator who ensures that the right information is reaching staff at all levels.

The staff developer who guides his or her immediate staff and ensures a staff development system for those staff out of his or her immediate orbit.

The standard setter who is increasingly important as services become more diverse and individualised.

The umpire who resolves disputes and co-ordinates activities.

The monitor who judges the right amount of information to oversee the task without being bogged down by trivia.

The line manager who ensures that daily work runs smoothly.

Creating heroes and heroines

"Every middle manager should spring out of the gate every morning as a dedicated, proactive 'boundary basher!'"
Tom Peters (1989)

"They can because they think they can."
Virgil

Innovative projects start with energised people at a local level and yet so many staff have only enough energy to stagger from one reaction to events after another, like the punch drunk British heavyweight boxer! However heavy the daily pressure, however massive the pile of paper slung into your in-tray, there is a necessity to put aside time for developmental work only. You must punch and knead and mould the stuff of life around you as a potter moulds clay. The clay doesn't mould the potter!

Heroes and heroines aren't plaster saints but people who can recognise their weaknesses and utilise their strengths. The message is that everybody who has the potential to push forward the parameters of the possible is encouraged to do so. The author John Buchan put it succinctly: "The test of leadership is not to put greatness into humanity but to elicit it, for the greatness is there already."

Conclusion

"The head of a college should be identified with the interests of the college . . . he should put forward the undergraduates, suggest thoughts and plans to the fellows, create a common spirit. He should be absolutely above personality. He should inspire a feeling of duty in the whole college. He should know how to 'put pressure' upon everybody".
Benjamin Jowett, master of Balliol (1870-93)

Leadership brings forth a number of seemingly conflicting concepts. Here are some of the themes running through this chapter.

Create a vision

"Our greatest need and most difficult achievement", wrote psychologist and concentration camp survivor, Bruno Bettleheim, "is to find meaning in our lives." All the ancient and modern writers on management urge the necessity for an organisation to create a vision for its people to strive for and a culture in which they can thrive. As Robert Waterman (1988) says: "The need for meaning runs so deep in people that organisations must apply it if they are to renew."

The singer and *the song*

The glamour of leadership writings should not blind us to the fact that organisations usually require a "how" as well as a "why" to operate successfully, and in local or central government, public accountability demands a structure. The leader, or "singer" is vital to the project at its inception, but unless this is a small commercial firm or something that is to remain a project and therefore essentially undeveloped, it will need to have the systems or "song" so that the vision endures after the singer has long since moved on. As the Audit Commission stated: "For vision to become important and influential, there are two prerequisites. First, there must be a strong and almost inspired leadership . . . Second, there must be a pattern of systems and structures which reinforces what is to be achieved, rather than militates against it."

Go out and win

Middle managers are the "meat in the sandwich". They are like the character in the cartoon who has a mound of paper in his in-tray and a sign on the desk with the legend: "Work hard and you will be rewarded". The second picture shows him with an even larger mountain of paper in his in-tray! Winning is often a matter of mental attitude and a determination to shape events rather than let them grind you into the dust.

One favourite military story is of the Union general Ulysses S Grant, at the edge of defeat after the first day of the battle of Shiloh. Urged by many to retreat he doggedly stood his ground, believing correctly that the tide would turn the next day. General Sherman was also about to request the withdrawal but changed his mind, observing merely that: "We've had the devil's own day, haven't we?" Grant reputedly took a pull from his cigar: "Yes", he replied, "Yes, lick 'em tomorrow, though". And so he did.

Graham Day, chairman of Rover Group, criticised British management in the 1970s for having a tendency to "duck the issues", and having an essentially passive response with the feeling that they couldn't do anything about external pressures. Andrew Leigh, in his book *Effective Change* (Institute of Personnel Management, 1988) suggests that teams might benefit from undertaking a "circles of influence" exercise where problems are tabulated and the team attempts to move problems from the circle where they have no influence to one where they do.

Influence over events is often a matter of attitude. Tom Peters (1988) quotes the president of Notre Dame University, enlarging on St Paul: "The very essence of leadership is that you have to have vision. It's got to be a vision you articulate clearly and forcefully on every occasion, you can't 'blow an uncertain trumpet'".

Celebrate success

Family life is a history of celebrations. Even funerals in a healthy society can be an evocation of a life lived fully, and family and community solidarity. Our puritan traditions, however, somehow make it unseemly to celebrate at work, except at the New Year binge when people celebrate far too much!

People get disheartened, however, if the events they deem important aren't recognised. Public service, especially, is notorious for taking exceptional effort for granted. A shared team meal is a good way of getting everybody together, and quite often the most imaginative ideas are thought of over lunch (or like Archimedes in the bath!), but don't forget to bring along the administrative staff who so often get left out. The American literature on management puts a great deal of emphasis on celebrating success, and although the manner offered may be a bit overblown and emotional for our taste, the basic idea is sound.

If the OTs put in their hundredth lift; or the community mental handicap team produces an information handbook; or a small satellite unit is opened, then these events should be celebrated with all due pomp and circumstance rather than British understatement. The bottle of champagne (or more likely the Sainsbury's sparkling wine), should always be in the manager's bottom drawer.

Be genuine

Practitioner students of Carl Rogers and Gerard Egan will recall that genuineness is one of the necessary attributes of the skilled helper. Despite Machiavelli's opinion that leaders need only appear to have good qualities (*The Prince,* XVIII), managers as well as practitioners must be genuine — pretence cannot be maintained for long.

Nobody should need to feel obliged to declare their weaknesses, but neither should they feel embarrassed by them. The good manager doesn't need to be a Daly Thompson, but rather somebody who recognises strengths in other people which complement his own qualities and develops them. As Francis "Buck" Rodgers, former vice-president of marketing for IBM, wrote, his mentors at IBM "considered *my* success *their* success" (our emphasis) (Rodgers, 1986). In the same way managers should allow their staff to be genuine with them: working on weaknesses rather than excoriating them, and allowing the expression of anger without retaliation. As Rodgers goes on to point out, "too many people work under insecure leaders, whose paranoia stifles the growth of everyone around them. A leader who runs scared fills the environment with tension, hostility and tentativeness. He batters the self-esteem of his people, frightening them just as he is frightened. He kills incentive in the very people he must motivate in order to achieve his prescribed goals".

Terence Kardong, commenting on the complexities of community leadership, opts for integrity and genuineness rather than mere cleverness. In the long run it is this which pays dividends: ". . . the abbot can always seek input from experts in the community. Though the role of the abbot . . . is to make wise decisions in the light of the available information.

"What seems essential in an abbot today is the personal strength and serenity to exercise authority in the midst of many leaders and experts. To do that without defensiveness or rancour the abbot must be secure enough in his own self image . . . to do what needs to be done for the good of the community. The abbot should recognise that the office is essentially one of unification and not domination" (T Kardong, *The Benedictines,* Glazier Inc, 1988).

The moral dimension in industrial and commercial firms, if not always in governments, is now becoming an important part of their image projection. Rosemary Stewart (1985) points out that "social responsibility" tends to appear in firms' public objectives in the late 1970s, and books on morality now figure on the commercial shelves (for example, Adair, 1980, and Blanchard and Peale, 1988). Integrity is one of the qualities most stressed by the services and it is the one that Rodgers picks out as absolutely essential — even for a salesman! Machiavelli, though, points out that the kind of integrity that sticks to an original proposal even though the circumstances have completely changed will lead to disaster.

Set the course, steer the ship

It was the Roman philosopher and politician, Seneca, who commented sardonically that "if one does not know to which port one is sailing, no wind is favourable". The leader has the responsibility to decide on the destination and then steer the course. Rodgers (1986) maintains that "you can't talk about leadership without talking about responsiblity and accountability." The leader has got to delegate responsibility and provide the freedom to make decisions. He or she has also to make clear that the ultimate buck stops with him or her, and that delegation without some form of monitoring leads to irresponsibility.

Power to the people

Self-advocacy, citizen-advocacy and empowerment are influential concepts today in the world of social care in terms of working with service users. But sometimes we do not accord the same courtesy to staff. When the Social Services Inspectorate undertook its 1988 study *Managing to Care*, it found front-line managers ill-equipped for the management role they were playing "either in human resource management or budget management". The level of autonomy afforded to these managers on the front line was largely accidental, and seemed to have more to do with their line managers being preoccupied elsewhere, rather than a purposeful devolving of power to those closest to the action.

Empowerment and delegation, however, does not mean an out-of-sight, out-of-mind attitude. Consistency and support are essential elements of delegation.

One might misquote Rousseau and say "middle managers were born free and are everywhere in chains"! Once the vision is enunciated, the objectives clarified and the equipment for the job set out, then the role of the leader is that of empowerment not embargo. As Tom Furtaldo, director of Prat and Witney put it: "The fundamental purpose of management is not to control but to get out of the way".

Power and paradox

It was both Karl Marx and a number of Christian philosophers who pointed out that weakness can be strength, and the success of Japanese companies in Europe and America would appear to rest partly on the Japanese success in motivating within task groups rather than through a traditional management style.

Failures in social care have led to a more autocratic style to sort out problems and set down clear objectives. Machiavelli, the

Figure 6.3.2: *Empowerment – The upside down pyramid*

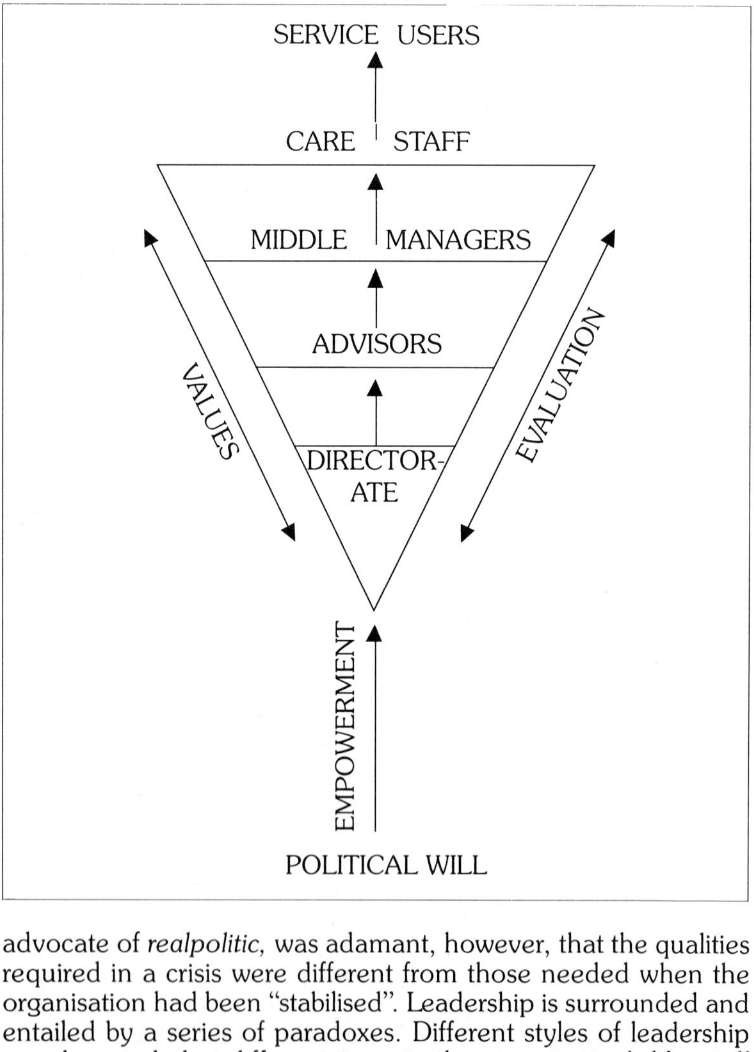

advocate of *realpolitic,* was adamant, however, that the qualities required in a crisis were different from those needed when the organisation had been "stabilised". Leadership is surrounded and entailed by a series of paradoxes. Different styles of leadership may be needed at different times in the organisation's life; staff need to be empowered but not abandoned; the leader must be personally secure but not complacent; projects need backing but without warping the overall direction of the team; staff development must develop innate abilities without going into the "blue-eyed boy" syndrome.

Just as the practitioner cannot afford to be a Dickensian Mrs Jellyby, who neglects her children in order to stimulate good works in distant parts of the globe, the practitioner turned manager should be thinking in terms of developing skills rather than simply jettisoning old ones, and creating a different equipoise. Sheila Cassidy, doctor and hospice director, acknowledges that having in the past "mocked the hierarchial barriers in medical . . . society" she now sees a value in them as "it is not easy to be in a position of authority, still less a good leader", and a difference in emphasis will be needed in the move from practitioner to manager. The Social Care Association's 1989 conference "Managing to care in the 1990s", put forward that learning about management should form part of basic social work qualifying training. Des Kelly, SCA's deputy general secretary, told the conference that many social care staff "continue to feel awkward about authority, and this has been a major obstacle to effective management development at all levels".

Toughness is an attribute much talked about but also much misunderstood. Adair talks about being "ruthless with time but courteous with people", and it is circumstance which must be coerced not people. When Graham Day, chairman of Rover Group, was appointed a member of the NHS Management Board in 1989, he was asked about his reputation for toughness. Day replied that he did not think he was tough with people, rather he was a person who was able to take decisions that needed to be made, and which many other people shied away from. Social care has traditionally produced women managers who have managed to combine mental strength, intuitive awareness of feelings surrounding the situation, and the demand for the highest standards in quality control. Wellington was known as the "Iron Duke", and yet he was moved to tears after battles, because of the human losses, and one of his subordinates said of him: "He has nothing of the truncheon about him; nothing foul-mouthed, important or fussy; his orders are all short, quick, clear and to the purpose" (quoted in Keegan, 1987).

Leadership is essentially a form of service and if it is not carried out in this way then it will be merely ephemeral. Just as the triumph of Granthamite political ideology is a graphic illustration of British post-war debility, so the Gorbals management style demonstrates only too clearly social work's nascent weakness.

One potent exemplar in recent times was Mikhail Gorbachev's attempt to democratise the Soviet Union. Despite the warnings of political philosophers such as de Tocqueville and Machiavelli that nothing is "more difficult to handle, more doubtful of success, and more dangerous to carry through than initiating changes in a state's constitution", Gorbachev largely set aside his armoury of powers in favour of persuasion. This was because he clearly recognised that to achieve *lasting* change he would need to energise the man and woman in the street.

As a social services director remarked recently ("Open Forum", *Insight*, 24 May 1989), it is the ability to cope with ambiguity and paradox that is the hallmark of the successful manager. The element of paradox is often more clearly felt in the field of social care than in the sometimes more simplified world of industry and commerce, because the political and public pressures are so very acute. Sometimes the only way to deal with complexity is to simplify and the manager who keeps the three circles of the task, the team and the individual in mind will not go far wrong.

The wisdom of the ancients may also be a guide, such as that of Lao Tzu, Chinese philosopher of the sixth century BC:

"The best of all leaders is the one who helps people, so that, eventually, they don't need him.
Then comes the one they love and admire.
Next comes the one they fear.
The worst is the one who lets people push him around.
When there is a lack of trust people will act in bad faith.
The best leader talks little, but what he says carries weight.
When his work is completed and his aim fulfilled, the people will say: "We did it ourselves".

J. Adair (1980), *Management and Morality,* Gower.
J. Adair (1983), *Effective Leadership,* Pan.
J. Adair (1988), *Developing Leaders,* Talbot Adair.
Audit Commission (1986), *Making a Reality of Community Care,* HMSO.
W. Bennis & B. Nanus (1985), *Leaders,* Harper & Row.
R. Black (1987), *Getting Things Done,* Michael Joseph.
K. Blanchard, P. Zigarmi & D. Zigarmi (1986), *Leadership and The One Minute Manager,* Collins.
K. Blanchard & R. Lorber (1984), *Putting the One Minute Manager to Work,* Collins.
K. Blanchard & N.V. Peale (1988), *The Power of Ethical Management,* Heinemann.
M. Clarke & J. Stewart (1988), *Chief Officers: Roles, Dilemmas and Opportunities,* Local Government Training Board.
D. Clutterbuck & S. Crainer (1990), *The Makers of Management,* Macmillan.
V. Coulshed (1990), *Management in Social Work,* Macmillan.
B. Dale & J. Plunkett (1990), *Managing Quality,* Philip Alan.
P. F. Drucker (1964), *Managing for Results,* Heinemann.
A. Fowler (1988), *Human Resource Management in Local*

Government, Longmans.
G. Forest (1986) in J. Boardman, *The Oxford History of the Classical World,* Oxford University Press.
W. Goldsmith & D. Clutterbuck (1984), *The Winning Streak,* Weidenfield & Nicholson.
V. Grocock (1988), *Women Mean Business,* Ebury Press.
C. Handy (1978), *The Gods of Management,* Souvenir Press.
C. Handy (1989), *The Age of Unreason,* Hutchinson.
J. Harvey Jones (1988), *Making it Happen: Reflections on Leadership,* Collins.
J. Hebden (1985), *She'll Never Do Anything Dear,* Souvenir Press.
Robert Heller (1972), *The Naked Manager,* Barrie & Jenkins.
Frederick Herzberg (1960), *The Motivation to Work,* Wiley.
S. Hook (1955), *The Hero in History,* Beacon Press.
F.F. Jacques (1983), *Verdict Pending,* Capistrano Books.
Rosabeth Moss Kanter (1984), *The Change Masters,* George Allen & Unwin.
J. Keegan (1987), *The Mask of Command,* Jonathan Cape.
J. Kotter, "What leaders really do", *Harvard Business Review,* May/June 1990.
J. Locksley & J. Fawcett (1989), "There is another way", INSIDE supplement, *Community Care,* 31 August.
M. Maccoby (1981), *The Leader,* Simon & Shuster.
D. McGregor (1960), *The Human Side of Enterprise,* McGraw-Hill.
K. Ohmae (1983), *The Mind of the Strategist,* McGraw-Hill.
Tom Peters (1989), *Thriving on Chaos,* Pan.
T. Peters & N. Austin (1985), *A Passion for Excellence,* Collins.
T. Peters & R. Waterman (1982), *In Search of Excellence,* Harper & Row.
T. Philpot (1986), "Values" in T. Philpot ed., *Social Work: A Christian Perspective,* Lion.
F.G. Rodgers (1986), *The IBM Way,* Harper & Row.
W.D. Rees (1984), *The Skills of Management,* Crown Books.
P. Ritchie & A. Ash (1990), "Quality in action", in T. Booth ed., *Better Lives: Changing Services for People with Learning Difficulties, Community Care* & Joint Unit for Social Services Research, University of Sheffield.
J. Ryan & F. Thomas (1987), *The Politics of Mental Handicap,* Free Association Books.
W. Slim (1956), *Defeat into Victory,* Cassell.
P. Smith & M. Peterson (1988), *Leadership, Organisations and Culture,* Sage.
Social Services Inspectorate (1988), *Managing to Care,* DoH.
D. Stewart (1987), *Handbook of Management Skills,* Gower.
R. Stewart (1985), *The Reality of Management,* Heinemann.

R. Tannebaum & W. Schmidt (1958), "How to choose a leadership style", in H. Koontz and C. O'Donnell (1976), *Management: A Book of Readings*, McGraw-Hill.
D. Torrington & J. Weightman (1985), *The Business of Management*, Prentice Hall.
D. Towell (1988), "Managing strategic change", in D. Towell ed., *An Ordinary Life in Practice*, Kings Fund.
R. Waterman (1988), *The Renewal Factor*, Bantam Press.
M. Woods (1988), *The New Manager*, Element Books.
Arthur Young (1986), *The Manager's Handbook*, Sphere.

7

The right ingredients: Building teams

". . . the successful team may look as if it happened by magic but you can be sure that it did not . . ."
Pauline Barrett in D. Stewart, (1987)

Most of the services that we work in are made up of groups of people working together, in order to accomplish much more than would be possible if activities were the responsibility of individuals. Similarly, teams do not exist in a vacuum, but are part of interdependent and mutually influential networks of services, where the behaviour of one part of the network affects that of others.

Teams need managing in order to achieve their goals, and these will vary depending on the type of service being offered. However all teams will possess similar characteristics. Payne (1982) offers a practical definition: "A group of people working together, trying to plan their work so that each individual's activities take account of those of others and who attempt to use their togetherness to improve their work."

The manager's responsibility is to use the skills of leadership with its team-building elements to enable the team to develop a shared commitment to a common purpose, and the recognition that a team needs the efforts of every one of its members to achieve this. When the team has reached this state it will see itself as a team, have a team direction and established ways of working together. If this is achieved then membership of a team that works well can bring benefits that cannot be overestimated. The sense of purpose from being clear about agreed goals, the sense of security from being part of a cohesive work group, the identity with team activities and aspirations, and the feeling of self-worth that reflects pride in personal standards that the individual team member sets themselves. Other benefits can include, knowing that mistakes can be made without recrimination, and that development is encouraged and new skills acquired that enhance the individual and overall team potential. Other important aspects of teamwork include the friendship, sharing and caring that is experienced where a team has developed good interpersonal relationships.

The reality of teamwork

With some of the high aspirations of teamwork clearly stated, what are the realities for staff in services? A number of common problems appear frequently in services and are described by staff as reasons why they find teamwork dissatisfying, and result in teams failing to achieve the clarity of purpose, interdependence and cohesiveness that exemplifies the successful team. The following problems are mentioned frequently by staff:

- poor leadership, either providing no structure or control, or dictatorial leadership.
- lack of clarity about roles and responsibilities.
- absence of, or infrequent meetings.
- poor communication about team functions, and between members of team.
- time not managed to enable members to meet.
- always given the "dirty" jobs to do.
- opinions not sought.
- lack of praise and recognition.
- lack of training.
- humour used to attack an individual.
- personal problems of members brought into team inappropriately.
- poor working conditions.

When asked to list good team experiences staff do not just describe the absence of the above problems, but a number of distinct features that have made team work fulfilling:

- time allocated to agree on team and individual values, team aims and objectives, procedures and ground rules.
- good leadership, that provides framework for practice, consults and listens to staff, and supports and rewards staff for efforts and achievement.
- team meets regularly, and where members feel confident to express their views, or question statements of leader or other members. A record is kept of meetings and all staff receive, or have access to the record.
- relaxed atmosphere, friendly staff, and where it is fun to work.
- good interpersonal relationships between team members, who are open and honest with each other, and where constructive criticism is welcome.
- a balanced team of staff in terms of experience, skills, age and sexes.
- avoidance of racist or sexist remarks.
- companionship in and out of work.
- recognition of stress and methods of helping team members.
- feeling comfortable in making mistakes.
- training and support to increase skills.
- support for temporary/agency members of team.
- awareness of other teams and their objectives.

The potential of teambuilding

From the responses of staff listed above, it is clear that effective team work requires considerable investment of time and effort on the part of the manager and team members. If the team is to achieve the effectiveness, creativity and energy that is said to characterise the best team, then specific team development activities need to be employed on the initiative of the manager.

A useful starting point in understanding the needs of a team is Adair's (1986) description of the interlocking needs of teamwork, where the elements of achieving the task, building and maintaining the team, and developing the individual overlap.

These three elements of effective team development constitute the core responsibilities of the manager. In Adair's model —task, team and individual — represent needs which if not met, will reduce the effectiveness of the team. Cormack (1987) describes the needs that should be met for the team to achieve success:

Individual needs (your own and others)

- to be accepted by the leader
- to be valued by the leader
- to be able to contribute to the task
- to know what is expected in relation to the task
- to be part of the team
- to know what is expected of you by the team

Task needs

- to set clear targets for the task
- to set standards of performance
- to make full use of resources
- to clarify responsibilities
- to ensure members' contributions are complementary
- to achieve the set targets and standards

Team needs

- to know and respond to the leader's style and vision
- to feel a common sense of purpose with members
- to have a supportive climate
- to grow and develop as a unit
- to have a sense of corporate achievement
- to have a common identity

Cormack sees it as unlikely that teams will have a correct balance of these needs, and it is more likely that there will be an imbalance for much of the time. This is natural as teams are not static, but are continually changing and responding to demands made on them, whether these are service users' needs, or staff and material resource changes.

Which of the three needs is dominant will be dependent on the life of the team, and the particular demands it is responding to at that time. For example, the new team, with members concerned about personal acceptance and assumptions about other members is unlikely to give its energy to task and group activities. Time needs to be spent helping new members understand what is expected of them, both individually and as a team, and enabling them to find their place within the team with their contribution acknowledged. Similarly, task orientation can mean the team is preoccupied with task completion, for example if the team has a specific project to complete, but this can be at the expense of individuals and the team.

Finally, a team oriented phase can result from a situation where team members are preoccupied with personal relationships within the team, regardless of the needs of a new member, or achievement of the task. In developing the team, the manager has to lead the team, and help it to balance the conflicting demands of these three needs. The application of Adair's model will enable the manager to begin to understand a particular stage of development of his team, and provide an invaluable starting point for team development.

Some key activities for team development

Writers on team development, when describing the "team at work", identify a number of key activities that are essential for team effectiveness. These are seen as important, no matter what the purpose, size, composition or structure of the work group.

- agreeing the purpose of the team
- clarifying roles and responsibilities
- promoting and maintaining communication
- managing team resources
- managing relationships with other groups
- reviewing team performance

Although these key activities are suggested as a basis for team development, they are in no way exclusive. Teams will wish to add to this list their own activities that they see as important, following a review of team performance and an identification of the problems that limit its effectiveness. These key activities can nevertheless be used as a starting point for assessing team performance.

Working on key activities

Agreeing the purpose of the team

The obvious starting point for a review of the team is an exploration of its purpose. The objective is to create a shared vision of the team and gain members commitment to it. A team needs to have a purpose or a "mission" which is a long-term statement of intent which describes how the team will meet the main goal of the service. Purpose or mission statements should be discussed among members, with differences explored and agreement reached as part of creating the shared vision. The statement should then be a working document which can be used whenever the team is involved in discussing the service it is providing, and how individual and team needs fit the goals of the service.

A useful example of the development of a mission statement can be found in Hoskins and Mansell (1988), which has a sample statement, with detailed guidance on creating a shared vision.

Clarifying roles and responsibilities

Team members often report being unsure of what they are expected to achieve with service users, and what are the limits of their responsibilities. Statements like, "I thought that was her responsibility" or "Nobody told me that was my job", can cause considerable insecurity and reluctance to take initiatives that can benefit users. An essential step is for staff to agree with the team leader the following points: What is required of me? What results am I expected to achieve to fulfil my role? What are the limitations of my responsibility? What specific short-term targets will enable me to integrate my work with other members of the team?

This is particularly important for a new member of the team. This will avoid the confusion that can be caused when responsibilities between members are not clarified which not only reduces the effectiveness of the team, but can damage relationships between team members.

Promoting and maintaining communication

Communication within the team according to Adair (1987) is important for three reasons: to achieve the common task, to maintain the unity of the team and to meet individual needs. The focus on these three areas can help identify the purpose of communication within the team. To achieve the common task means that communication will focus on the purpose, objectives and targets for the service, and how the team and individual members can enable the service to achieve its aims. The unity of the team will require communication concerned with team effectiveness in practice and the maintenance of standards. Individual needs will relate to conditions of service matters, individual job performance and career development within the service.

Effective communication means that the manager has to develop a system that is designed to aid understanding and commitment to the purpose of the service. In the context of the team this will mainly take place through team meetings. Regular team meetings should be scheduled to enable all staff to attend, and have a degree of formality in order to make most effective use of time and the contribution of individual members. These meetings would emphasise reaching agreement on decisions by consensus and generating a commitment to decisions agreed by members. Again material by Hoskins and Mansell (1988) mentioned above offers managers and team members activities and exercises that can improve team communications.

Managing team resources

Team development needs to take place within the context of efficient use of resources. The contribution of members is invaluable and unique, therefore the manager needs to ask a number of questions about how the human team resources are being used. Cormack (1987) suggests a number of factors that the manager can use as a focus for reviewing the use of resources:

- ○ How well is the talent of the team being used?
- ○ Are all members contributing?
- ○ Are all active?
- ○ Have you any passengers?
- ○ Are team meetings too long?
- ○ Would any members be better redeployed?

A number of other major resources are available to the team. The following checklist can be used to "rate" the team in terms of use of these other resources:

Managing relationships with other teams

A further important area is relationships between teams and other groups. Services for people with learning difficulties are complex and often depend on the co-operation of multiple agencies and their staff, as well as users of services, their relatives and carers. The success of the team can be dependent on external relationships, as this is an area of practice that is less under the influence of the manager.

Cormack (1987) sees one target of the team's development as the creation of open communication and harmonious activity with the main teams around it. Teams need to be aware of the risks of focusing inwards and ignoring external relationships and communications that are crucial for the overall success of the service.

In addition teams can increase their effectiveness by building formal and informal networks with individuals who matter to them and can help and support them. Teamwork should not lead to insularity which cuts the team off from comments and contributions of others. Cormack warns that team development can fail to take account of the fact that the team has to exist in an environment which can be hostile or at least uninterested in its activities.

Reviewing team performance

The team needs to regularly check the progress it is making in

RESOURCES ASSESSMENT CHECKLIST			
Resource	Assessment		
	Deficient	Adequate	Strong
1. **Physical assets**			
Buildings			
Equipment			
Skills			
Money			
Numbers of members			
2. **Intangible assets**			
Good will			
Commitment			
Reputation			
Team spirit			
3. **Systems and organisation**			
Financial control			
Planning methods			
Review procedures			
Organisation, authority and structures			
Quality control			
Training methods			
Reward systems			
4. **Team relationships**			
Formal relationship			
Informal relationship			
Communications			
Group relationships			
Climate			
Satisfaction			
5. **Team identity**			
Sense of who we are			
Understanding of why we exist			
Knowledge of how we are seen			
Understanding of how we want to be seen			

(D. Cormack p.116-117)

working together to accomplish tasks. A first stage of reviewing a team has been described by Everard and Morris (1985). Here a short time is set aside at the end of each meeting on team development to review progress. This "process review" time provides an opportunity for members to explore the way they work together (for example, the team's response to a member who had strong views about users' involvement in decision making) from which it is possible to identify the successes and difficulties. When important points arise they can be processed into group decisions, to be worked on between meetings if urgent, or included as targets to be included in action plans for the next or a subsequent meeting.

A second stage is the more substantial task of evaluating team development in relation to the longer-term goals the team has set itself. One way would be to use the idea of strengths and needs, to generate a list of factors that are contributing to, and detracting from, the team's effectiveness, based on the key activities. These could form the basis of the evaluation. The following questions could be used as a starting point for a thorough team review:

- What progress has been made in achieving the targets the team set itself?
- Is the work of individual members contributing to the work of the team as a whole, and in turn the purpose of the service?
- Are communications within and outside the team effective? What is the level of trust and openness between members, and does it allow good communication?
- Can members give and receive feedback, and thereby help each other to learn from individual and group experiences?
- Is the team making effective use of all its resources, particularly its staff?
- Once the team feels secure enough to evaluate the contribution of the leader, then this can be helpful in providing the leader with feedback on his/her performance. It can then enable teambuilding to focus on leader/member issues where necessary.

In addition the manager could make use of a number of texts on team development which provide examples of checklists that can be used by teams to evaluate their progress, including Woodcock (1979), Adair (1987) and Cormack (1988).

Putting teambuilding into action

With some understanding of the issues that need to be considered when setting out on the path of team development, how can the team get started? If team development is to be effective then the main need is for a regular meeting where every member of the team is expected to attend. At the initial meeting problems can be identified, analysed and a plan made, with dates, that indicates what issues will be addressed at subsequent meetings. The manager will need to create a climate at these meetings where staff feel free to express their viewpoints about the team, and do not feel that their candid statements will be viewed negatively. A climate of openness and trust is essential for good team-building, and this will need to be experienced by members if their commitment is to be secured.

The following stages have proved useful to managers and their teams we have worked with:

Stage One: Gathering information about your team This can be achieved through bringing members together and reviewing the team's performance, ideally in small groups. This can provide members with a greater opportunity to contribute to discussion, and reduce the anxiety of individuals who are asked to comment on the performance of their team. Once information has been gathered it can be displayed visually using a flip chart or overhead projector.

Stage Two: Reviewing information gathered Following collection of information on the team, this needs to be reviewed against the purpose of the service. Here the team can begin to examine how much the strengths and needs of the team support or hinder the achievement of the team's work, and how strengths can be used to support action to overcome the difficulties identified. This stage of the exercise will enable the team to focus on those problems that require action, because they are vital for the achievement of the purpose of the team. Problems can be prioritised in order to give more time to crucial problems that need urgent attention.

A word of warning! This stage can easily become protracted with analysis undertaken for its own sake, and action avoided. Although getting more information is a plausible activity, making it happen is more important.

Stage Three: Agreeing an agenda for action Information has been gathered, and problems identified. The final step is to look ahead to what you want to achieve. This is the action plan stage, where the team moves from analysis to action, with an agreed timetable of team-building activities based on a vision of the future. Identify where you need to begin work, for example, by discussion and agreement on introducing initially those small changes that would make a significant difference to you, to team members and to the overall achievement of the team's purpose. Later when the team develops trust and confidence in itself it can work on more difficult long-term problems.

J. Adair (1987), *Effective Teambuilding,* Pan Books.
D. Cormack (1988), *Team Spirit,* MARC.
K. Everard and G. Morris (1985), *Effective School Management,* Harper & Row.

S. Hoskins and J. Mansell (1988), *What Matters Most: Quality Assurance for Front-Line Staff,* South East Thames Regional Health Authority.
M. Payne (1982), *Working in Teams,* Macmillan.
D. Stewart (1987), *Handbook of Management Skills,* Gower
M. Woodcock (1979), *Team Development Manual,* Gower.

8

Supervision and staff development

"Help people reach their full potential — catch them doing something right".
Blanchard & Johnson (1983)

"If you *don't* hear from me you'll know you're doing alright".
A senior social services manager

"It is essential that management offers positive and constructive leadership and guidance".
The Wagner report (1988)

The fortnightly supervision session with the senior is so ingrained in the field of social work tradition and practice that it is still a shock to come across heads of establishments who hardly ever see their managers. If they are fortunate enough to get a visit then there occurs a one-sided conversation, which is rather like the one related to one of us by an SEC manager: "Just dropped by to see how you are Brian, everything alright? Good, good. Thank God *you're* okay, it's chaos everywhere else and county hall are breathing down my neck over the attendance stats. Any chance of a coffee?"

This kind of "ask the questions quickly so nobody can give me an answer I don't want to hear" is all too common, and beautifully encapsulated in the title of Beth Barker's article: "When did you last see your manager?" (*Insight*, 28 February 1989).

Residential and day care establishments are often geographically and administratively isolated from the local community and their professional colleagues. Many residential workers expressed a feeling of being "second class citizens" in the personal evidence submitted to the Wagner committee (1988). The community mental handicap team members sometimes sacrifice close relationships with their own profession when they gain the added richness of multi-disciplinary teamwork. Managers need to bear in mind the context in which staff development operates, especially in teams where members come from different disciplines and varied cultures.

"Most people, whatever their work, feel the need to talk over the special problems with which they are faced if they are to get and keep them in perspective", maintained the Williams report, *Caring for People,* written over 20 years ago. "This is particularly important", continued the report, "for residential workers because of the nature of the job. Most such workers feel, and with some justification, that outsiders do not appreciate the day-to-day problems of their close intimate relationships with difficult residents and to have the opportunity of constant discussion with an adviser . . . would be of real value." Frontline managers and middle-managers have to be the cement which binds together groups of staff with many different backgrounds and pre-conceptions about their work, give them a common purpose and opportunity to discuss their work, and an exploration of the way forward.

The word "supervision" bears unfortunate connotations of the factory foreman scrutinising workers on the assembly line. Partly for this reason, while in fieldwork it is put into adverts as a selling point, in residential and day care it is often regarded with suspicion (see Atherton, 1987 and Porterfield, 1987, p.20). Once, when one of the authors was introducing supervision into some residential and day care services, he met with each individual member of staff at a social education centre, together with their respective seniors, to talk through the purposes of supervision. Some staff were immediately positive, others regarded it as a form of "Big Brother" overseeing their work. A patient discussion of the purposes of supervision removed a considerable amount of the suspicion. Positive benefits happened almost at once as staff gave feedback to seniors as to what they found helpful or unhelpful. For example, one new day centre officer was able to say that he would really welcome his senior coming into the base group, to observe and give advice as to how to move the group forward; before the meeting both had been "standing off" the issue. Others sought for guidance or support in various different ways.

What's in a name?

As we saw above, supervision has a problem of association, but other alternatives also run into difficulties. Consultation implies a near equality which may not exist, and plays down the need for accountability. Staff support emphasises only one part of the process and implies staff need propping up! One-to-one narrows the range of methods down to the two-person discussion.

It is, therefore probably best to keep "supervision" as a generic term, but move away from the rather one-paced effect of the dictionary definition: "To direct or oversee the performance or operation of", and, rather, view it as an over-arching vision of what the organisation, team and individuals can achieve through clear objectives and guidance.

What is supervision?

Dorothy Pettes defines supervision as "a process by which one social work practitioner enables another . . . *who is accountable to him* to practise to the best of his ability" (author's italics) (Pettes, 1979).

This is very much the traditional casework model, but it is too narrow for our purposes. Supervision is not just about professional practice, nor is it only possible in one-to-one interaction. Chris Payne and Tony Scott (1982) more recently considered supervision in field and residential social work and give the concept a much wider parameter: "Supervision . . . is a process that is integral to the working life of every operational unit. It is to do with the working practices of team members, and the ways and means of mobilising and making use of the total resources placed at their disposal to meet their service objectives. 'Supervision' can take place in a number of contexts, formal and informal. It can select from a range of methods and arrangements; selection depending on needs and circumstances."

How supervision works in practice is dependent on the task, the setting, the type of team and the mix of individuals, but it can be both formal and informal; with individuals and groups; involving outside consultants; and with or without accountable managers.

The aims of supervision

When the DHSS looked at social services teams in the late 1970s, the authors of the report, Parsloe and Stevenson, (1978) found that there was considerable confusion as to what supervision was all about. They concluded that there were two main purposes of supervision. One was to "establish the accountability of the worker to the organisation", while the other main purpose was to "promote the worker's development as a professional person".

Parsloe and Stevenson also go on to say that "since accountability is concerned not only with whether a task is performed but also with the quality and standard of the work, the two purposes of supervision are practically and conceptually interwoven".

We can therefore identify three main functions of supervision:

- the *managing* function.
- the *educative* or *coaching* function.
- the *supportive* or *enabling* function.

The functions of supervision — managing, educating, and supporting and enabling — overlap. The elements of these functions are:

Managing: Getting the job done; ensuring the operation is consistent with the vision; defining roles and responsibilities; quality control.

Educating: Training in the job; expanding the role; bringing in consultants.

Supporting and enabling: Attending to personal problems; giving encouragement; career development.

Objectives in supervision

The objectives stem from the aims and may consist of the following:

Managerial

- Ensure the operation of individuals and teams is consistent with the overall aims and vision of the organisation.
- Define roles and responsibilities so that individuals and groups have a clarity of purpose.
- Aid responsiveness to changes in legislation, practice and organisational and external influences.
- Develop a suitable environment for purposeful creativity and initiative.
- Review work in a non-threatening setting.
- Get the job done through ensuring targets are met.

Educative

- Induct the individual into the culture of the organisation and how it operates.
- Inculcate core skills to enable individuals to fulfil their roles.
- Assist professional development in terms of gaining and developing basic skills; and training to take on new roles in a changing world.

Supporting/enabling

- Reduce dysfunctional stress while energising people's full potential.
- Defuse unhelpful personality clashes.
- Aid the individual's career development.
- Ensure that staff are stretched but not stressed.

Payne and Scott (1982) provide a useful checklist for the supervisor/manager in looking at major objectives in practical terms.

Team work

The type of supervision will and should vary according to the situation. Much will depend, when we look at groups of staff, on how coherent the group is as an entity.

The Wandsworth study of fieldworkers in various settings (1988) demonstrated that "supervision was carried out almost entirely on a one-to-one basis . . . and supervisors tended not to see staff when they were working with clients". In residential and day care work it is relatively easy to observe staff working with clients but difficult to organise a one-to-one discussion between supervisor and supervisee.

One-to-one formal supervision may appear rather artificial in a residential or day care setting, but, as Atherton (1987) points out: "the very deliberateness of supervision is some hedge against the development of sub-cultural systems. For example, those

which are based on grumbling and are more interested in the grumble than in doing anything to change the situation."

Payne and Scott have a useful diagram (Payne and Scott, 1982, page 5) with a sporting anology between different kinds of sporting teams and social care teams. The football team is akin to a patch office, hostel or small family group home, while the athletics team, with the skills of each member unique to a specific event, is likened to a large area office, social education centre or multi-disciplinary staff of a hospital ward. Some commentators refer to the athletics team as a network rather than a team because the members are so individualised.

Community mental handicap teams might come at either end of the continuum depending on whether they are a fully integrated team with their own co-ordinator, or a loosely formed network of professional groups who work in separate settings and meet occasionally to allocate and review work.

What is definite, however, is that all teams need a mandate by which to operate, so that the team knows to whom it is accountable and what boundaries it has in which to operate.

The need for supervision

In chapter 5 we quoted the recent South East Thames Regional Health Authority survey, which recorded the views of people with learning difficulties, carers, staff and managers. Staff "saw managers as essential in enabling them to give of their best. They needed close guidance and support in their work". Unfortunately, the results of the survey showed that managers did not live up to their staff expectations of them. Other studies, such as the CCETSW staff development conference of January 1986, and the UKC report of 1988 (Peter Allen, Jan Pahl and Lyn Quine, *Staff in the Mental Handicap Services: A Study of Change*, Health Services Research Unit, University of Kent, (1988)) show that staff are crying out for clear guidance and support.

Allen *et al* found that different kinds of stress affected staff in hospital and in the community. "Frustration in the community was produced by staff feeling uncertain about their expanded professional role, whilst in the hospital it was produced by staff feeling unable to do the job in the way advocated by professional training and ideology".

Performance feedback was experienced as low by all groups of staff. In the new community service staff gained positive affirmation from the dramatic changes in the residents' abilities following discharge from hospital. When this tailed off, however, there was a lack of impetus. The importance of effective supervision in new small-scale community developments is stressed by Alaszewski and Ong in their description of the Barnardos Intensive Support Unit in Liverpool (see N. Malin ed., *Reassessing Community Care,* Croom Helm 1987).

The Wandsworth study, probably the most comprehensive of its kind in a social services department, shows the vital contribution of supervision in ensuring that work is carried out to the satisfaction of the agency; enabling staff to critically review their work and gain satisfaction from increased professional expertise; and avoiding the pathological effects of stress. As one respondent wrote: "I receive an excellent standard of supervision, and feel this is a very important factor indeed in making my job so enjoyable and rewarding".

What staff want from supervisors

The limited studies completed so far give a reasonably consistent idea as to how staff would like their supervisors to be and what they want from them. They would like:

- The supervisor to be relaxed and friendly. Over 80 per cent of the Wandsworth study wish their supervisor to be more friendly and less detached.
- More availability in between planned sessions.
- Regular sessions which are kept to and not interrupted.
- Consistency, and the containment of the high emotion engendered by the work.
- Supervisors to be more proactive in contributing to the agenda (see M. Clare, 1988) and more specific in goal setting.
- Increased co-working or observation of "live" work.
- Better advice on cultural, race and gender issues.
- More attention to stress identification and reduction.
- A stronger client, as opposed to agency, orientation.
- More positive feedback.

Clearly there will be some differences in perspective between the imperatives on supervisors and the needs of supervisees, and indeed there are some inherent inconsistencies in the supervisee's view.

While the supervisee may wish their supervisor to be less detached, social distance is a factor which the supervisor has to think very carefully about. It is less easy than usual to demand the tightening up of sloppy working practices if the person you are trying to move forward is your drinking companion! Likewise the supervisor will need to preserve a careful balance between the needs of consumers as the staff member sees them and the objectives of and constraints on the agency. What is clear is the importance of expectations in supervision being discussed openly and the aims clarified, for otherwise, as Nixon points out, "there is a risk of poor communication . . . yet effective communication is so essential in the practice of supervision in social work".

The essential ingredients

"Ideally, I see the supervisor's role as helping social workers to manage their caseloads, cope with stress, look in depth at particular cases and develop their skills. I also see the supervisor acting as a 'container', offering space, emotional and thinking, and a 'holding' capacity in order to promote understanding and a sense of progress in their work and professional development."
Wandsworth Study

The environment

Time Enough time to ensure that the work can be done without undue pressure or so much time that it becomes merely a chat.
Space for the individuals or groups to gather without the phone ringing or other people passing through.
No interruptions Tell people you want no phone calls or people popping their heads round the door and saying: "It's not really important, but as you're here . . ."!

The supervisor

The supervisor should have a clear model from which to work and the necessary skills to make it effective.

One such model sees the supervisor: giving support; managing the supervisee's work; and helping the supervisee to grow (the development function). To undertake these he or she must explore, understand, take action and review what has been achieved and set new goals.

The skills needed for this are:

- Exploration: active listening skills (attending, paraphrasing, summarising, use of questions);
- Understanding: facilitation (making issues concrete and specific, setting goals, devising strategies, and deciding means of evaluating achievement).
- Action: supporting/holding-to-account (checking out, providing resources, giving encouragement and praise, acknowledging and celebrating success).

The supervisee

should *share the same model of supervision* as the supervisor. Supervision is not a game where only one side knows the rules!
stick to the agreed arrangements.
Accept that the supervisor is accountable for his or her work.
Take a full part in setting agendas etc., rather than saying: "You're the boss, over to you"!
Be prepared to be open about how work is proceeding, especially in settings where direct observation is difficult.

Other ingredients

Consistency Whether the sessions are one-to-one for an hour or on-the-spot coaching the approach should be consistent and the staff member should be able to rely both on the regularity and the supervisor's mode of working.

Preparation All concerned should think about the session beforehand rather than starting "cold".

An agenda Both parties should contribute to and agree on an agenda of items for discussion.

Recording Any records should be open and agreed, and a focus for review at the next session.

Review Review the last session and how any agreed action has been implemented.

Confidentiality The supervisee must know that she or he can trust the supervisor especially in any personal matters related during supervision.

Accountability Supervision does not take place in a vacuum. Both supervisor and supervisee are members of an organisation which is itself accountable to clients, politicians and legislation. Staff must see their work in this wider context.

The pit and the pendulum

There are a number of "pits" which we are all liable to fall into and many issues in which we ride a delicately balanced pendulum. A good example is confidentiality when the staff member needs to know that what is shared is confidential, but the supervisor mustn't get trapped into a confessional where he or she is told vital information, for example, financial chicanery, or ill-treatment of residents, which gives into a conflict of interests. The nature of the confidentiality must be defined at the start.

Some do's and don'ts of supervision and staff development are:

Do

Appraise continuously and in a positive way so that the possible resentment at an annual heavy binge of appraisement is avoided.

Criticise the behaviour, not the person.

Make any criticism specific and as appropriate as possible (see Blanchard & Johnson, 1983).

Listen actively. Keep your talking to hearing ratio at 30/70.

Use the department's supervision and staff appraisal forms constructively. If there isn't a system then set one up which positively meets local needs.

Be open to changes in job focus and the use of task groups to give people new impetus.

Delegate more as individuals become more confident.

Encourage and inspire.

Don't

Get trapped into doing the supervisee's job for him or get drawn into a "piggy-in-the-middle" role. If there is a conflict between

two staff members get them together and don't let them out for a smoke break until you've all thrashed it out and reached a solution!

Approach appraisals with the attitude that staff are underworked, overpaid and inclined to contemplate their collective navels rather than get down to the work in hand.

Play the therapist. If an individual needs counselling then that should be done by a trained counsellor and not in a supervisory session by a line manager.

Get drawn into a negative cycle of "Isn't it all awful"!

Underestimate the effect of other team members and the environment on an individual's performance.

React defensively to complaints about your management style. We all need to change and grow!

Apologise for making a criticism. An apologetic manner raises doubts about your right to evaluate performance.

Compare the person's behaviour with that of others. Comparisons are odious and will destroy your efforts at team building.

Catch your staff doing something good

"We shall love and we shall praise"
Augustine of Hippo

There is a story told of the novelist Charles Dickens, that once, when out walking with a friend, he stopped, clapped a hand to his forehead and exclaimed: "I am not praised enough." Many of our staff probably share the same feeling, and indeed the only praise they may receive is during their leaving party, when the boss either lies through his teeth or tells them all the good things that they have done, and which he should have told them all the way along!

Partly because the British find giving and receiving praise embarrassing and partly because British management has put the stress on avoiding mistakes rather than achieving excellence, the style in nursing and social care has often been what Americans called "seagull management" — the seagull manager flies in, makes a lot of noise, dumps on everyone and flies out again! As we said in chapter 6, managers in disability services have to ensure that their staff are doing the right things, when they the managers, *are not around.* The best way to ensure this is to have staff who are well-orientated to the task and highly motivated.

Jan Porterfield's excellent and succinct booklet, *Positive Monitoring* (1987) is "based on the concept that staff will do a better job when they know exactly what is expected of them and their work is recognised and supported than they will when their job descriptions are unclear and their good work ignored. This seems to be commonsense but the concept is rarely applied in service provision — or in life! It is very common for staff to be left to 'get on with the job' as long as they are working well and for them to be reprimanded when something goes wrong".

Porterfield's positive monitoring system is made up of six components:

- Defining the aims of the service.
- Specifying clearly what staff should do to achieve service aims.
- Helping staff to work in the specified way.
- Regularly watching staff work and looking at records and other aspects of the service.
- Giving specific feedback to staff on their work and listening to staff comments and suggestions.
- Reviewing individual job performance.

Kenneth Blanchard's work on situational leadership (1983, 1984) follows a similar theme based on learning theory. It may sound somewhat cut and dried but it actually gets down to the basics of effective supervision. Otherwise praise or criticism is too often random and based on the supervisor's state of mind. How many times has a staff member come out of a session with the boss and thought: "I know I need to improve X, Y and Z so why did he shout at me over W, when we both know I did everything he asked me to?"

In each case the supervisor's reaction to staff's action should be immediate, specific, genuine, and constructive.

Improvements should be noted and frustrations acknowledged. When setting goals they should be what Blanchard terms SMART: Specific, Measurable, Attainable, Relevant, Trackable.

Peter Gilbert recently asked a nursing colleague at a conference, what his new unit general manager was like. "Demanding" was the reply, "but good to work for. With this manager everybody knows what they're meant to do." Which implies that nobody did know what to do when his predecessor was in post!

A question of style

Winston Churchill once remarked that he enjoyed learning but couldn't stand being taught. Most of us are irritated at being told things we already know or reminded about tasks we already have in hand. As we said in chapter 6, the manager's/supervisor's style should depend on the circumstances and the commitment and ability of the staff. When new people come into jobs their skills may be uneven or lacking but they will probably be enthusiastic — even too enthusiastic(!) and need guidance. After a time, "Jane" or "Harry" will realise that they know even less than they thought they did and lose confidence and motivation. With coaching their skills will improve and then positive monitoring will boost their confidence as well at a time when the supervisor should be delegating parts of the whole operation to "Jane" or "Harry" so they are given a real responsibility for what goes on in the unit.

Table 8.1.1 *Leadership styles appropriate for the various development levels.*

Development level	*Appropriate leadership style*
D1 Low Competence • High Commitment	S1 DIRECTING Structure, control, and supervise
D2 Some Competence • Low Commitment	S2 COACHING Direct and support
D3 High Competence • Variable Commitment	S3 SUPPORTING Praise, listen, and facilitate
D4 High Competence • High Commitment	S4 DELEGATING Turn over responsibility for day-to-day decision-making

(From K. Blanchard *et al*, 1986)

From style to mode

The 1978 DHSS Survey found that some practitioners complained that they never saw their supervisors and felt unsupported, others made clear they saw formal sessions as a waste of time. Some managers proclaim an "open door" policy, yet give plenty of non-verbal signals that anyone dropping in for advice is a nuisance; some staff dislike the accountability of one-to-one sessions and try and harry their supervisor into an off-the-cuff decision while she's on the way to the coffee machine!

Although the formal session is essential for in-depth discussion and getting down to project work, career development etc., the wise manager will be flexible, especially in residential and day care settings, where there may be suspicion of new methods and/or difficulty in sitting down for a set period.

As Payne and Scott (1982) point out: "'Good' supervision practice . . . should blend formal/informal, planned/*ad hoc* activities as needs and objectives demand. An important supervision skill is the ability to make appropriate and full use of all the opportunities presented for supervision purposes".

Supervisors should be aware that their perceptions and those of their supervisees may differ greatly. In the Wandsworth study (1988) 52 per cent of staff spoke of essentially unplanned supervision, while only 28 per cent of their supervisors perceived it like that, most asserting that they planned the sessions jointly with the worker.

Table 8.1.2: *Workers and supervisor reports of the extent of planning for sessions*

	Workers' perceptions	Supervisor's perceptions
Sessions not planned in advance; parties discuss what seems appropriate at the time	52%	82%
Supervisor and worker plan jointly	34%	65%
Worker plans alone	10%	2%
Supervisor plans alone	0	5%

(From the Wandsworth Survey)

From mode to method

The 1978 research (DHSS, 1978) on supervision found a predominance of one-to-one "discussions"-type supervision in fieldwork, and ten years later the Wandsworth study confirms this.

Payne and Scott's work on developing supervision in teams, and their companion volume on practical exercises (1982), are so good that they are a must for any middle manager and establishment manager. Suffice to say we all need to gain more skills and confidence in different methods of supervision, and this flexibility of approach should also be used in other areas such as training (see chapters 15 and 16) where formal courses are by no means the only way to gain knowledge and skills.

There are perhaps a small number of basic precepts in regard to methods:

- Think flexibly.
- Choose the method which suits the circumstances and gets the job done.
- Don't be arrogant — staff have a great deal to teach managers and the more they move into general management the more managers need to be aware of other people's expertise.

Some of the methods which could be employed are:

One-to-one discussions These need to be purposeful rather than simply a chore to be gone through by both parties. The main problem with this method is that the supervisor relies on the supervisee's ability and willingness to recollect accurately what happened in practice.

Clear agendas, action identification and prioritising, can make the one-to-one both supportive and dynamic. Every so often a wide-ranging discussion is helpful for developmental purposes.

Task-centred work Individuals or groups working on specific projects for set periods so as to enable the individuals or organisation to move forward in a new direction (see also the concept of quality circles in chapter 17).

Live Supervision Joint work; Managing By Walking About; coaching on the move; shadowing an experienced worker; imitation and modelling; observation and intervention, for example, through the use of one-way mirrors.

At secondhand The use of process records, videos and tape-recordings.

Peer groups Useful for developmental learning, especially in a specialist setting. Honesty is needed to avoid sessions becoming self-congratulatory and flaccid.

Lateral thinking "Brainstorming" and nominal group technique to aid thinking around obstacles to progress.

Group supervision For example, supervising three residential managers or community mental handicap team co-ordinators so as to enrich the discussion, improve communication and move people forward simultaneously. Helps avoid manipulation by supervisor or supervisee.

Don't just do something, sit there!

At some stage a manager may well decide to delegate an area of work. This should be *real* delegation, with the knowledge, skills and resources to do the job. It should not be an abdication of responsibility or a situation where the manager is continually pulling people back to check and, therefore, undermining their confidence.

The successful directive manager who has been effective in setting up a project and guiding it in its initial stages, may find delegation particularly difficult, but practise sitting on your hands!

The more social work moves to a model where there are consultants in various specialist areas of work and staff working in dispersed residential and day care settings the more genuine delegation there will need to be. John Adair (1973) quotes Abraham Lincoln's letter to General Grant in April 1864, as a good example of the kind of confidence of delegation to a proven subordinate: "Not expecting to see you again before the Spring campaign opens, I wish to express, in this way, my entire satisfaction with what you have done up to this time . . . the particulars of your plans I neither know nor seek to know. You are vigilant and self-reliant; and, pleased with this, I wish not to obtrude any constraints or restraints upon you. While I'm very anxious that any great disaster . . . shall be avoided, I know these points are less likely to escape your attention than they would be mine. If there is anything wanting which is within my power to give, do not fail to let me know it.

"And now with a brave army, and a just cause, may God sustain you."

To record or not to record

All that we have said before leads to the conclusion that there should be a written agenda and record of supervision where that is possible. Recording could take a number of forms. Between a team manager and a care manager it could be progress on individual personal profiles; developmental project work; team issues; and developmental issues with planned action on each. Between a service manager and a team manager the issues might be broader and concerned with task-centred issues; team issues; and developmental issues. This latter would include matters about staff and projects. Any form would include what was discussed and tasks allotted to both supervisor and the supervisee.

Supervision between team manager and unit manager may need a regular agenda with more detailed headings because of the diversity of headings under which an establishment manager has to organise his or her work. These headings could include clients; staff and staffing; building and equipment; budgets; future planning; liaison with other agencies; working together as a service group; and any other business. Each heading should allow for an action plan.

Come on down – the price is right

The three *One Minute Manager* books (Blanchard & Johnson, 1983; Blanchard & Lorber, 1984; and Blanchard, Zigarmi & Zigarmi, 1986) are worth reading in sequence for a stimulating, easy-to-read and practical guide to motivation and supervision. Much of what they and what we have talked about can be summed up in the following diagram:

Modern management has a tendency to jump from one concept, system, or guru to another in an attempt to find a panacea. The social services and health services are particularly prone to fall for the latest fads and fashions and run lemming-like towards a sea of troubles of their own making. Supervision is essentially about accurate and active listening, clarity of thought,

Figure 8.3.1: *A Summary of the price system*

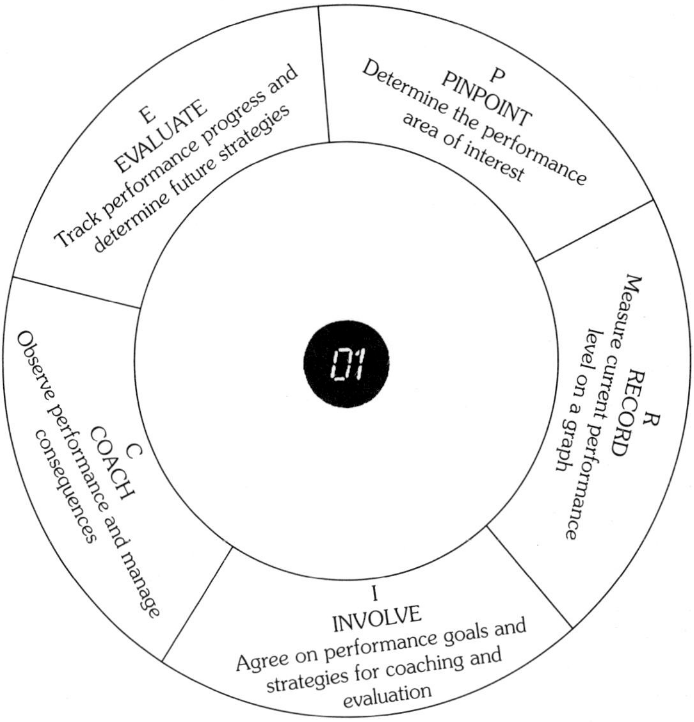

(From Blanchard and Lorber, 1984)

agreed goals, purposeful action and effective review. Do the simple things right and you will achieve a great deal.

Developing staff

"A prince should also show his esteem for talent, actively encouraging able men, and honouring those who excel in their profession."
Niccolo Machiavelli, *The Prince*

"You must not abandon a ship in a storm because you cannot control the winds."
Sir Thomas More, *Utopia*

Leaders "should look for the teaching possibilities in every situation and the basic attitude should always be 'what can we learn from this?' Rather than the issuing of instructions and prohibitions". Hawdon Hague (1975)

A hospital charge nurse once remarked that he had been nominated by his nurse manager to go on a course. "Does this mean she thinks I've got expertise to contribute" he ruminated, "or does she see me as so awful I need to go back to school!?" Just as in supervision so in staff development, there should be no hidden agendas between staff member and supervisor if they have worked together over a period of time. Supervisors need to ask themselves some hard questions, such as in Table 8.1.3.

Table 8.1.3: *The supervisor's "Have I?" checklist*

	Yes	No
Have I agreed with each of my subordinates the main targets and continuing responsibilities, together with standards of performance, so that we can both recognise achievements?	☐	☐
Do I regularly review performance in a way that enables people to move forward?	☐	☐
Am I helping staff to grow or holding them back because I need them more than they need me?	☐	☐
Am I compiling and assessing individual and group training needs?	☐	☐
Do I make sufficient time to talk and listen in order that I understand the unique (and changing) profile of needs and wants in each person, so that I can work with the grain of nature rather than against it?	☐	☐
Am I "talking up" my good people to others in the department or "talking them down"?	☐	☐
Am I doing "positive monitoring" and "management by wandering around"?	☐	☐

As Hawdon Hague points out, staff development appraisals are often resisted both by managers and staff who feel uncomfortable with them. However, questions like "have we the right to sit in judgement on people?" are self deceptive. Appraisal takes place whether it is formalised or not, and Hague turns the question round and asks whether everybody does not have a right to know the yardsticks against which they are being measured. Formal staff development appraisals minimise the amount of subjective assessment which takes place all too often even in "people services"! If the appraisal is a list of criticisms, a mere formality or a discussion of personal characteristics then it serves no useful purpose and may be destructive. On the other hand, if it is very much about two adults getting together in an atmosphere of mutual respect, setting down agreed goals which will benefit the organisation and the individual, then this is likely to lead to greater motivation.

Managers can usefully chart staff's individual needs in the context of the establishment or group along the line of knowledge and skills required in certain roles. An action plan for unit training can then be established (see chapter 16) and worked on in conjunction with the training section.

What is clear is that the modern manager must be proactive. While in the past managers were told by training officers, finance and personnel that they had a problem or needed to change direction, today's manager identifies these issues himself or herself and uses specialist sections as consultants. If, sadly, disciplinary action is required with the staff member then the first thing the enquiry will look at is the effectiveness of supervision. Line managers need to consider staff training and development as an integral part of managerial responsibilities, making a direct impact on the quality of service provision.

Supervisors need to know what they are aiming for in terms of developing staff for the organisation's requirements and the individual's developmental progression. A group of service managers were once asked by a divisional trainer as to whether they would find it useful if she set up a management course for their frontline managers, "Oh no, they've all done management courses", came back the reply. Indeed they had but often ten years ago. When the trainer asked them whether any training was needed for their junior management staff she received a list of items which could neatly be summarised as a management course!

Kent SSD has a staff development and performance review system which looks at the individual and his or her relationship with the organisation and its goals and objectives. The action plans agreed are an integral part of the department's planning process, and the staff development interview identifies the training specific to work in the coming year. If your organisation has no formal system then it should be possible to devise one. If the staff development programme is not a corporate one then there is all the more need to gain staff's acceptance. The Industrial Society suggests (Lawson, 1987) that a minimal organisation policy would include:

- All employees shall have a discussion at least once a year with their manager about their performance. The discussions should recognise good performance and address weaker areas. Most of the content should relate to the future and should result in a specific plan for targets, training and development, to help the individual improve.
- The immediate line manager is responsible for seeing this done.
- The discussion should take place *at least* once a year.

- Both parties should prepare for the interview and have an input on previous performance and priority for the future.
- The conclusions of the manager after the interview shall be written on the form and individuals shall have the opportunity to add written comments if they wish.
- Either then, or soon after, a limited number of important targets shall be set on areas of work where progress is needed during the coming period. The person accountable, the timescale and result required should be clearly indicated.
- Performance against these targets and key result areas should be reviewed regularly throughout the year.

There is a danger of formalism in staff development. As one departmental guide puts it "there is little point in 'appraising' just for the sake of it. This may not only be a waste of time, but may actually be counter-productive. If judgements are made and communicated for no apparent purpose, the people who are judged may rightly feel resentful" (J Jeffrey, *Dartford and Gravesham Supervision Policy,* 1988).

Good supervision is a function of effective leadership. It is the platform for training and staff development, and the stem on which the flower of good practice is nurtured.

J. Adair (1973), *Training for Communication,* MacDonald.
J. Adair (1988), *The Effective Supervisor,* The Industrial Society.
J. Atherton, "Linking the chain", *Insight,* 20 February 1987.
B. Barker, "When did you last see your manager?", *Insight,* 28 February 1989.
K. Blanchard and S. Johnson (1983), *The One Minute Manager,* Collins.
K. Blanchard and R. Lorber (1984), *Putting the One Minute Manager to Work,* Fontana.
K. Blanchard, P. Zigarmi and D. Zigarmi (1986), *Leadership and the One Minute Manager,* Collins.
M. Clare (1988), "Supervision, role strain and social services departments", *British Journal of Social Work,* Vol.18, No.5.
M. Couldery, Internal London Borough of Croydon *SSD,* paper on professional supervision in a residential home for elderly people, October 1981.
R. Douglas and C. Payne (1988), *Organising for Learning,* NISW.
G. Egan (Third edition), *The Skilled Helper,* Brookes/Cole.
A. Forrest (1971), *Delegation,* The Industrial Society.
A. Fowler (1988), *Human Resource Management in Local Government,* Longman.
H. Hague, article in *Industrial and Commercial Training,* September 1975.
Kent SSD *Staff Development and Performance Review Procedure.*

I. Lawson (1987), *Target Setting,* The Industrial Society.
R. Middleton (1983), *A Briefer's Guide to Team Briefing,* The Industrial Society.
NISW (1988), *Residential Care: A Positive Choice,* Wagner report, HMSO.
P. Parsloe and O. Stevenson (1978), *Social Services Teams,* HMSO.
C. Payne and T. Scott (1982), *Developing Supervision of Teams in Field and Residential Social Work,* Parts I and II, National Institute for Social Work.
D. Pettes (1967), *Supervision in Social Work,* George Allen and Unwin.
J. Porterfield (1987), *Positive Monitoring: A Method of Supporting Staff and Improving Services for People with Learning Disabilities,* BIMH.
T. Thorne (1989), *The New General Manager,* McGraw Hill.
Wandsworth SSD (1988), *Social Work Supervision in a Local Authority: Wandsworth Study and Review of Supervisory Practice.*
Wandsworth SSD (1989), *Learning Supervision,* Wandsworth SSD/Tavistock Institute.
C. Whittington (1989), *Exploring Staff Development,* CCETSW.

RESOURCES

M. Brown and P. Ferns (1990), *Staff Supervision in Services for People with Learning Difficulties,* South East Thames Regional Health Authority.

9

Coping with stress

"We want to avoid unacceptable levels of stress, but at the same time we may seek challenge and diversity".
Peter Warr and Toby Wall (1975)

"I was much further out than you thought, and not waving but drowning".
Stevie Smith (1902-71)

Staff working in the helping professions are particularly vulnerable to stress. Although stress can affect anyone who is faced with the complex organisational and personal demands common to the caring services, staff are particularly at risk where they have high ideals, are attempting to develop high quality services and are under pressure in services with limited resources.

What is stress and how can it be defined? Although there are many descriptions of what constitutes stress, one useful way of looking at it is by the idea of pressure. Pressure can be defined as all those demands that are made on you, or that you make on yourself. These would include physical demands, such as noise or change in the environment, or psychological demands such as the need for support or dealing with difficult people. Using this approach stress is seen as the response to inappropriate levels of pressure. Too much pressure can result in stress, and too little pressure can also be stressful. Pressure is not in itself stressful, except where the level of pressure is inappropriate. What is appropriate depends on the individual. What could be stressful to one person, could be energising to another.

Stress: Where does it come from?

Six main sources of pressure have been identified by staff in the helping professions who have attended stress management workshops (Gardner and Lancaster, 1987):

Pressure from the organisation

The conflict between the demands of the organisation for orderliness, standardisation, uniformity, public accountability and the authority of rules and regulations.

There is the professional ideal which emphasises the uniqueness of people; the need to be sensitive to special needs; individual initiative; flexibility and experimentation and the authority which comes from professional skills.

The pressure from management

- ○ to carry out agency policy without including the worker in the decision making process;
- ○ to respond appropriately to an unpredictable volume of work without adequate resources;
- ○ to do a difficult and demanding job without sufficient relevant training or competent supervision;
- ○ to offer an effective service to clients without well-established lines of communication, well-defined goals and clear boundaries of responsibility;
- ○ to set priorities that do not coincide with their own, without adequate recognition or appreciation.

Pressure from clients

- ○ to take on board their anger, hostility and possibly aggression;
- ○ to respond to unreasonable or impossible demands and to offer solutions to every problem;
- ○ to respect their individuality, but to take the responsibility of problems from them, yet leave them feeling adequate to life's demands.

The pressure from colleagues

- ○ to cope with breakdowns in communication and relationships and to deal with competitiveness and apathy;
- ○ to continue to provide an effective service when trust and respect have broken down.

The pressure from other organisations and agencies

- ○ to be able to provide an immediately responsive service without their appreciation of the problems or constraints;
- ○ to succeed where *they* have failed and to respond to *their* unrealistic expectations.

The pressure from within ourselves

We need to recognise that external pressures hook into personal needs to create internal pressures.

The need to:

- ○ respond to every demand or risk rejection;
- ○ succeed and to be able to measure success in situations in which "success" is difficult to measure;
- ○ effect change in clients, the agency and the social structure;
- ○ be liked and appreciated by colleagues and management;
- ○ be seen to be efficient in dealing with people whose difficulties cannot be overcome;
- ○ be able to say "the job is finished";
- ○ be liked and appreciated by every single client;
- ○ be seen to be thoroughly competent in every situation.

We often expect more of ourselves than others expect of us and the internal pressures create greater stress than those that come from outside.

The signs of stress

One of the main difficulties individual staff face is that they may be unaware of how stressed they are, because they are spending so much time looking after the needs of others. Brandon (1989) describes stress creeping up on the individual over a period of time. The worker can lack support; can be dealing with difficult situations; can feel uncared for; can be handling the suffering of service users and relatives. The result can be the Fawlty Towers syndrome - the smiling tension thinly overlaying repressed hysteria.

Helping others can mean that individual staff fail to look to their own needs. They are far too busy helping others to attend to themselves. All of us experience some of the signs of stress at some time, but when these persist over days and weeks, or when they are not part of our normal pattern of feelings or behaviour, then we should be concerned. Fineman (1985), who conducted a two-year project that identified patterns of stress among workers in a social services department, lists some of the signs and symptoms of stress. These are psychological, behavioural and physical. Their manifestations may include:

☐ *Psychological:* tension, worry, anxiety; anxiety-depression; panic; stewing over difficulties; frustration; loss of confidence; self-doubt; tearful; inability to relax.

☐ *Behavioural:* constant questioning of own actions; not eating; insomnia; freezing; running round in circles; distancing; too aggressive; too impatient; taking tranquillisers; unrealistic expectations of others.

☐ *Physical:* High blood pressure; heart racing; coughs and colds; skin disease; backache; muscle tension; migraine; asthma; nausea; gastric upsets; fatigue; exhaustion; breathlessness.

Turning to the specific needs of staff in community-based services, Firth and Myers (1985) describe some of the difficulties staff experience as a consequence of stress, particularly in terms of low morale and burnout.

- They have difficulty completing tasks; they are threatened when asked to respond to new situations, or some change in the service; they may hide behind the manager's responsibility and fail to take decisions that they should be capable of making.
- They may lose initiative and be unable or unwilling to find ways round problems; challenges become insurmountable obstacles; and they cease looking to the future and remain stuck with present practices.
- Experienced staff find their work unrewarding or lacking in

personal accomplishment and may lose confidence; they may become defensive towards new ideas, and to younger members of staff and subordinates, they may appear rigid and negative. Loss of concern about the lives of service users can be mirrored by lack of concern for colleagues. Criticising and running down other staff, particularly those in other disciplines, departments or agencies, can be a result of overwork or frustration.

Firth and Myers are concerned that because these problems are not life threatening and are often insidious, managers may not regard staff morale as a high priority.

One example of extreme stress experienced by a worker has been documented by Hegarty (1987). "Mary" had been in charge of a therapy unit for adults with profound handicaps for three years, during which time she had attempted to run a high quality service. She eventually became so emotionally depleted that she left the job and needed to enter psychotherapy. Mary described her feelings on leaving her job:

"By the time I did leave it was for my mental health as I had been chronically depressed for 11 months. I found myself creating new projects just to keep going. When I did leave I felt worthless and useless and that anyone could do my job (trained or not). I felt threatened by one of my junior staff members who was better than I was (or seemed to be) in dealing with behavioural problems with clients and I could not tolerate this ... although I voiced my difficulties the threat and feelings of worthlessness still prevailed and I felt like a failure".

Hegarty states that when an individual who is hard-working and creative, and who has a strong commitment to developing high quality services leaves the service as a result of extreme stress, this results in a valuable resource lost, that could have been avoided if support and encouragement were provided. Incipient stress needs to be recognised and steps taken to prevent it, before valuable elements of the service disappear. He sees staff who are idealistic and who are attempting to be innovative at particular risk, and if wanted in organisations, then they must be actively supported, certainly before signs of extreme stress appear.

How can stress be managed?

The organisation's responsibility

In any analysis of the causes of stress, the manner in which the organisation creates a climate that recognises that caring roles are inherently stressful, and as a direct consequence has systems for responding to the needs of staff is crucial. Where there is little or no recognition of the impact of stress on the individual (and writers on stress suggest that few organisations make anything like adequate provision for their staff), then it is hardly likely that staff can be expected to maintain the necessary level of commitment necessary to build high quality community services.

Before examining those issues, there are some factors related to working conditions that are basic requirements that are worth emphasising. Staff need to be well paid, with duty hours that enable them to live civilised lifestyles and their off-duty respected. They should be encouraged to develop or maintain a full and active life outside the service, and have holidays that are of sufficient length to enable them to renew their energies. They need to feel they are doing a vital and unique task for which they are appreciated (Dunham, 1978).

The Wagner report on residential care (NISW, 1988) clearly points to the essential requirement of the manager to take the lead and offer positive and constructive guidance to staff. This will include developing conditions that enable staff to share problems and work on the resolution of issues before they become unmanageable. Here the role of regular staff meetings, held as frequently as the pressures and complexity of the work require, is suggested. The report also recommends that support for staff through the development of guidelines on practice is important, particularly in areas such as risk taking and users' rights. These are areas of considerable concern to staff, but often they search in vain for support.

The report also suggests that staff need access to independent counsellors. This is particularly important where staff are unable to discuss their difficulties with their line manager. As Brandon (1989) makes clear if you fall out with your manager, you effectively lose a large element of your support system. Here he recommends that managers should support the establishment of supervisory/counselling sessions from someone completely independent of management.

Firth and Myers (1985) describe some of the essential elements needed by a service if it is to offer the level of support required by staff, and avoid the loss of morale that can lead to the difficulties described earlier.

The service needs a "mission" or purpose, and objectives that are clear to all staff. Staff working with service users need resources in order to meet the desired objectives of the service. For example, individual programme planning as a mechanism for developing goals for service users.

Staff need job descriptions and guidance, but in addition they need personal discussion about what is expected of them which avoids any ambiguity. They suggest the following questions may help reveal the degree of role ambiguity:

- how clear are you about the central objectives you should be working towards in your job?
- how clear are you about what your superiors expect from you? What would represent a satisfactory achievement, or a

considerable achievement?

- how clear are you about the limits of your authority and responsibility in your present position?
- how clear are you about how satisfied your superior is with what you do?

Role clarity is seen as a major influence on morale. Discussion between staff and managers can lay out the overall service priorities, and describe what is expected of each member of staff. An example would be the priorities needed to run a staffed house that are drawn up against the purpose of the service. This would then enable achievements to be identified.

A further area of concern is the need to avoid the risk of staff becoming emotionally drained, due to lengthy face-to-face contact with service users without a break. Firth and Myers suggest that staff should have a variety of tasks, some of which do not involve direct contact with users. This is seen as particularly important, for example in residential settings, where every task can involve teaching users domestic, personal and social skills. These can be very demanding emotionally.

The individual's responsibility

Just as the organisation has responsibilities for avoiding stress among its staff, so the individual has to consider what they can do to avoid becoming stressed as a result of the way they manage their lives. Here we are talking about those actions which a member of staff can take, that can help them to manage stressful situations more effectively.

A useful starting point for the individual who is stressed is to begin to examine the way they work, and what steps they can take that lead to greater effectiveness and greater self-understanding. This means avoiding instant action, unless of course the person is in extreme stress and needs immediate help, but identifying what elements of the job, interacting with personal factors, are causing stress that is unmanageable.

It is helpful to think about stress in an holistic way. What factors are operating in the work setting which result in a response that leads to the person feeling stressed? We have seen what organisations need to do to reduce or eliminate stress in staff. Are any of these factors present in your work situation possible causes of stress? If there are, can you identify where you might be able to influence the situation through discussion with your manager and colleagues? Managing stress means that you will need to develop assertive strategies, where you begin to revalue yourself and take control of your situation. Gardener and Lancaster (1987) describe a series of demands you may need to make:

Trying to remove or reduce external pressures. This could involve you in asking for support and supervision; relevant in-service training; realistic goals that you have been able to influence; an effective communication system; participation in decision-making; adequate resources; clearly defined boundaries of responsibility; better workload management, including help with time management.

This may involve confronting managers, colleagues and service users. It could also mean checking exactly what management expects. "Am I really required to do . . . ?"

Trying to change the way we respond to pressure by reframing a problem by looking at it in a different way. Where we are faced with a demanding situation that creates stress, changing our perception to a positive one, in order to turn the energy tied up in stress into action.

It may also mean taking control of the situation. This could mean taking control through the use of time, through planning priorities and tasks and avoiding getting diverted.

Staff may need to withdraw from the pressures at least on a temporary basis, recognising that there may be times when the only course of action is to withdraw from a situation.

Emotional stress will need to be discharged on a physical activity in order to displace pent up feelings, such as playing a high-activity sport.

Emotional support may need to be found through the development of good personal relationships. This includes building opportunities for support through good supervision, but also supportive groups of colleagues meeting regularly.

We need to recognise that much of our stress is self-inflicted. This can include our inability to say "no"; making unrealistic demands on ourselves, like listing all the things we are going to do, but have no hope of achieving, or filling our diary full of appointments which we haven't got time to keep.

We need to acknowledge that stress is common and a by-product of a demanding job, and the need to work within a set of realistic and clearly defined goals, working on what we can change and admitting that there are things we cannot change — that there are a limited amount of hours available to us and that there is only so much that can be achieved.

A lifestyle should be developed that acts as a buffer against the effects of stress. This could include stopping or reducing smoking, drinking in moderation, eating a healthy diet, by going easy on sugar, salt and saturated fats, and eating more fibre. Taking regular exercise and maintaining your recommended weight.

Staff should be clear about their values, life goals and objectives. Until it is clear what is important, staff will find it difficult to establish personal goals.

These are just some of the approaches that can be taken to manage stress. In addition more specialist help may need to be considered, such as workshops where you can learn about stress management techniques, or help from a counsellor either through the workplace (if this facility is available), or from a professional counsellor (The British Association for Counselling, 37a Sheep Street, Rugby CV21 3EX, can provide a list of counsellors).

D. Brandon, "Sinking into The Fawlty Towers Syndrome", *Care Weekly*, 17 February 1989.
D. Brandon, "Falling out with your boss", *Care Weekly*, 24 February 1989.
C. Cooper and R. Payne (1978), *Stress at Work*, Wiley.
J. Dunham, "Staff stress in residential work", *Social Work Today*, 25 July 1978.
S. Fineman (1985), *Social Work Stress and Intervention*, Gower.
H. Firth and M. Myers, "Supporting staff in community services", *Mental Handicap*, September 1985.
D. Gardener and R. Lancaster (1987), *Stress Management for Workers and Managers in Helping Professions*, PEPAR Publications.
NISW (1988), *Residential Care: A Positive Choice*, HMSO.
P. Warr and T. Wall (1975), *Work and Well-Being*, Penguin Books.

10

Care management

"Enter the Honest Broker".
Ken Edwards (1989)

Care management is a method of service provision that has been extensively developed in North America, and is now beginning to be introduced into this country. Warner (1989) has described care management as "a set of arrangements that assess individuals in their social context; identify the service elements they need in an individual service plan, and then secures the provision of an appropriate package of services". The impetus to introduce this service system has been provided by the recommendation in the White Paper, *Caring for People,* that social services departments should appoint case managers who will "take responsibility for ensuring that the individual's needs are regularly reviewed, resources are managed effectively and that each service user has a single point of contact".

Care management is described in the White Paper as an effective method of targeting resources and planning services to meet the specific needs of individual clients. This claim is based on the evidence gathered from care management projects that have been piloted in this country, for example in Kent SSD. To achieve the effectiveness claimed for care management the White Paper recommends some key features:

- identification of people in need, including systems of referral;
- assessment of care needs;
- planning and securing the delivery of the service;
- monitoring the quality of care provided; and
- reviewing the client's needs.

The White Paper also suggests that care management could be linked with delegated responsibility for budgetary management, although this need not be pursued down to individual client level in all cases. Nevertheless, it is clear that considerable emphasis will be placed on individual care managers' awareness of the costs of services and that care packages will need to be developed within a fixed budget. These new responsibilities will enormously extend and change the role of social workers and home care organisers, who are most likely to be appointed to care manager posts, due to the lead role that local authorities will take in community care. The White Paper also suggests that community nurses would also be particularly suitable professionals to fulfil this role.

Care management in action

From the reports of care management projects some essential features emerge that enable us to begin to paint a picture of the new role. Although these projects have been in services for elderly people (the Wakefield Study (Richardson and Higgins, 1990) is an exception) and for people with a physical disability, they nevertheless describe a system which will be similar in most other respects to arrangements made in services for people with learning difficulties.

In Kent a community care scheme for frail elderly people employs the care management system. Here a care manager is an experienced worker, who has responsibility for approximately 30 clients, for whom he assesses the needs and designs care packages. Services contracted typically include home help, locally paid helpers and equipment to increase independence.

In order to provide the care package within agreed financial limits the care managers are provided with detailed costing of the services they coordinate. Services are charged against a client-specific budget, set at two-thirds the cost of residential care. Care managers have to "purchase" services within their client-budget, although they are able to use the budget flexibly to create novel ways of meeting need within the financial target set.

In designing the care package the care manager has to describe what care can be provided directly by the social services department and what services need to be purchased from other agencies. The client is provided with a contract which outlines the provision arranged, and includes a diary that workers and the person receiving the service use to comment on progress and satisfaction with the standard of service provided. Following the introduction of the services, the care manager is responsible for monitoring and reviewing the package. Managers are given considerable autonomy, and are able to work flexibly in order to develop imaginative solutions to the needs of clients.

The emphasis in this care management scheme is the design of a service package that reflects the needs of the person, rather than fitting the person into existing services. This needs-led approach to service provision offers an opportunity to use a range of services that draw on the resources of the local neighbourhood, with the aim of reducing clients admissions to residential care or the risk of such admissions. This system piloted some years ago, continues to operate in Kent. An evaluation of the care management project in Kent can be found in Challis and Davies (1986), whilst King (1990) has a description of care management in practice.

Care management and individual plans

Reading a description of care management one would be forgiven for thinking that there was something familiar about the process.

Staff who have worked in services where individual plans have been introduced will see considerable similarities between the two approaches. Already Kent SSD has begun to bring together individual service plans and care management, as this new system extends into services for people with learning difficulties.

An individual plan (IP) is a process which enables professionals who deliver services to focus on the unique needs of individuals receiving those services, and to ensure that they have a major say in planning their life and determining the help they need (see Blunden *et al*, 1987). IPs consist of three stages. There is a preparatory stage, where the worker and person concerned, and where appropriate other people, spend time identifying the person's needs. The second stage is a meeting where a plan is drawn up based on the needs of the person, with goals set for a specified period of time (ie, up to six months). The third stage is where individuals work on their agreed responsibilities, with or on behalf of the person. The action is then reviewed at regular intervals, and the entire process repeated at the end of the previous planning cycle.

Figure 10.3.1 : *Care management cycle*

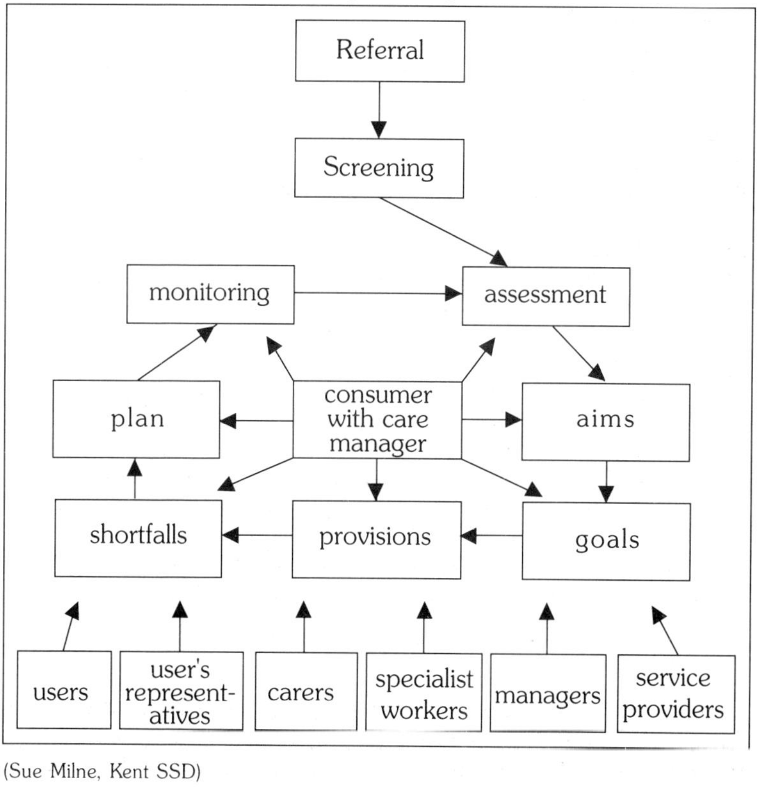

(Sue Milne, Kent SSD)

Where care management differs significantly from individual planning is the additional responsibility for a devolved budget that is used to purchase services in order to meet the user's needs. The care manager would undertake many of the same tasks to a coordinator of an IP, but would have additional responsibilities, including knowledge of pricing policy for a range of services, designing a care package, based on the expressed needs of the service user, establishing contracts with service providers, and monitoring the implementation and quality of the services provided that constitute the package, and arranging for services to be changed and updated as necessary. The overriding responsibility will be to design a package that can be delivered within the financial allocation for the service user. The only exception to this firm financial control is where service users have particular needs that demand greater budgetary flexibility in view of the complex package of services required, where some financial discretion will be necessary.

Concerns about care management

Care management has proved effective in North America and in the small number of schemes operating in this country, with service packages tailored to the individual needs of the user. Nevertheless, fears have been expressed about the ability of care managers to deliver all that is promised, due to a number of severe constraints.

Local authorities will have an obligation to assess potential users without charge, but Warner (1989) has suggested that issues of eligibility and levels of charges for services should not be left to individual care managers, but will require local political decisions, as no national guidance will be given.

Care managers will have conflicting roles. They will be responsible for the assessment of need, but also have budgetary control as an employee of the local authority that holds the funds. Combining these roles risks vested financial interest. This is very different from the North American scene, where Thomas and Towell (1990) reported that no care managers held budgets themselves.

Assessment is a professionally dominated procedure that could mean needs being defined to fit into available resources. The care manager has a potentially powerful gatekeeping role that could result in service users being denied services they believe they require. To avoid this risk some form of advocacy, complaints procedures and access to a second opinion is suggested (Barker and Peck, 1989, and Kings Fund Institute Briefing, 1988).

Will budgets allocated to individual care managers for use on behalf of service users enable them to purchase a high quality range of services? The example from Kent where care managers had a budget for their elderly clients set at two-thirds of the cost of residential services, has been questioned.

Care management will still depend on services being available, and of the right quality. In the project documented by Pilling (1988), the unavailability of services was one of the main reasons why some elements of plans were not completed. Similarly Thomas and Towell (1990) argue that one of the minimum conditions for an appropriate care management function will be the commitment by public authorities to develop a variety of services, so that choice becomes a reality for people with learning difficulties.

Future requirements

The development of care management will be critical in the new three-way relationship between purchasing authorities, provider services and the service user contained in the White Paper. It is clear from the North American experience and reports of projects in this country that certain preconditions are necessary for the establishment of care management on a large scale. These include, first, recruitment of skilled and experienced professionals as care managers, who have the necessary personal qualities to work in an autonomous manner and devise new solutions to complex problems. Second, there need to be limited caseloads to enable sufficient time for comprehensive assessment, monitoring and evaluation of services provided. There must also be access to computer systems that provide up-to-date financial information, with services available, and costing levels. Fourth, there should be comprehensive training for care managers in assessment techniques, purchasing skills, budget control, case monitoring, quality control and service costing. Last, sufficient autonomy must be given to care managers to be able to act flexibly in constructing care packages that meet user needs, including using budgets to make spot purchases where necessary.

I. Barker, E. Peck and H. Smith, "Safeguarding service users", *The Health Services Journal*, 7 December 1989.

V. Beardshaw and D. Towell (1990), *Assessment and Case Management*, Kings Fund Briefing Paper 10.

R. Blunden, G. Evans and S. Humphreys (1987), *Planning with Individuals: An Outline Guide*, The Mental Handicap in Wales Applied Research Unit.

D. Challis and B. Davies (1986), *Case Management in Community Care: An Evaluation Experiment in the Home Care of the Elderly*, Gower.

K. Edwards, "Enter the honest broker", *New Statesman and Society*, 15 September 1989.

J. King, "A helping hand", *Community Care*, 22 February 1990.
Kings Fund Institute Briefing, *Care Management*, No. 1. November 1988.
D. Pilling (1988), *The Case Manager Project: Report of the Evaluation*, Rehabilitation Resource Centre, City University.
J. Renshaw, "Care in the community: Individual care planning and case management", *British Journal of Social Work*, 18, 1988.
A. Richardson and R. Higgins (1990), *Case Management in Practice: Reflections on the Wakefield Project*, Nuffield Institute.
D. Thomas and D. Towell, "Common goals across oceans", *The Health Services Journal*, 4 January 1990, pp. 22-23.
N. Warner, "Community care: How do we make it work in social services?", paper presented to the National Association of Health Authorities, 12 December 1989.

Consumer's view: A life of one's own

Judith Wood

Lack of choice is the biggest problem people with learning difficulties face today. People think that, because you have Down's syndrome like I have, or because you can't speak well or need a wheelchair to get about, that you don't have views or wishes. That's why I joined the movement People First - because I believe people have a right to stand up and say what they want.

Some friends and I started a self-advocacy group about five years ago. We meet in Camden, north London, every month to talk about what we're doing and to support each other. I'm a very confident person with a strong will, but there are others who find it hard to speak out for themselves. It's all new to them. They've never tried it before because they're afraid they might get a nasty reply back or that someone will take the mickey.

Some people do treat you badly, especially school children. They call you names, laugh and swear. I feel angry, but I never ever answer back - I walk away. Names can't hurt me. In the end they stop because they realise what they're doing.

We don't like to be called "handicapped" people - it gives the wrong impression about people like me. We have learning difficulties. That's the kind of thing we discuss in our group. We also didn't like some of the posters done by MENCAP, which we thought made people like us look pathetic. We wrote to MENCAP and complained. The group gives you the support and confidence to say what you think and do what you want. I go around the country now talking about People First and get others to set up their own groups.

I've been living away from my parents for eight years. My mum and dad don't mind really - they support me in what I want to do - but not all parents of children with learning difficulties are as understanding. They try to hang on to their children and not give them a chance to do what they want. It's very hard for them to become independent.

I was about 14 when I decided that I had to make my own life, and I got my social worker to help me. I left school at 17 and took a two-year course in independent living in a MENCAP home in North Wales and then lived in a south London hostel for another three years. I moved into this group home 18 months ago and I'm happy here. There are six of us in the house. We all work, do our own shopping, cook. We all have learning difficulties but there's a full-time member of staff around if we need advice or help. We have a weekly house meeting to discuss who does the cleaning and so on. We live our own lives.

I'm working in a nursery two days a week at the moment, and I want to take a course next year on working with children. I went to meet the other staff at the school, and told them all about myself, that I had Down's Syndrome - which they could see from my appearance. (My parents didn't realise until I was two). I got interested in children because of my nieces and nephews - my sisters both have children. The other three days a week I work at the Job Assessment Centre learning various skills including how to use a computer.

I'm critical of the government. We need more money for group homes so that people like me can live independently rather than being stuck in institutions. And we need more opportunities, so people with learning difficulties can make their feelings known.

Reprinted from The Observer *with permission of the editor.*

11

"The right stuff": Staff selection and induction

"It is vital that staff with the right personal qualities and skills are recruited and selected; that they are adequately paid, and have conditions of service and training opportunities which match the job . . . Also, as residential provision becomes more closely integrated into local services networks, we should expect staffing patterns to reflect the social and multi-cultural characteristics of neighbourhoods and communities".
The Wagner report (1988)

"What has become strikingly clear is the need to have well developed skills and the right attitude among staff at all levels. Unless the human resource is properly developed and well managed, tinkering with structures and systems will be to no avail . . . "
Annual report of the Local Government Training Board (1986)

"The Right Stuff" was the expression used by the United States space programme about the successful astronauts turned out by its rigorous selection and training process. Staff in social care may feel that they have to be as resilient as astronauts as the job becomes progressively harder and more demanding, with service users in all client groups becoming increasingly more frail and more dependent, or more challenging in their behaviour.

Managers are often caught between the knowledge that they need to employ supermen and superwomen on less than super wages, and yet also being desirous of recruiting a wide range of staff with special interests and aptitudes, including mature entrants to the profession. Despite the tough challenges in social care, the Wagner report remarked that "its strongest asset" was that it was able to attract "people of different ages, from various walks of life and ethnic backgrounds, possessing a rich assortment of personal qualities, skills, interests and experiences".

As practitioners and teachers we have always been struck by the quality of staff we meet day-to-day and their abilities to produce what the NASA programme controllers call "routine magic"!

The recruitment mountain

We all know that the right care worker or charge-nurse, officer-in-charge or middle manager, can transform part of a service.

Getting the right staff in the right place is going to be increasingly difficult as the year 2000 draws on, and employers can no longer rely on vague appeals to the "job satisfaction" of working in social care.

The factors that militate against recruitment, especially in certain areas of the U.K. are:

- An increasing unwillingness to work unsocial hours (for example sleep-ins and weekends).
- A shortage of some professionals, especially amongst the therapies, due to a squeeze on training places and secondments.
- Competition from less psychologically rewarding but more financially rewarding jobs, so the new DIY store may be attracting your care workers on to its staff!
- Prohibitive house prices for young home buyers in certain parts of the UK, often areas of concurrent increases in population, social need and family dislocation.

On the more hopeful side, however, the ADSS survey (1989) indicates a move towards a more stable workforce, and a continuing desire from people to enter the service. Over 60 per cent of field social workers have been in their present post for over three years, and 40 per cent for over five years. The vacancy and turnover rate is particularly high in some sections of the workforce, but there is a good level of intake in the annual start rate. The York University study of health authorities, found a turnover rate for nurses of 20.2 per cent, and this may be higher among RNMH qualified staff in health districts where a clear role has not been given post-hospital closure.

What do applicants look for?

As in so many matters concerned with management and service delivery, the best way to start looking at how other people might view the job you are offering is to put yourself in their shoes. What do I look for in a job? How would I like to work here? Would I like to work for me!?

Over the past few years professional journals have set up job forums for prospective employers and applicants to meet explicitly at a marketstall. *Community Care's* survey, conducted in July 1988, showed the following factors were deemed by respondents to be the most important when choosing a new job:

Table 11.1.1: *Important factors when choosing a new job: social services sector*

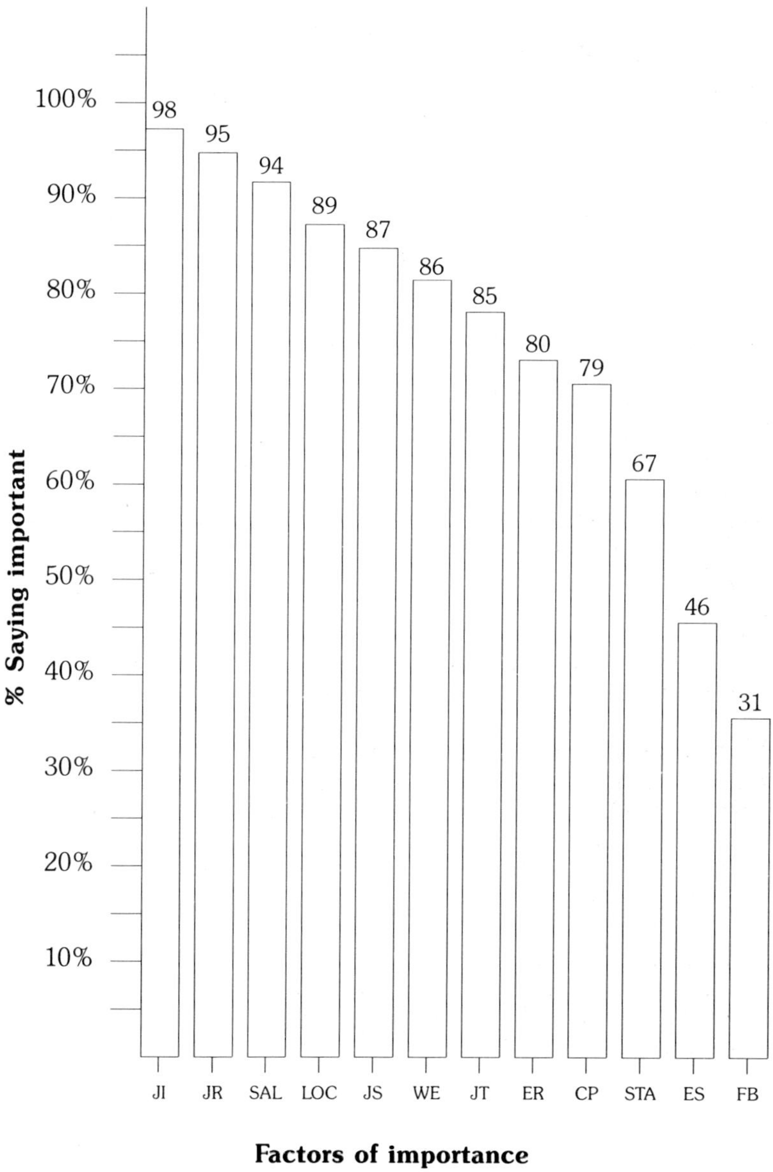

Key:

JI = Job interest
JR = Job responsibility
SAL = Salary
LOC = Location
JS = Job security
WE = Work environment
JT = Job type
ER = Employer's reputation
CP = Career prospects
STA = Status
ES = Employment sector
FB = Fringe benefits

Another obvious source of information is our own staff. Why did they join this outfit? Did the image we project fit with what we are like in practice? Would the people they know in their neighbourhood be good at this job, for example, residential work? If so, would they be interested? If interested, would they want to work for us? How do we need to shape ourselves to the labour market? The manager needs an overview to ascertain whether the staff group are inclusive or exclusive. If visitors/prospective staff/new staff are viewed with suspicion then you won't attract new people into the service.

Everybody needs a recruitment strategy

"Blankshire for Better Child Care" and similar messages are now increasingly portrayed in the professional journals, as the employers attempt to counter the Audit Commission's judgement that "little effort is being made by local government . . . to capture an adequate share of the market".

While it is vital for an SSD or a health authority to have its recruitment strategy, it is also important for the divisional director, middle manager, charge nurse, community mental handicap team co-ordinator and establishment head, to have a recruitment hat as well as a management and training one. Each should look at their own domain and consider:

● *What kind of jobs the unit has:*

☐ How appropriate are they for the service?

☐ Are there clear job descriptions?

☐ Are there possibilities of career progression?

● *If people are leaving, why are they leaving?*

☐ Lay yourself open to a leaving interview, and encourage honesty.

☐ Are all the people with bright ideas leaving?

● *What is attracting people to work in the unit and what retains them?*

☐ Are some people staying too long for their own and the unit's good?

☐ What are you offering in relation to the competition?

☐ Are we staying ahead of the market?

● *Methods of advertising*

☐ Are we relying too much on advertising in the media?

☐ Why not try posters in colleges, schools, newsagents, public places; leaflet distribution; or local recruitment forums and displays?

● *Community contacts*

Some of the best staff are those who have come in from local courses, for example, PCSC, RMNH, NNEB and so on, and have returned after qualifying.

Contacts with local sixth form colleges and training courses, allied with well supervised placements, can reap dividends. Don't treat students like "an extra pair of hands", but people who need space to learn and develop.

● *Courtesy at all times*

Each unit is an ambassador for the authority and its strategy, and the image it projects needs to be closely allied to that of its parent body. Applicants who are not suitable for one part of the service might be ideal for another and should be courteously redirected.

● *Be proactive*

It isn't enough to "leave it to the personnel department". You have to bring your service up to a level of excellence and then get out and get the staff you need.

● *Develop your own resources*

The ADSS survey (1989) states that "relatively few authorities" are trying to make "the best use of existing staff". Staff development and training (see chapters 8, 15 and 16) can increase the skills of the staff you already have, with their local knowledge and commitment to the service.

In a situation when you have service users from one or more cultural or ethnic group, your own staff from those groups are likely to be the best ambassadors to gain staff from that ethnic group so as to make yours a more ethnically sensitive service.

● *The selection process*

During the selection process the manager should be working with the personnel department through a series of logical steps:

● *Think through the job* and ascertain whether there should be any changes to the job, and to the conditions attached to it.

● *Write or rewrite* the job description to make it a broad statement of the purpose, scope, duties and responsibilities of the job, together with the post to which the job is accountable to.

● *Add in,* under a separate heading, any specific tasks attached to this job in particular.

● *Construct a "person specification"* so you know the type of person you are looking for and won't be unduly swayed on the day by shiny qualifications but little experience.

● *Attract suitable applicants.* In the *Community Care* survey, respondents to the questionnaire put the following as most important:

Description of the job	36%
Job title	18%
Location	18%
Salary	9%
Employer's name	5%

Lyrical descriptions of sand, lakeland walks, the cultural benefits of living in a metropolis and so on, on their own, tend to make the people feel that the job itself may not be up to much!

● *Give additional information.* In an effort to be fair to all applicants, many equal opportunities employers tend to allow no pre-interview contact with the service. Unfortunately, this often results in a distinct advantage given to internal candidates who already know the service and the issues it is currently grappling with, and a form of magical mystery tour for external candidates.

Applicants must know what the job is they're applying for and the service in which it is set. Each applicant should be sent an information pack with items such as an outline of the service and the geographical area in which it is placed; job description; structure of the department/division/service group; structure of the team or establishment; mission statement/operational policy; consumers' charter; policy documents (or excerpts from them); details of schemes, e.g. lease car etc; and literature showing house prices, leisure facilities etc.

● *The day itself* could see a variety of methods used depending on the post. It is vital to involve the immediate line manager of the post to be filled and the service users. An applicant may be very able, but if he or she will clash with the line manager, or cannot relate to users of the service then it is not right to appoint.

Methods which can be used in combination are:

☐ Analysis of the CV and follow-up of references.

☐ Informal interviews with service users and possible colleagues.

☐ Individual or group tasks.

☐ Testing of aptitude and/or personality.

☐ Formal one-to-one or panel interviews.

Experience has shown that formal interviews on their own, are not very reliable as a judge of quality of aptitudes. A combination of methods is best and this may include a personality test, especially where close team work is concerned. Teams need to be aware of how they operate and the make-up needed to become and remain effective.

If you are tempted to appoint subordinates you can control or manipulate, then you need to read the chapter on the Pygmy Syndrome, in Flamholtz and Randle's, *The Inner Game of Management* (Hutchinson, 1989).

● *The follow-up* after the decision has been made is a stage often mishandled. Waiting for police and medical checks can be nerve-racking for the successful applicant and contact must be maintained so that the momentum, and indeed the potential staff member himself isn't lost.

● *Be aware of bias and discrimination* at all stages, and either know the law yourself or have back-up from specialists in personnel.

Induction

"Induction is one of the great neglected areas of management policy".
Alistair Graham, director, The Industrial Society

"I care not if we have a right to make them miserable: have we not an interest to make them happy?"
Edmund Burke (1729-97)

People usually start a new job with a burst of enthusiasm and a twinge of apprehension. An organisation can build on that initial desire to do well by a good induction programme, or produce in that individual an impression that the organisation doesn't know what it's doing, or at least doesn't care whether the new member of staff discovers this well kept secreti Stories abound of social workers and community nurses arriving to find their line manager on a course and a pile of thick case files on their desk, or the care staff left to fend for themselves in a ward or residential home. One residential manager once recalled to one of us the experience of her first day as a care assistant in a hostel. She was greeted by the officer-in-charge with the words: "Hello. Why haven't you brought your overnight bag? You'll have to stay overnight for a few days as you're in charge now - we're off on holiday"!

People who have had a good induction programme, however, are often heard to say after a few months: "It's hard work here, but at least I know what I'm doing, and who to contact when I get stuck".

Rooting people in the service

The Texas Instrument plant in Bedford, compared ten new recruits receiving a full induction programme with a control group who received "the normal treatment". After one month's working the differences were clear:

Table 11.1.2: *Differentials of induction*

	Experimental group	Control group
units produced per hour	93	27
absence rate	0.5%	2.5%
number of times late	2	8
training hours undergone	225	381

(quoted in J. Adair, *The Effective Supervisor*, 1988)

The University of Kent study of a staffed housing scheme found several important effects associated with induction training. Staff who had benefited from it reported a greater feeling of confidence and autonomy, had a better view of how they contributed to the service as a whole, experienced less ambiguity in their role and were less likely to leave prematurely. Those that did leave that particular scheme were more likely to consider joining another form of community-based social care than those that had had no induction. The study stated: "Clearly any new community service should give priority to mounting and maintaining such a training programme" (P. Allen *et al,* 1988).

One group that is often left out are clerical staff. One of the authors was recently involved in a diagnostic workshop on training with frontline staff. A staff member from a children's home had not been able to attend and the establishment's clerk stood in. She was most apologetic about coming, but was reassured that her presence was most important.

Clerical staff are often left feeling that they are only bit players on the stage of social care, and yet, in many instances, they are the person around whom service users, carers, staff and outside agencies revolve. Their attitudes and knowledge of how things operate, and their commitment, are most important. In a study of clerical staff in a social services area, a questionnaire survey found that only 23 per cent of all clerical staff in the area had had an induction programme of some type arranged for them. The great majority of the staff would have welcomed a properly arranged and supervised induction programme, continuing supervision and appraisal and training. It was felt that after a few months in post, clerical staff should have the opportunity to visit other establishments to see their place in the wider picture, and to gain greater insight into the significance of their work (from Buss, 1989).

The aim of an induction programme is to:

- give a new staff member a firm grip of their new job;
- inculcate a sense that each member of staff is a significant part of a vital service; and
- obtain clear information on the administrative practices of the organisation.

Putting it into practice

Practical induction should start with a combination of Maureen Lipman's "How was it for you?" and Rudyard Kipling's "Six honest serving men"

> They taught me all they knew
> Their names were What and Why and When,
> and How and Where and Who

The manager's first task is to ask himself or herself what joining that particular organisation felt like. Who told him how the computer operated? Did anyone tell her that the team went to the "Rose and Crown" at Thursday lunchtimes. The informal "rules" are as important as the formal ones.

Why and who? We know why, and the "who" devolves very much on the line manager who should be the fulcrum whereby selection moves on to induction, supervision and staff development.

The line manager may, however, wish to involve others with specialised knowledge in the process where appropriate, for example, the personnel officer, the person responsible for health and safety on site, the training manager, the computer systems staff, and the finance officer.

When and how The manager will need to assess how much staff need to know at any one time and how much they can absorb. For preference new employees should have a copy of their induction programme before they report for work on the first day, and a clear idea where to go, what time to arrive and who will greet them.

If the staff member is part of an establishment team, then a practical format should be drawn up along the lines of that used by Merton's Employment Assessment Centre in Wimbledon (see also chapter 22). To become aware of the wider service in which they operate the new staff should meet with staff from other teams within the specialism; and other useful people, for example, county hall staff or consumer and voluntary groups. They should understand the divisional and departmental philosophy, and understand the organisation in which they operate, and meet the bosses' boss.

The service manager will want to agree with his or her unit heads that certain specific items will be covered, and check with unit managers this is being carried out. He or she should also talk with individuals when visiting establishments and teams to ensure induction is working in practice, and that staff feel orientated within the service.

It is enlightening to invite a small group of people from each unit in for beer and sandwiches at about three to six months after they had arrived in post, to share experiences and remedy omissions.

Induction should be part of a systematic plan; clearly set down in writing; recorded at each stage as completed; constantly monitored; and an integral part of the selection, supervision and staff development process.

What As unit teams get smaller, as hostel care moves into dispersed housing schemes, social education centres move toward neighbourhood day activity programmes, and fieldworkers move into locality teams, there is a need to bring this dispersed group of staff together for an induction day which gives them a sense of being part of the whole organisation.

The Industrial Society proposes that there are five main categories of information which should be given to new employees:

Organisation information. This should include information about the organisation, including size, history and details of the wider organisation. It is important that new employees know exactly who it is that they are working for.

Procedural information. This comprises information concerning organisational procedures which affect all members of staff. The information provided should include:

- ☐ Terms and conditions of employment.
- ☐ Disciplinary and grievance procedures.
- ☐ Fire and Health & Safety procedures.
- ☐ Standards or codes of dress or conduct.
- ☐ Rules on entering and leaving the premises.

Job information. This relates to what is necessary for a new employee to know in order to do a job effectively. The information provided should include:

- ☐ A job description detailing the major tasks and accountabilities of the job.
- ☐ Details of any training which is involved.
- ☐ Procedures for obtaining equipment, etc.
- ☐ A copy of relevant sections of an organisation chart, as it is important to inform recruits of not only what they have to do, but also why it is important and how it fits into the department and organisation.

Personal information. This is the area which affects a new employee's private life and personal needs, for example, how salaries are paid, where to eat, the location of the toilet facilities, and sporting and social opportunities. Everybody has anxieties on starting a new job and having to ask about these fundamentals only adds extra stress.

Team information. Team information provides knowledge of all those things which will encourage employees to integrate into the working group. This category needs to cover the informal, as well as formal aspects of working life, for example, "the fact that we all go for a pint at lunchtime on Fridays", can be more important to this process than knowing who the shop steward is (Watts-Davies, 1973).

Managers should think about making up an induction pack, like the one that goes with the Employment Assessment Centre programme.

At the end of the induction process, the individual staff member should have started the process which results in the committed workforce. The individual will be informed, involved, beginning to share in the success of the organisation and with a sense of belonging.

J. Adair (1988), *The Action-Centred Leader,* The Industrial Society, Chapter 8.
J. Adair (1988), *The Effective Supervisor,* The Industrial Society, Chapter 5.
P. Allen *et al* (1988), *Staff in the Mental Handicap Services: A Study of Change,* UKC.
Association of Directors of Social Services (1989), *Survey of Social Services Employment,* LACSAB.
C. Buss (May 1989), *Induction and Staff Development of Secretarial Staff,* unpublished project.
Cary L. Cooper and P. Makin (1984), *Psychology for Managers,* Macmillan, Chapters 10 & 11.
K. Edwards, "Assessing the psychometric factor", *Insight,* 30 August 1989.
A. Fowler (1988), *Human Resource Management in Local Government,* Longman, Chapter 4.
D. Hancox (1981), *The Supervisor's Pocket Guide,* The Industrial Society.
Open University, *Effective Manager Course,* Books 4 and 6.
T. Philpot (1989), *The Residential Opportunity? The Wagner Report and After, Community Care,* Chapters 9-15.
D. Roach, "Employment and recruitment of black staff", *Community Care,* 4 May 1989.
Dorothy M. Stewart (1987), *Handbook of Management Skills,* Gower, Part II.
P. Thorne (1989), *The New General Manager,* McGraw-Hill, Chapter 7.
R. Watts-Davies (1973 - Third Edition 1989), *Induction,* The Industrial Society.
C. Wright (1973), *Selection Interviewing,* The Industrial Society.
Codes of Practice by the Commission for Racial Equality and the Equal Opportunities Commission.

VIDEO

More than a Gut Feeling (1987), Melrose Film Productions (describes behavioural interviewing).

12

Women do it differently
Alexis Waitman

"Of course, when we are elected or promoted to leadership, we lead as victims of the conditioning. We set up our organisations to be aggressive rather than problem-solving, as competitive rather than co-operative, as task-and-achievement-orientated rather than having concern to improve how things are done. We tend to have a central concern with control rather than with enabling and empowering people to think for themselves."
Michael Simmons (1986)

In the 1990s "it will be considered legitimate for women to be different. This will affect women's behaviour in terms of the pride and dignity of feminine values and standpoints."
The Henley Centre for Management Studies

First lady Has he got over his divorce?
Second lady I think so. His wife got custody of the stereo and they sold the children.
First lady And do you ever see your daughter-in-law?
Second lady I do, funnily enough - she's our window cleaner.
First lady That's women's lib for you.
Second lady No, she's under a man. He's the skilled half, she just dunks the chammy. Anyway what about you?
First lady Oh me? Same as ever.
Second lady Still on that diet?
First lady Still on my diet, still married to Ken, and still General Secretary of the United Nations.
Second lady No gossip then.
First lady No . . .
Victoria Wood, *Barmy* (1987)

The quotation above from Michael Simmons will serve to reinforce the underlying messages in this chapter, whose premise is that, unless women and men can find a way to redress the imbalance of power that exists in our organisations and institutions, not only economic life, but social, cultural and personal life, are doomed.

Organisational culture and values are predicated on the behaviour, philosophical standpoint and value systems of those who find themselves in key leadership positions. Despite the acknowledged, considerable, and increasing growth of women managers and senior executives, their advancement to the most enviable, prestigious positions is, to understate, not happening at an impressive rate of growth.

So long as we have a leadership that is predominantly male, and of the traditional conditioning patterns outlined by Simmons, where boys are reinforced for being strong, brave, manly and distanced from their feelings, and men are epitomies of endurance, discipline and warrior-like qualities, it is unlikely that any significant changes will occur. It is also unlikely that women, whose conditioning is of a different order, will feel comfortable in such a culture, and so will choose for the most part, to remain outside it. This will pose a dilemma for organisations over the next five years — a critical period in organisational terms — since, demographically, women are likely to return to the workforce in great numbers, offering an array of skills and knowledge. To suppress this talent at point of entry, by preventing its rise through male-dominated (and created) hierarchies, because of patriarchal attitudes that are not conducive to free thinking and creativity, is nothing short of criminal.

Women have not only been raised in a different tradition to men - they have also been subjected to a different conditioning which has freed us to be able, in adult life and, therefore as managers, to choose to operate to a different set of priorities. That's not to say that the conditioning has been a wonderfully positive experience: it hasn't. But in the struggle for freedom from our own oppression which tends to make us passive and subservient, we learn to establish and believe in our own strengths *and in each other.* It is in this latter expression of emotional value, that perhaps our greatest strength lies. And that is the one that can be perceived as threatening.

Not only are we sexual and sensual beings, increasingly aware of our own powerfulness and therefore increasingly able to cope with workplace harassment, but we are also laying claim to those things that are also ours by right, like training and preparation for advancement, and personal action plans which include a developmental component pointing the way towards a constructive career. But it is not only that. It is also the wherewithal to enable us to act on our desires. Even the government now sees the wisdom in loosening restrictions on workplace nurseries - a small step but not one that will help the thousands of women (and men) who need nursery places located safely in their communities and offering high quality at low prices. If women's needs are different - and we are arguing that they are - then different means of meeting them must also be available. And our needs go far, far beyond the provision of crêches for our children. That is an expectation, not a gift.

Latterly, or at least since the 60s and its highly overt resurgence, the women's movement has, like women themselves, learned to opt for disguise or to become invisible when this seems appropriate for confirmation or safety. Women have learned how, and found the confidence, to make greater demands, in greater numbers. By joining unions (and what a battle that was - male bastions of political intrigue and power that they were), by forming groups, by talking, training and working together, women have pushed through some of the barriers to success in the "real world", the world that is immediately accepted as being valuable. But the power is still vested within the confines of the minority group; women now comprise in total, in excess of 52 per cent of the total workforce in SSDS, yet still we hold only 25 per cent of management jobs and only 14 per cent of top management jobs. Assuming that no-one actually believes in phrenology any longer (or will openly admit to it!) this has, by definition, to be a socially constructed phenomenon.

Where we are now

This short chapter is about the *perception* of these differences. It is about the life-scripts that women are given, and which we learn, like our multiplication tables and French verbs, by heart. We do a lot of things by heart - and our rewards are often felt elsewhere. This chapter seeks to redress the unreal balance, to restore equilibrium by restating the rules; and by offering a model for the reconstruction of the way in which women enter the workforce and the paths that are open to them as they pass through. We want to offer a way of getting there without giving in. This is not to acquiesce in the male dominance that insists on autocratic rule; or conformity to a set of rules that completely impugn our integrity; or passive acceptance of a management style that represents everything we want to change. We are the change mistresses - no longer the mistresses of men. We are our own people and we want to invite you all to do it differently, too, because together, we can create a force for change so positively powerful that it will be irresistible.

Men who are threatened tend to be self-seeking and competitive and feel safe only if they select other men who are like themselves. It is our contention, however, that these false "leadership skills" are totally inappropriate to meet the demands that will be placed on organisations during the next 10 years.

Simmons suggests that our society is anti-male in its conditioning approach and cites the male as beast, warrior, and uncontrollable entity, aspects that render men "less than human" which then leaves them open to the abuses of "exploitation and expendability". This, he asserts, is not only men's conditioning, it is men's oppression.

As the opening quotation from Simmons suggests, this is all a self-fulfilling cycle of deprivation, humiliation and, ultimately, defeat. Or is it? Could it not also be said that this very "oppression" also allows men to continue to be reinforced for being arrogant, abrasive, aggressive and autocratic: the big four A's of traditional male management practice?

But who does this to men? Without entering into a deeply psychoanalytical discourse around the Oedipal and preoedipal years, it does seem reasonable to suggest that men are not, in any systematic, institutionalised way, oppressed by women. Men tend to be their own oppressors. They "nurture" each other. Grit breeds grit.

By the same argument, and taking patriarchy as the cornerstone of oppression, it seems fairly clear that women's oppression has been, and, to a lesser extent, still is the direct result of a patriarchal ideology that has held political and economic force since the beginning of the Industrial Revolution.

Women's oppression is based on a model of domesticity, rather than the male one based on aggression and the notion of expendability (the warrior syndrome). Constantly and consistently forced into the role of mother, carer, domestic servant and nurturer, a woman learns where her rewards lie. The moment she begins to think about encroaching onto male territory, she faces abuse, harassment, impediment and tribulation. Every entry point to the world of work, at whatever level, is strewn with hoops to jump or walls to climb. Whether typing-pool (or word-processing room), lecture hall, shop-floor or print-room, she must deal with the bastions of male power that will surely greet her. From recruitment ("Girl Friday wanted") to interview (gender-specific psychometric tests and all male interview panels), she is dealt the blows of maleness. If she retaliates, she is aggressive; if she responds, she is over-assertive; if she caves in under the constant barrage, she is hysterical and weak; if she stares back, she is insolent. And, the most unfair one of all, if she dares to look good, cross her legs, or exude confidence, she is "anyone's". Unfair? Exaggerated? Spiteful? Feminist clap-trap? Whatever might be thrown at such a list, it is difficult to refute. So long as men are taught not to cry, not to allow their emotions to inform who they are and how they feel, women (and some men) will find it difficult, if not impossible, to trust or confide in them.

This analogy created by a psychiatrist colleague, neatly expresses our feelings: imagine an ordinary domestic toaster - see the thermostat turned right up so that the toast comes out blackened and inedible. That is one extreme of the organisational cultural overload on maleness: hot, angry, aggressive, sweaty, unapproachable and uncaring. At the other end, there is the "low" section: pale, thin, colourless, crisp, unwieldy and snappy toast comes out, not very appetising and certainly not efficient. Now, put the dial in the middle, and somehow the emotional and environmental rheostat will facilitate a perfect piece of toast: brown, warm, right thickness, right texture, perfect for buttering and eating.

That is what could happen - an amalgam of power, male and female, strong and calm, warm and caring, working together to provide an environment conducive to creativity and development both for individuals and the organisation.

Women are socialised and conditioned to be men's help-mates. We go from being "Daddy's girl" to being somebody's "other half" or "the wife", always defined in terms of someone else. At work we are "Mr Brown's secretary" or "that girl with the legs" or, if we are very lucky, "the MD's PA". Women are no longer satisfied with being an extension of a male person's ego. Imagine it the other way round.

I want to focus on looking at ways in which the model of competitiveness and self-seekingness - which promotes stress and management burn-out - can be converted into a model that is gender neutral and enhances people as well as the organisation. No magic, nor mirrors, not even a witch's broomstick - just a simple model of empowerment. Yes, it is a much-abused word, especially in the post-Griffiths, public sector world, where everyone from cooks to consumers are about to be "empowered". However, we are going to stick our female necks out and suggest, firmly and in the safe knowledge that there is sound evidence to back our statement (Handy, 1985, Kanter, 1985, Peters, 1988), that there is a great deal of ground to be made up: women's position in the workforce, although around 52 per cent in number, is insignificant in terms of *power*.

What can be done

Women are different. Everyone knows that, but if that is so, why is most organisational culture so hostile to women? How is it that we are, at work, as in most other settings generally, not appreciated *because* we are different. Rather, we are reviled for not being the same - not being "as good". The epitome, to many men, of a "powerful woman", is an Eastern European athlete on a diet of growth-inducing steroids. Power, to a man, is manifested in strength and external competencies. Rugger-playing, cigar-smoking, jet-setting, club-going "chaps" are OK. Women are not really "chaps" and present difficulties like needing special loos and time off in the school holidays. Why are men, at work, so insecure? Are they truly caught on the petard of their own inadequacies?

Women entering the world of work *know* they are in for a rough ride. For many, the wrench from home to work is almost unbearable, especially after childbirth. For many women returners the concept of 'letting go' is both a necessity and a painful aspect of economic life. Yet, like other painful experiences it can also assist development and growth for everyone concerned.

Heider (1985) offers this offering of Taoist philosophy: "When I let go of what I am, I become what I might be. When I let go of what I have, I receive what I need."

These are feminine paradoxes: by yielding, I endure; the empty space is filled; when I give of myself, I become more; when I feel most destroyed, I am about to grow; when I desire nothing, a great deal comes to me.

Women often feel pressured not only to do well, but "to do better than", to push themselves beyond all reasonable expectations or standards of acceptability. Trying too hard can produce unexpected results:

- ☐ the "flashy" leader lacks stability;
- ☐ trying to rush things gets you nowhere;
- ☐ trying to appear brilliant is not enlightened;
- ☐ insecure leaders try to promote themselves;
- ☐ impotent leaders capitalise on their position;
- ☐ it is not very holy to point out how holy you are.

All these behaviours stem from and feed into, insecurity. None of them helps the work and none contributes to the leader's health. The leader who knows and understands how things happen has no need for such behaviour.

Autocratic leadership, whether perpetrated by women or men is, ultimately, debilitating to both people and organisations. It is one of the games managers play. But isn't sharing better than competitiveness in decision-making? Isn't influencing better than manipulation? The risk involved is in the potential giving up of (some) power. By giving some away, the empowerment of others' process begins.

Women enter the workforce with many management skills already available - running a home (sometimes two); a family, an executive partner and a social existence is no mean feat - although there are those who would argue women are well able to think about a dozen things at once - and well. We do it all the time! We can think on our feet, see out of the backs of our heads (a particularly useful skill when knives are out), and we are good with our hands. We have these scripts for working life firmly in place. Those that we need to acquire are learning to say "no", firmly but politely (this has a double meaning: "no" to sexual harassment, assertively; "no" to yet another dumped, not delegated, task; "no" to the date/invitation/compliment not wanted.)

Organisations need balance, homeostatis, for energy and efficiency. Women are good at maintaining balance - we have had so much practice at being in the middle, at holding things together.

Men are often isolated at the top. The participation of women could facilitate a series of changes that release such powerful energy within people and organisations. We have natural vitality and people skills. We do not allow the home/work split to get in the way of efficient practice for we develop a style that encompasses all our needs - that is how we cope. Male management skills have traditionally been those that are accepted, expected, rewarded. They differ from women's styles, which are based on empowerment and enabling, the nurturing of domestic life converted into organisational material.

There are two groups of skills. The (male) management skills are accepted, expected and rewarded. The domestic (management) female skills are expected, negated and rejected.

By balancing out the value in each, and encouraging a combination of these skills in the workplace, a sense of organisational homeostatis can be engendered. In this way, women gain by "getting there" without giving in to the power-relations of the dominant (male) model and men gain by enjoying the assimilation of women's skills, gentleness, and by validating their differences. There *is* another way. Unless we find and use it, the present debilitating climate will continue, and then we shall all be losers. Men and women must work together to lay foundations for a model of management that facilitates and welcomes an approach that empowers people.

For women's part, now is the time when we need to think in earnest about acquiring two more essential, yet specifically gender-neutral organisational skills. As defined by Marilyn Davidson (1985) these are "political nous" and "the visibility factor".

The first one - political nous - is politics with a small "p", yet it can make the difference between aiming for the top or hovering, wraith-like, in the middle ground. However, this latter is neither a comfortable, nor an impressive place to be, especially if *not* from choice. Being a middle-manager involves a great deal of skill and judgement: it is also the position that creates the essential tension caused by being pulled from below and pushed from above.

For many people, especially women who have become firmly socialised into, and reinforced for being in, subordinate, lower-paid positions, there is not only a crisis of confidence about 'moving-on', there is also a conflict between the head and the feelings about "letting-go". This may mean relinquishing practice for a professional teacher, social worker or nurse; it may mean changing the focus of work to a new, more challenging area; it may mean entering a more traditionally male-dominated environment. Whichever of these is true, it is important to acknowledge the feelings and, in some way appropriate to the person and to the situation, mourn the loss before moving on to celebrate the change. The more people become able to behave in these ways - to celebrate and validate the emotional component

Summing up

The intention has been to motivate, for the next five years will bring many changes and many rewards for women's patience and tolerance, for that is what we have shown. Now the time is come for action. Legislation is creating possibilities. Demography is on our side. Economic imperatives are beckoning (if not pleading) and organisations are struggling to convince themselves of our value right through the structure for the first time ever. What a combination of factors for empowerment. Michael Simmons (1986) was right when he stated that "we must develop a new leadership for men and we have to develop a new management development that will develop those leaders". Men in management must themselves begin the process of examining their conditioning and assumptions if they are to assist other men to change.

Barbara Tuchman (1984) wrote that "three outstanding attitudes - obliviousness to the growing dissatisfaction of constituents, primacy of self-aggrandizement, (and the) illusion of invulnerable status - are persistent aspects of folly." Women do it differently.

M. Davidson (1985), *Reach for the Top,* Piatkus.
C. B. Handy (1985), *Understanding Organisations,* Penguin.
J. Heider (1985), *The Tao of Leadership,* Wildwood House.
N. Josefowitz (1980), *Paths to Power,* Columbus.
R. Kanter (1985), *The Change Masters,* Counterpoint.
J. Laborde (1987), *Influencing with Integrity,* Syntony.
M. Loden (1986), *Feminine Leadership - How not to be one of the Boys,* Times Books.
T. Peters and R. Waterman (1986), *In Search of Excellence,* Harper Row.
T. Peters (1988), *Thriving on Chaos,* Pan.
H. M. Rosin, "Consequences for men of dual career marriages: Implications for organisations", *Jnl. of Managerial Psychology,* Vol.5.No.1, 1990.
M. Simmons, "Undoing men's gender conditioning", ICT, Nov/Dec 1986.
B. Tuchman (1984), *The March of Folly: From Try to Vietnam,* Alfred A. Knopf.

The author expresses her thanks to Kath Johnson in the preparation of this chapter.

13

Finance
David Claridge

"The devolving of budgets to front-line managers increases accountability but decreases flexibility."
A local government finance officer

"'Two added to one - if that could be done',
It said, 'with one's fingers and thumbs!'
Recollecting with tears how, in earlier years,
It had taken no pains with its sums."
Lewis Carroll, *The Hunting of the Snark*

"Most officers-in-charge have no idea how much money they are expected to spend, though they all know that if they spend too much 'someone will come down on them like a ton of bricksı'"
Paul Brearley, Social Services Inspectorate

Sources of funding

To support its services local government receives cash from a variety of sources. Broadly, these are:

- Revenue Support Grant from central government
- uniform business rate (set by central government)
- community charge (set and collected locally but which is to be abolished)
- income from charges (for example, for services provided)
- interest from balances (cash can also be taken from balances, but it is not likely to be a regular source of funding)
- specific grants (including joint finance, section 11 mental illness specific grant and so on)

The Department of the Environment decides each year on the level of expenditure for local government that will enable a standard level of service to be attained by each local authority. Standard spending assessments (SSAs) are calculated on a complex formula of indicators some of which are based on historical data and others on current information. On this basis the DoE can make assumptions about the overall level of expenditure that will be supported and the level of RSG that is allocated to each authority.

In practice there are often marked differences between the SSA for each authority and its actual budget. Often, spending is in excess of the SSA. Given that the DoE sets the level of the RSG and the uniform business rate, those authorities spending above

Figure 13.3.1: *Where the money comes from*

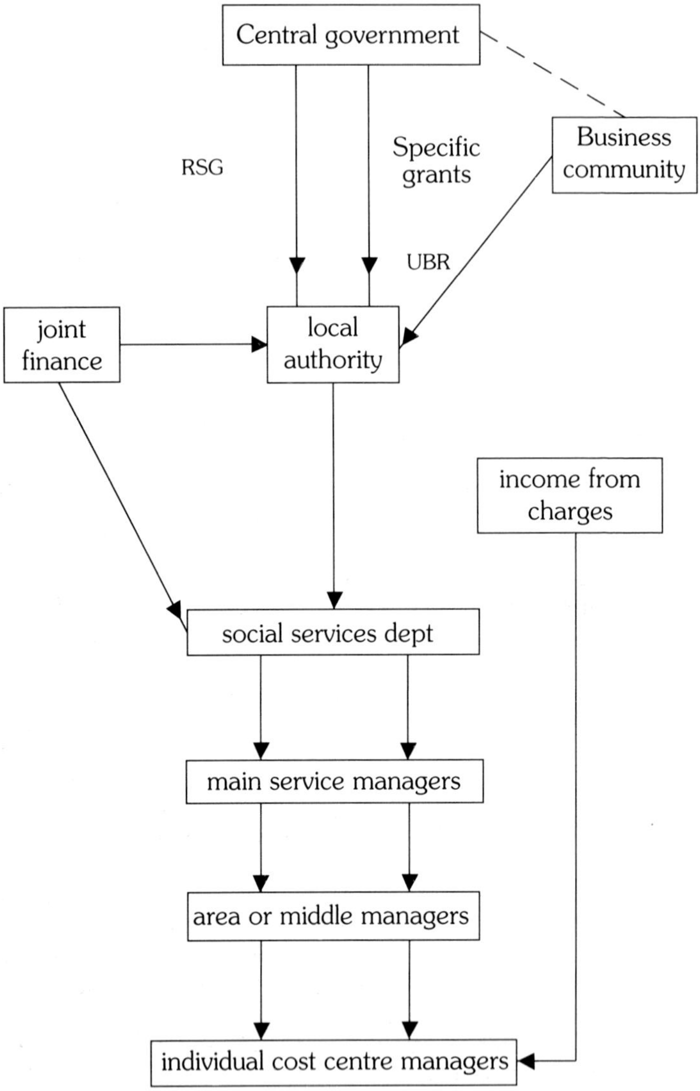

their SSA will have to raise any cash shortfall through the community charge, other income or by drawing from balances. In practice the community charge bears the brunt of funding such shortfalls.

The Secretary of State for the Environment has the power to cap the spending of any authority that is considered to have too high a level of community charge. Charge-capping has the effect of forcing an authority to reduce its budget. Almost inevitably capping means hastily conceived cuts in service.

The RSG is a non-specific grant and thus it is for each SSD to make its case locally for a share of the resources. The DoE also constructs SSAs for each SSD but in practice only a little of the information is used in the construction of the main SSA for each authority. SSD-level SSAs are based very substantially on historic data and it is unwise to use them in any local bid for additional resources. Equally, any cuts in budgets based on the fact that the SSD was spending above its SSA would be using a spurious assumption. It remains to be seen if the SSAs for SSDs will be used in the process of transferring Community Care funds.

Figure 13.3.1 shows the route by which cash flows from the various sources to the budget manager.

NHS and Community Care Act

The implementation of the legislation will not change the sources of funding already described. The main intention is that some of the funds currently used to support people in residential care will be transferred to local authorities over time. The sum to be transferred will be based on a prediction of the numbers of people that might otherwise have sought support from Social Security towards their residential care costs. Such cash will only relate to care costs. The RSG is to be used as the method for allocating the transferred cash. At the time of writing this chapter, there was no intention to separately identify the amounts added to the RSGs of each authority save for specific grants for training and mental health service developments.. It is therefore going to be very difficult to validate the additional amount derived from the transfer of social security funds that is actually received at a local level let alone by each SSD.

It is also intended to change the rules relating to Housing Benefit for those people who are placed in residential care after April 1991. In future, it appears likely that those people in private or voluntary registered homes who are eligible for support towards their costs will receive it from up to three sources. Income Support will meet food, clothing and other personal costs, Housing Benefit will cover accommodation and the SSD will meet the costs of care. The new arrangment will be similar to those that have existed for people admitted to hostels since October 1989, although DSS rule changes in 1990 altered this situation.

Joint finance, which is to be reviewed, is money made available through local health authorities. The intention is that it facilitates the development of new services that will reduce pressure or demand for health services, sometimes where a health authority has been providing social care and wants to withdraw from it.

The funding can only be applied to schemes which are agreed jointly by the respective local health authorities and SSDs. Funding can be used for either capital or revenue schemes. Revenue schemes are generally supported for seven years (three years 100 per cent and four years tapering) although provision exists for 10 year 100 per cent schemes directed at discharging people from long-stay hospitals. Until the future of joint finance is determined, authorities may not wish to commit themselves to large long term projects.

Finally, community care brings with it the concept of care management. This concept will inevitably mean a further devolution of budget accountability and management. In the past few years we have seen the role of service managers at first line level encompass budget responsibility for their respective service units (cost centres). To this group will be added the role of purchasing services (whether from an internal or external service provider sometimes known as a contractor) for clients. This implies a new budget manager who will not be responsible for the provision of specific services but instead for purchasing them to meet the assessed needs of clients. New, more sophisticated, budgetary and financial information systems will be required to make the care management job feasible.

The budget manager's perspective

For budget managers to exercise effective control over their budget they must be able to:

- ☐ identify clearly those items for which they alone are responsible (for example, staff, running costs and so on
- ☐ confirm that the budget is adequately funded to meet the agreed, or intended level of service
- ☐ receive regular reports on the monthly expenditure being incurred against their budget
- ☐ maintain a commitment system for items they have agreed but not yet showing on their budget
- ☐ receive regularly non-financial information that will assist in interpreting the budgets performance (for example, occupancy levels and staff vacancy rates)
- ☐ determine easily the extent to which they can act autonomously (that is, rely on clear ground rules which will establish what he or she can or can't do)
- ☐ have a clear understanding of the key points in time when bids for cash can be made and the overall budget is reviewed
- ☐ participate in the annual review of their own budget.

As devolved budget responsibility is increasingly being introduced the trend is towards cost centre-based budgets. This approach enables separate budgets for individual staff teams or units of accommodation to be developed. It is not uncommon for an SSD to have several hundred different cost centres to enable budget managers to be made clearly accountable.

Even the more modern financial information systems (FIS) are not particularly user friendly, having been developed primarily for the accounts within the organisation. The trick is not to be put off by this. Also, do not assume that the finance officer for your organisation is not interested in helping the budget manager get to grips with their budget. Finance officers are just as concerned about good budgetary control at individual cost centre level as they are with the overall budget. In most cases you will find a helping hand rather than a stumbling block.

It is important for the budget manager to understand how the FIS works and ensure that maximum use of any facilities are made. These are some of the questions that should be asked of centrally based finance staff of the organisation:

- Is it possible to divide the budget in a way that will more accurately reflect the pattern of spending? Unless profiled, most systems divide the budget into 12 equal parts.
- What price base has been used and will any inflation allowance be automatically added during the year?
- Is the budget cash limited? (Does it already include an inflation allowance to cover the whole year?)
- What level of virement is permitted? Virement is the ability to transfer money from one (underspent) budget to another (sometimes overspent) one.
- Can budget variances be turned into percentage to assist in scaling the significance of the under or over spend?
- How are budget queries dealt with (for example, apparent overspends researched and budget miscodings corrected?)

The next step is for the budget manager to systematically review the budget. Budgets can be a reflection of the pattern of consumption rather than the level of service ostensibly available. For example, residential accommodation which has had low occupancy over a long period may have inadequate provisions budgets if say, high occupancy is suddenly attained for a consistent period.

There may also have been a failure to adjust all budgets when changes in service level were agreed. Car allowances are quite often overlooked when additional staff are funded. The priority should be to focus on staffing costs, moving on to the other headings when this has been completed. The review should be completed as soon as possible in the financial year and ideally before the Autumn when there is usually a corporate budget review.

There can be a great degree of satisfaction from exercising control over a well-managed budget. This can only be achieved however, by the acquisition of knowledge about how the FIS works and from confidence in the fact that the base budget is accurate.

These processes should also help to identify the weaknesses of the FIS. For instance, many systems do not have adequate facilities for monitoring commitments. This can be overcome, but may require a degree of sophistication. For small items such as furniture for a unit a simple manual system will do. But for others such as private and voluntary residential placements a micro computer-based system may be the only answer. Such a system holding named individuals should be able to tell the budget manager at any time how much of the budget is committed. It should also be able to project the full year effect of new placements taken on part way through the year. It can also keep track of the inflationary increases, thus helping to justify what might otherwise appear an abnormally high level of increase. Such systems, when fully developed, can be more value than the information derived from FIS, but should never be regarded as a substitute for it.

There is a further level of budgetary review that can be undertaken. This is more about service audit than individual budget headings and their accuracy. The work of the Audit Commission has, in recent years, done much to assist managers in the self audit of services. The concept of value for money has become a byword and is a major part of the thrust behind *Caring for People.* Value for money reviews are essentially about the economy, efficiency and effectiveness of service delivery. *Effectiveness* means providing the right services to enable policies or objectives to be implemented. *Efficiency* means providing a specified volume and quality of service with the lowest level of resources capable of meeting that specification. *Economy* means ensuring that the services are procured at the lowest possible cost consistent with a specified quantity and quality. Professor John Stewart of the Institute of Local Government Studies, Birmingham University, has always argued that there are four Es. He adds *Equity* to the list: whether the available resources have been distributed fairly.

The three Es (or four Es) combine to form the basis of performance measurement or value for money. There are two distinct activities involved: monitoring and analysis. Monitoring is looking at what is done, requiring the regular and systematic collection of data. Workload levels or occupancy rates are just two simple examples. Ideally the measures should be quantitative, but this is not always possible. Analysis looks at how things are done. It involves asking the question: "would the service be better if it were provided in a different way"? Whilst monitoring should be a continuous activity, analysis is an occasional one.

The Audit Commission has undertaken a number of value for money reviews of aspects of the personal social services. These reviews are usually based on sample surveys of a representative group of SSDs. These national studies are used to emphasise areas of particular concern and are followed up at a local level by the

District Audit Service or, where appointed, external auditors. The last such review of services for people with learning difficulties was in 1989.

In essence the budget manager should be looking to ensure that resources are being deployed cost effectively. There should, for example, be an overall service objective or mission statement. This should provide a context for the objectives to be set for a specific service. For instance it is not enough to say that a hostel is there to provide residential care. It is necessary to clearly identify the purpose in order that performance can be measured. For instance, is the hostel long-stay provision or somewhere to acquire skills to enable people to live independently? Do the staffing levels and the physical resources meet the requirements that will enable the stated objectives to be met?

Unless these sort of questions can be answered easily and unit costs compared with others for similar units (both within and without the organisation) it will not be possible to audit the service. Remember, value for money is not about obtaining a service at the lowest possible price regardless of quality. That is cost efficiency. Value for money is about ensuring that the given level of quantity and quality with the desired outcomes are achieved for the lowest possible price.

In general five comparisons are made as part of performance review. These are:

- *Time* for example, last year's performance against this year's.
- *Standards,* comparing actual performance with a standard that might be locally or nationally derived.
- *Intra service,* which is comparing the performance of two or more different units within the organisation that provide the same service.
- *Private sector,* where possible comparing performance for the same services.
- *Inter-authority,* making comparisons with all other authorities; all authorities of the same type; specially selected authorities that have similar characteristics; and neighbouring authorities.

There are a number of sources of data that will assist in making comparisons. The Chartered Institute of Public Finance and Accounts produces considerable information on the personal social services based on both estimates and actual expenditure. These are helpful with unit costs. Annual returns to the DoH produced as "feedback documents" give levels of provision. More recently the Social Services Inspectorate has produced Key Indicators which combine the CIPFA information with feedback material making comparisons much easier. The main drawback is that often information is two to three years old before it is readily available as Key Indicators. The SSI is, however, attempting to shorten this time. Finally, the Audit Commission has done some work on grouping authorities with similar characteristics into families making it easier to make comparisons which have real relevance. Figure 13.3.2 is a diagram of performance review when considered as a process.

Figure 13.3.2: *Performance review — The process*

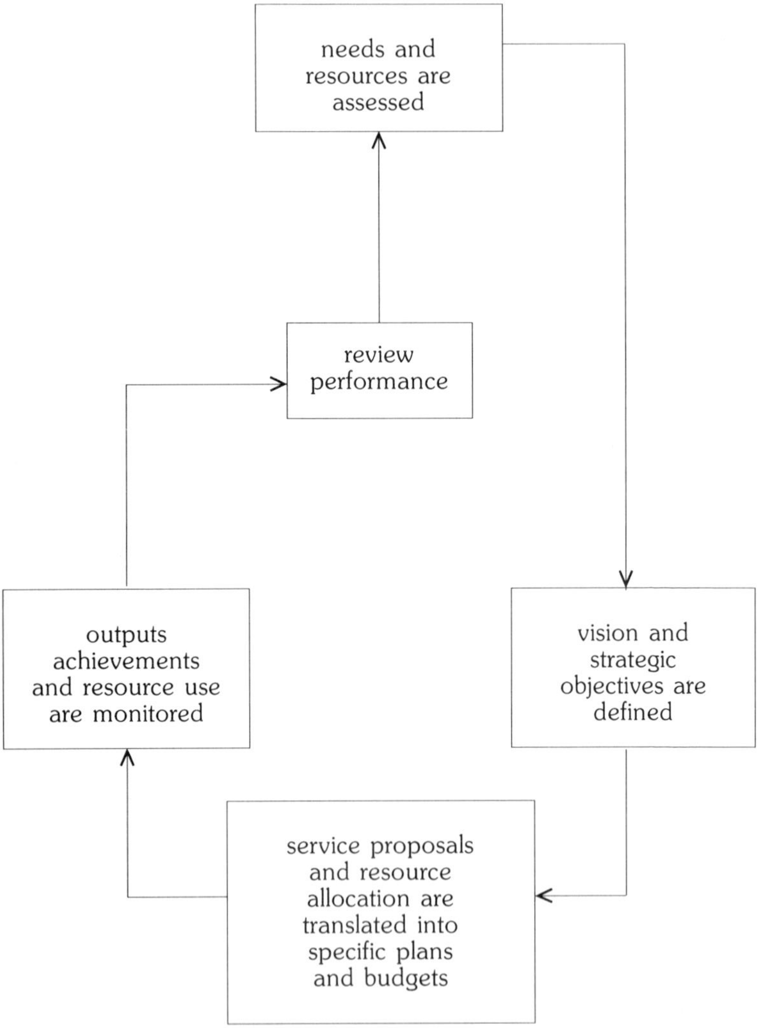

The problems related to performance review are threefold. First, effectiveness cannot always be measured in quantitative terms. Second, some information although quantifiable, may not be available because it has not been collected before. Third, there may be no single measure that can be looked at sensibly in isolation. Value for money is not a precise science. The results need careful interpretation. The benefits of careful, methodical work will be well worth the effort involved.

For many finance is often perceived as a mysterious process more often misunderstood than understood. Finance is at the heart of much of what managers do. Money has the ability to make things happen and budget managers in the 1990s will have a responsibility to make their budgets work for them in the most effective way possible. Given time and an enquiring approach every budget manager should be able to master the mystery of budget management.

Audit Commission (1986), *Making a Reality of Community Care,* HMSO.

Audit Commission (1986), *Performance Review in Local Government - A Handbook for Auditors and Local Authorities,* HMSO.

Audit Commission (1987), *Community Care: Developing Services for People with a Mental Handicap,* HMSO.

Audit Commission (1989), *Occasional Paper - Developing Community Care for Adults with a Mental Handicap,* HMSO.

J. Glynn (1985), *Public Sector Financial Control and Accounting,* Blackwell.

C. Miller, "Keeping track of the action", *Insight,* 10 January 1990.

C. Miller and N. Flynn, "Budgeting from the bottom up", *Insight,* 16 August 1989.

G. Mott (1987), *Management Accounting,* Pan Business.

D. Norman, "Taking up the gauntlet", *Insight,* 19 July 1989.

D. Rawlinson and B. Tanner (1989), *Financial Management in the 1990s,* Longman/Local Government Training Board.

W. Warburton, "Outlying principles", *Insight,* 5 July 1989.

P. Whiteley, "Stumbling block or helping hand?", *Insight,* 25 October 1989.

P. Whiteley, "Working to new formulas", *Insight,* 28 March 1990.

14

Managing change

"Change is not made without inconvenience, even from worse to better."
Richard Hooker (1554-1600)

Change is one of the forces competing for the manager's attention, and is a task which they are expected to fulfil while at the same time maintaining the day-to-day stability of the service. The strains imposed by this work can place considerable pressure on the manager, as services experience increasingly rapid cycles of change. Change can take the form of a large number of small adjustments, as well as overt and systematic attempts at improvement. These can be internally driven with staff striving to develop better services, or major organisational change that is externally imposed. Whichever form and scale change takes, the manager needs to understand the dynamics of the change process, in order that it is managed more effectively and has a greater rate of success in achieving the goals identified for the service.

In understanding the process of change it is helpful to put aside orthodox thinking about how change happens. This view assumes a consensus among staff in terms of values and interests. The manager's task is seen to be one of clarifying purposes and goals, and then discovering ways of achieving them, monitoring performance and providing staff with appropriate skills and training. The management of change can then be carried out vigorously, since values and interests are not in serious dispute. With a hierarchical structure and authority relatively unquestioned the management of change can proceed smoothly. This view tends to be over-optimistic about what can be achieved by management power and authority in initiating and managing change.

Reality can be very different! In our work with numerous organisations which are introducing change and innovation, it is clear that in spite of considerable initial investment in the formulation and implementation of plans for change, that services often continue more or less as before. Many services do not develop to anything like the extent originally envisaged by those managers initiating change, or where change is imposed considerable staff resistance can be experienced, with staff seeing new ideas foisted on them by insensitive management, with potentially damaging consequences for those individuals involved.

Problems of introducing change

What are the reasons for the difficulties in bringing about change in services? A brief scenario loosely based on similar examples which we have met quite often will help illustrate some of the issues more clearly.

Jane has recently been appointed manager of a day service, and wants to introduce changes in the way the centre operates. She would like to see activities developed that are more relevant to the needs of users. This would mean changing the long-established programme that is organised around contract work, social skills training and recreational activities, and encouraging staff to design more relevant activities, based on the individual needs of service users. This would increasingly take place in the community as part of the process of building a range of diversified community-based activities. Jane consulted with colleagues, and held a meeting of all staff and outlined how she saw the service changing, and gave a suggested timetable for action.

Some months later, in spite of further meetings and discussion about how the changes would be beneficial to the users, little had happened. A handful of staff have shown a commitment to change, but the majority seemed unconvinced and described numerous reasons why the changes would not work, and how it would be detrimental to the service users by exposing them to increased risks, and failure in more demanding social situations.

If we now analyse this brief snapshot of the manager's attempt to initiate change, why did most staff show little interest in what appeared to be a positive development that would benefit service users? To understand this question we have to recognise the central role of resistance to change. Plant (1987) has described how resistance to change can take many forms, and is usually a complex mix of traditional, factual and emotional issues. The following list is some of the most frequent examples that will be familiar to staff working in services for people with learning difficulties:

- fear of the future
- lack of information
- historical factors
- threat to core skills and competence
- threat to status
- threat to power base
- no perceived benefits
- organisational climate of low trust
- poor relationships
- fear of failure
- reluctant to experiment
- custom bound
- strong peer group norms

Just listing the possible causes of resistance to change can help the manager begin to identify why staff may be unwilling to respond positively to the benefits of service change. Some issues such as low trust among staff may require considerable long-term work rather than concern about specific skill deficits. Plant identifies two main forms of resistance to change. First, systemic - which arises from lack of appropriate knowledge, information, skills and managerial capacity, and secondly, behavioural - which is derived from reactions, perceptions and assumptions of individuals and groups in the organisation. One being cognitive and the other emotional. Recognising the different forms of resistance can enable the manager to identify those forms that will be easier to correct and minimise than others.

Identifying resistance means the manager can use the above approach to increase the potential for successful change. For example, the manager in our scenario might have overcome some of the problems associated with systemic resistance, through the provision of more information and a better communications flow about some of the key issues, during the uncertainty of the change process. Similarly, resistance based on a historical perception of users could be approached by staff training. Staff could re-examine their views through case examples of change, which demonstrate the achievements of people with learning difficulties to both cope effectively in situations of "ordinary life", and increase their range of skills and achievements.

Of course, it is important not to overstate the resistance to change. Some staff will welcome change, and see opportunities that will encourage them to support new initiatives. Resistance to change is more likely to be a response to the method of introducing change, rather than the change itself. Many staff we speak to would welcome change in their services. Where change is resisted, it is likely to be seen as "change for change's sake", or where change is imposed without prior consultation.

Preparing for change

In preparing staff for change in services, the following steps adapted from Torrington *et al* (1989) offer one approach to managing the process sensitively:

Establishing the need for change

It is first essential to establish a felt need for change in all those staff who will be affected by it. This could arise from a common understanding of the need for change in the service, or from a crisis, or because of an opportunity to make improvements. For example, staff in day services may need to be made aware of the changes taking place in residential services, that affect the lives of users, and requires a response from day services. This could mean recognising that users are increasingly unlikely to be willing to attend a centre that offers little in the way of activities that meet their aspirations for an ordinary life. At this early stage the manager needs to spend sufficient time creating the rationale for change, before developing an action plan for the implementation of the change.

What's in it for them?

If staff can see that the change with its new approaches, procedures and techniques will make their work easier, more interesting, and be fun, they are more likely to be enthusiastic. If they cannot see any benefits, they are likely to resist it; or may pay lip service to the ideas behind the change, but might not help to make it work, or even behave in such a way as to undermine it. For example, the development of community-based day activities could mean new roles in job finding, employment support, community education and recreation for staff outside of centres, who have previously had little autonomy and decision-making power.

Our experience has been that staff respond positively to these challenges, if consulted and given sufficient information and support, but we also recognise that some staff will be sceptical and need convincing that the proposed changes will benefit themselves and service users.

Have they had a say in the changes?

If staff feel they have helped in creating the ideas behind the change they are more likely to be committed to making it work. There needs to be genuine opportunity to participate in the creation, design and execution of a new programme, in order that a sense of ownership exists that reflects shared values and a shared professional identity. For example, the development by a social education centre of a shop in the local town making and selling high quality ceramics gave staff and users new opportunities. A member of staff with both pottery expertise and business skills, was given considerable discretion to establish the shop, within an agreed framework, including financial targets, staffing, user's role, and evaluation of the business.

Is it clear what change is envisaged?

In expecting staff to change, they need to have a clear vision of what the manager wants them to achieve. This vision needs to be practical, with a detailed explanation about why, what and if possible how, it is to be done. It needs to be explained in language that everyone involved understands. It is important that the manager avoids painting a confused picture because the change envisaged has not been fully thought through. An example of a clear programme of change was where the manager of a day service who wished to introduce individual plans for users, consulted with staff about the inadequacies of current assessment procedures, which they felt poorly served the needs of users. A workshop was organised for staff, which introduced them to the use of individual planning techniques, and through subsequent consultation staff were identified who were willing to undertake pilot projects using knowledge and skills gained in the workshop. Discussion took place each week at a staff meeting on the progress of the project and individual staff involved directly were supported through resources, encouragement and back-up by the deputy manager who was given the responsibility to lead the project.

Identifying factors that can influence change

In introducing change the manager needs to ask some key questions about those individuals and groups of staff who will need to be influenced and whose support will be needed if change is to take place, and be maintained over time.

Who will benefit and who will lose out?

Turning again to the example of the day service, some staff will see change benefiting them, through better job prospects, promotion, more interesting work or a realisation of their aspirations for users. Others will perceive the reverse, through loss of power and control as old jobs disappear or spheres of influence contract. Similarly, staff who have established what they believe is good practice, will not necessarily welcome comments that they have not been effective.

The manager needs to recognise the good things that happened previously in the service. Change should not be presented in a manner that suggests what had been undertaken previously was of no value, with the implied criticism of competence and practice. If staff see themselves losing out, then they may need extra support to enable them to understand the benefits that will come from change, and how these build on past achievements. This will probably need to focus particularly on beliefs and assumptions about the future direction of the service that may be inaccurate. Information communicated by the manager that corrects misunderstanding is vital, particularly if the staff who see themselves as losers contain opinion shapers, who are influential among colleagues.

Who has power?

Although the manager needs sufficient power to see the changes through, it is also important to identify those staff in the unit and the wider service whom the manager will be able to work with in the change process. The manager will need to develop their interests systematically, or identify the support of others who are opinion shapers. This is necessary so that individuals and interest groups do not attempt to veto proposals, because they suspect the validity of the change envisaged. Identifying staff who are influential through length of service, experience or personal qualities, and gaining their support can be crucial.

These activities may appear time-consuming and frustrating to the manager who is impatient to get on with introducing change. Nevertheless, they are critical to the ultimate success of planned change. They also suggest that the process of change is much more complex than many managers realise, and require a perspective that challenges the conventional viewpoint which assumes a consensus will exist among staff about the way services need to be developed. Rather this view sees change focussing around conflicting interests, bargaining and compromise. In other words the micro-political life of an organisation, which is likely to be stronger where organisations are loosely coupled, with staff having a high degree of autonomy, supported by professional norms which inhibit the exercise of authority by the manager. As a consequence the manager's control will depend to a considerable extent on the exercise of latent power and influence.

This view also challenges the notion of managerial authority, where staff may be willing to respond compliantly to the manager's exhortations. The manager is no longer totally in control of the change process, and can only influence it to a greater or lesser extent. The manager needs to understand the dynamics of change and the work needed to be done to support and convert sceptics if the desired changes are to be achieved. So instead of the manager initiating the change process in a well ordered and purposeful way, we see the manager engaging with staff who all have their own personal interests and needs which have to be recognised and considered when introducing change.

Using this approach we can see that the manager is just one of a number of participants, although a key figure as a result of authority conferred by position or personal characteristics, who can influence the outcomes by involving different participants, influencing the nature of their interest and bargaining with them. In order that the manager can achieve the change intended it will mean using management power, not to bulldoze through organisational and individual defences, but to work with participants in the change process, identifying individuals and issues that are pushing for or resisting change. This perspective implies that the manager needs to have a close understanding of the interests of staff who are likely to be affected by change, and to develop improvements to maximise gains and minimise losses. Consequently it is useful early in the change process to identify how staff perceive the changes affecting them.

service development.

National Vocational Qualifications

Although many staff working in care roles participate in in-service training as part of organisational and personal development, it remains largely true that the majority of care staff receive little training, and the largely female workforce is marginalised within the structure of the caring services. One writer estimates that there are over one million people working in care roles who have no formal qualifications (Bartlett, 1990). Certainly, compared with qualified staff and managers, front-line staff receive few training opportunities. Messenger (1990) states that this situation is the result of organisational attitudes that isolate and make invisible the work of care staff. The work is seen as domestic in nature which can be learned on the job as part of day-to-day practice. As there is no requirement for training once in post this assumes that the wide range of skills involved in social care can be performed without any particular preparation. Because staff are unable to obtain training as of right, the impact on the quality of care and the ability of staff to respond to complex situations is unrecognised and undervalued. The consequences are to put staff at risk of stress and burnout as they take on increasingly complex tasks without adequate support. Where training does exist it tends to be ad hoc, and does not lead to qualifications that staff can accumulate to influence their conditions of service, pay or career prospects. Anecdotal evidence suggests that the lack of a career development structure is one of the factors in the high staff turnover in services.

Part of the response to this problem is the introduction of the National Vocational Qualification (NVQ) on a national basis in spring 1991. The system will be employment-led, and based on a credit accumulation scheme, with four levels of NVQ. Staff will be assessed following training or as the result of prior experience, and will be awarded "units of competence" and accredited with an NVQ at an appropriate level. Some of the unique features of NVQ are:

- ☐ assessment will be work based.
- ☐ it will operate independently of any training needed.
- ☐ NVQs should be accessible to as many people as possible.
- ☐ it should be possible to gain an NVQ without formal training, and be able to demonstrate competence which has developed as a result of previous work or life experience.
- ☐ line managers will be expected to take on the assessment role.
- ☐ assessment will be by direct observation of practice, with the member of staff being assessed against a "performance criteria".
- ☐ once the person has carried out the practice consistently, they will be assessed as competent and that aspect of practice recorded.

NVQ will provide access to training for staff who have traditionally had little opportunity to train. It also offers care staff the opportunity to have their current skills recognised and to develop further skills that enable them to accumulate credits towards a vocational qualification.

But in spite of the prospects of providing training for a large number of previously untrained and marginalised staff, the advent of NVQ is not without its critics. A number of concerns have been expressed about this approach to training staff. These include:

- how realistic will it be to assess social care activities based on general functional analysis of tasks, which are too narrowly based to produce acceptable standards for social care.
- in an attempt to escape from course-based pathways to qualifications, no reference is made to the learning process, and knowledge is viewed as an additional extra dependent on the level of activity.
- the role of the manager is crucial in the NVQ system. Consequently managers will need to develop skills in assessment as part of their overall management function. To do this work effectively they will need considerable training in staff development and training functions. This is of particular concern considering the relatively poor level of management training for first-line managers in social care. They will also need more time within an already crowded schedule!
- significant costs can be anticipated as this system will be expensive in money and staff time. For example, costs will be incurred in developing the infrastructure to implement and manage the NVQ, the work-based assessors, as well as developing and providing the learning curriculum for staff who require skills development prior to assessment. There will also be the cost of registration with the National Council for Vocational Training for staff who wish to undertake NVQs.

Qualifying training

Staff who wish to train for a professional qualification in services for people with learning difficulties face the obstacle of segregated and specialist training that reflects the historical structure of services. Staff in the health services can train as Registered Nurses for the Mentally Handicapped (RNMH), while staff employed by social services departments, voluntary and private organisations usually complete the Certificate in Social Service (CSS).

Both these forms of training have their strengths and weaknesses, and attempts have been made to overcome their respective deficiencies in the joint training schemes that have been established (see Walton, (1989) for a detailed discussion of the joint ENB/CCETSW courses). But, just as a limited number of joint training schemes have got off the ground and have begun successfully to bring together the professions of nursing and social work, changes are beginning to take place in nurse education, with the development of Project 2000, which will eventually replace existing nurse training. Similarly, social work training is also changing, with the decision by the Central Council for Education and Training in Social Work to phase out the CSS, and replace it with the Diploma in Social Work (which will also combine the current Certificate of Qualification in Social Work). These new courses for nurses and social workers will continue to have considerable structural differences and this will create difficulties in the future where joint training is envisaged.

Nurse training continues to see itself playing a role in preparing staff to work in services for people with learning difficulties, with the development of "branch programmes" in the Project 2000 courses. But, with the continuing run down of long-stay hospitals, and the contraction of nursing roles, it is likely that prospective staff will no longer see this as relevant training, particularly with social services departments assuming lead responsibility for community services. Many staff will seek social work qualifications, as more relevant to their needs, and providing greater career choice in the future, but there is continuing concern at the low priority given to disability issues in social work education.

Although staff may wish to acquire a professional social work qualification, currently through the CSS route, this requires a post in one of the agencies that subscribes to a CSS scheme, with limited opportunities to train as a result of restrictions on places due to financial restrictions in employing agencies. This situation is unlikely to improve with the introduction of the DipSW, as this will be a full-time course, with considerably higher fees, although the "advanced status" of the course means it will be eligible for local educational authority mandatory grants. This should at least remove one of the current impediments to direct secondment as the only route to a CSS qualification. Concern has nevertheless been expressed that this new form of training will mean a reduction in staff able to pursue qualifying training due to the increased costs and agencies' inability to release staff for a full-time course.

One solution to the problems of separate training, has been suggested by the Independent Development Council (1988). This would be a single qualifying training, that would replace the separate training courses, based on social work and nursing. Although this course would be approved by CCETSW, it would have to meet certain requirements of the 1982 RNMH syllabus, in order to retain those specialist components found in nurse training. It is argued that this is the only logical way forward with local authorities, and voluntary and private agencies assuming the role of major service providers rather than the NHS. Although this idea has considerable attraction, its adoption would need to overcome the objections that would arise from the suggested demise of the RNMH, and increased funding would be necessary to make training based on a social work model available to all those who wish to train.

Post-qualifying training

The development of post-qualifying training has not been plagued with the difficulties that have surrounded qualifying training. At post-qualifying level a number of courses have been established that bring together staff from different settings who have learning needs in common. The English National Board for Nursing Midwifery and Health Visiting and CCETSW recognise that nurses and social workers have shared interests in developing advanced skills in practice, and have issued guidelines for the development of such courses (CCETSW/ENB, 1988).

CCETSW and ENB are jointly promoting three broad programmes of study:

- programmes which enable participants to develop skills and expertise in managing community services;
- programmes which provide the opportunity for participants to develop advanced practitioner skills in working directly with clients and their families;
- programmes which enable skills and practices used in teams to be developed.

Examples of courses approved by either the ENB or CCESTW are the ENB course 705, "Behaviour modification in mental handicap nursing", and the CCETSW course, "The certificate in disability studies". In addition to courses approved by CCETSW and ENB, a number of other educational and training organisations have established post-qualifying training programmes, including the University of Kent's MA in applied psychology of mental handicap services, which provides training for staff who are in leadership roles in services for people with learning difficulties.

In the future post-qualifying courses are increasingly likely to move towards a system of credit accumulation, with more flexible guidelines issued by the validating bodies, which recognises the large volume of in-service training currently available to staff, that can be credited towards national awards offered by CCETSW, ENB or the Council for National Academic Awards.

Finally, as in discussion about other forms of training, financial considerations in agencies mean that relatively few staff are likely to be released for extended periods of post-qualifying study. This in spite of the critical need to extend the skills of front-line staff with particular responsibilities, and develop the next generation of service leaders, who will be able to see beyond the horizons of current thinking and policy (CCETSW 1988).

How effective is staff training?

Although services are increasingly recognising the importance of training, questions should none the less be asked - is training effective, with changes in the behaviour of staff, who in turn are able to improve the lifestyle of the people they serve? Mittler (1985), asks "six awkward questions" about training, which are designed to question the touching faith some people have in the effectiveness of training:

- What evidence do we have that courses have any effects at all on the participants, on service settings, and, above all, on the users with whom they work?
- If staff learn new skills, do we know whether they can use them in their own settings?
- Even if they start to implement skills which they have learned, how long do they continue to do so?
- What do we know about the obstacles to implementation - in the individual, in management, in the organisation?
- How can the effectiveness of staff training be evaluated by the participant, by sponsors or employers, by those who design and deliver the training?
- In the light of the available information, what changes should be made in the nature of the training courses and in helping staff and organisations to make the most effective use of the resources put into them?

One of the traditional methods of examining the effectiveness is through evaluation of training by staff on the completion of a programme. Although these can provide trainers with valuable feedback on the usefulness of the content of a programme, and the knowledge and skills participants have developed, they do not answer the most important question - has training led to any changes in the service provided, and has this change made a significant impact upon the lifestyles of the people served? (Mansell *et al,* 1987).

Despite the lip-service paid to the vitally important task of training in helping staff to work effectively in services, training programmes are often unable to present any direct connection between training inputs and service outcomes. It has to be recognised that no matter how well designed a training course, it can suffer from the fundamental misconception that this activity by itself can have a significant impact on staff. As Cullen states in describing the impact of training in a long-stay hospital, "there is little point in trying to change the quality of life of those who live in an institution by focussing on only one aspect of the organisation. Too many components are inextricably linked together to make this a sensible approach" (quoted in Mittler, 1985).

This suggests that no matter how effective staff are in terms of personal skills, if the service does not provide the resources, then the training can be in vain. We have often witnessed staff developing a high level of skills in a training context, only to learn subsequently that those skills were not used for the benefit of the users, due to the misplaced optimism of the trainer that the service would recognise the contribution of the newly trained member of staff. This means that trainers need to be much more clear at the early stage of setting up programmes that skills developed will be supported in the service. They need to build in means of evaluating how much the training has been put into practice, through an explicit contractual link with the service employing staff who will participate in training.

The future direction of training

Whatever its future direction, the structure and processes of training are changing. A recent report of a working party representing the statutory, voluntary and private sectors of social care described the changes taking place in training (*Joint Initiative for Community Care/ADSS,* 1990). Whether at in-service, vocational, qualifying, or post-qualifying level, training will increasingly have many of the following features:

- ☐ *Modular,* with self-contained units of study, that can be taken in combination with other units of study, and accumulated to form a whole.
- ☐ *Employment led,* with employing organisations taking a lead in identifying training needs, and designing programmes individually or with training providers.
- ☐ *Work and learner centred,* with training designed specifically to meet the needs of individuals and organisations. Much of this taking place in the workplace.
- ☐ *Integrated into work,* with theory translated into practice in the work situation, with a likely shift to on-the-job training and coaching used, drawing on newly designed learning materials.
- ☐ *Outcomes based on assessment of competence,* with standards of ability and skills attained assessed in the work situation. Performance appraisal systems will be a further contributory factor.
- ☐ *Varied training methods,* no longer relying exclusively on traditional college-based courses, but with distance and open learning materials, using peer group settings in the workplace.
- ☐ *Credit accumulation,* with staff able to build up units of study over time, and with "credits" recognised widely and transferable from one training and employment situation to another.
- ☐ *Career progression will be facilitated* as learning is transferable and built up over time.

N. Bartlett, "Getting to grips with NVQ", *Community Care,* 8 February 1990.

CCETSW (1985), *Mental Handicap, Progress and Prospects in*

Staff Training, CCETSW.
CCETSW/ENB (1988), *Co-operation in Post-Qualifying Studies for Nurses and Social Workers,* Central Council for Education and Training in Social Work/English National Board.
D. Felce, J. Mansell, J. de Kock, A. Toogood and A. Pumphrey (1982), *Staff Induction Training,* University of Southampton, Health Care Evaluation Research Team.
Guys Health District (1981), *Report of the Development Group for Services for the Mentally Handicapped,* Lewisham and North Southwark Health Authority.
IDC (1988), *Next Steps in Qualifying Training for Staff Working with People with Learning Difficulties,* Independent Development Council for People with Mental Handicap.
Joint Initiative for Community Care/ADSS, *Training for the Caring Business* (1990), *Insight.*
J. Mansell (1988), *Staffed Housing for People with Mental Handicaps: Achieving Widespread Dissemination,* South East Thames Regional Health Authority.
J. Mansell, H. Brown, P. McGill, S. Hoskin, P. Lindley and E. Emerson (1987), *A Staff Training Initiative in Mental Handicap,* South East Thames Regional Health Authority.
Messenger, "National vocational qualifications", *The Journal of Training and Development,* Vol 1, No. 1, April 1990.
P. Mittler, "How effective is staff training?", in P. Farrell ed. (1985), *EDY, Its Impact on Staff Training in Mental Handicap,* Manchester University Press.
NIMROD (1980), *Procedural Guides,* NIMROD, Cardiff.
A. Shearer (1983), *An Ordinary Life: Issues and Strategies for Training Staff for Community Mental Handicap Services,* King's Fund Centre.
I. Walton (1989), *Workforce Needs and Training Resources,* Department of Social Policy and Social Work, University of York.
L. Ward (1984), *Planning for People: Developing a Local Service for People with Mental Handicap. 1. Recruiting and Training Staff,* King's Fund Centre, London.
L. Ward and J. Wilkinson (1985), *Training for Change: Staff Training for "An Ordinary Life",* King's Fund Centre, London.
A. Wertheimer (1989), *Building on Positives: Staff Development in Community Services,* King's Fund Centre, London.

16

The manager as trainer

"We don't believe in a hierarchial structure but very much in a horizontal-type system . . . I believe very strongly that if somebody is very good at market research that we should invest in them as people and let them run their own sections . . . It's the best way to give people incentives".
Female entrepreneur, quoted in R. Goffee and R. Scase, (1988)

"Education makes a people easy to lead, but difficult to drive; easy to govern but impossible to enslave".
Lord Brougham (1778-1868)

It is an increasingly change-ridden and pressured world for the front-line and middle managers, and at a time of policy changes or staff demands for new skills the temptation is to reach for the 'phone and call the training officer. This is to miss the point, however, that the on-the-spot operational manager is the most effective trainer: by example, encouragement, coaching, and taking the opportunity to draw in outside skills if need be. As Tom Peters and Nancy Austin (1985) put it: "Coaching is face-to-face leadership that pulls people with diverse back-grounds, talents, experience and interests, encourages them to step up to responsibility and continued achievement, and treats them as full-scale partners, and contributors".

The front line and middle manager is in an excellent strategic position to influence training, and this will become even more manifest with the introduction of National Vocational Qualifications. Training sections in large organisations are often too distant to influence events at the level of the service user, though this is in no way to deny that, to be effective, the training section will need an overall view of the services linked firmly to the central values and policy objectives of the department. "The remit for trainers" claimed Jim Mansell, director for learning difficulties studies at Kent University, at a conference, "is to do what you like as long as you don't change anything".

The remit for the manager, of course, is to change things constantly. Often managers nowadays feel like the British Olympic marathon runner who prepared for the Seoul Olympics on a moving belt in his garage - running fast to stay still?

It is always right for the manager to take a keen interest in the training and education (for he or she must think of the future as well as the here-and-now) of his or her staff, and also worth trying to influence events. When Peter Gilbert went to Forest Hospital,

Horsham, West Sussex in 1981, he was fortunate enough to meet with Barry Spooner, a man who had been appointed to set up a community nursing service but had had the vision and courage to insist on forming the first community mental handicap team in West Sussex (see chapter 20). As the senior social services member of the team Peter Gilbert discussed the social work contribution with the senior tutor at the nurse education centre who showed him the new placement requirements for the RNMH course in the light of the 1982 syllabus. Apparently a meeting with the social services' training section at county hall had resulted in many promises of community placements in social services settings, but a whole year later nothing had come of this. The perplexed tutor sought guidance as to how to proceed in a delicate inter-agency negotiation. Sometimes the Alexandrian method of problem-solving (cutting the Gordion Knot) is the best and the CMHT simply set up the placements and told the training section afterwards that they had implemented their excellent ideas!

This project has been written up (see T. Meeajun, *et al*, 1985) and led to intakes of students demonstrating a strong skill-base and commitment to people with learning difficulties and their families. As one student put it: "This was our most interesting placement so far. I couldn't feel superior as I didn't have all the answers." This experience was the first of a number of instances which led us to agree with writers such as Alan Fowler (1988) that staff development is "a central function for all managers" and not simply a peripheral activity or the preserve of training and personnel officers.

The fresh ideas of the students were a constant stimulus both to the CMHT and the various community placements they were involved with. Having students around keeps you young! Unfortunately for the students they so often return to a traditional work setting where their still small voice is usually drowned in the hubbub of institutional practice.

"Training" says Mansell (1988) "is too often narrowly defined as improving the skills and attitudes of individuals outside the context of organisational change". Perhaps one of the saddest examples of this is when the registered nurse (mental handicap), after three years undertaking the progressive 1982 syllabus, goes back onto a traditional ward and is soon falling into reactionary practice and using terms like "boys" and "girls" for men and women twice his or her age. Just as likely, of course, is the CSS holder who is seen by his or her manager as a hero-innovator in a large hostel or day centre but soon becomes discouraged when, like Sisyphus, he or she is condemned to rolling the rock of their new ideas and values up a hill of indifference. The task of the trainer, therefore, is to find a way of *intervening* in services which opens up the prospect for change.

The intervenor or change-agent must, therefore, be a trainer working closely with those who hold power, a manager co-operating with trainers who have specific skills, or a "subversive" who infiltrates new ways of working into an organisation - but whose neck is as safe as a John le Carré spy with all the moles based at his own HQ.

Working in a small borough such as Merton can have advantages in that a flat hierarchy and an integrated service group necessitate clear thinking on how training should interlink with the service. There is also delegated authority for middle managers to get out there and move things along. Training is part of the function of the policy, development and inspection group (P D & I) and close working between managers and "developers" can utilise unit budgets both to produce some individual packages (in conjunction with the London Boroughs Training Committee) but also to create group training within and/or between units. In the case of learning difficulty services the care in the community proposals to reduce the long-stay hospital service, and the imminence (or immanence?) of the Griffiths' philosophy meant that the service manager (learning difficulties) had a policy development role which in turn had a knock-on effect on training.

In many local authority services for adults one finds a low level of professional qualifications; a lack of professional supervision/staff support; very little sense, if any, of staff development/training priorities; and often no real idea as to what the service is striving to achieve. Added to this, ethnic and gender issues are often ignored. In the absence of any central congruence and guidance Peter Gilbert found, when working in Merton, that each establishment was using or not using its budget as it saw fit without any reference to wider service issues. The first objectives seemed to be, therefore, to formulate service principles; bring different parts of the service together as a cohesive team; and undertake a training audit. Here of course is the classic chicken and egg situation: to produce a long-term plan training needs have to be assessed, but to create the right climate of regeneration some staff development has to be introduced straight away.

Jim Mansell (1988, *op.cit.*) believes that the traditional rationalist approach of creating a service-wide value base as a first step risks defeat by reactionary elements and institutionalised resistance. He goes for a spearhead or *blitzkrieg* method of reinforcing good practice as a model of what can be achieved. The trouble with this can be an Arnhem effect whereby successful elements are isolated, and thus neutralised. Also the new service/establishment may become elitist and self-satisfied while the more established service falls into despondency rather than being inspired. The best approach, therefore, may be both *simultaneously* shaking the service system; planning long term; encouraging individuals who wish to develop; and getting groups of staff together to learn both the values and the skills they need in order to provide the service the users want and need. With this in mind David Wright, the principal officer from P D & I, and Peter Gilbert put in some training on such matters as staff supervision and team building which an initial assessment showed were a vital pre-requisite to further progress. In fact the training audit could not be compiled effectively and fairly if frontline managers were not skilled in supervisory techniques.

An audit form was used and was successful in eliciting information, provoking thought on the job each individual was carrying out and setting out priorities. People were conscientious about completing the task and supervisors began to coalesce the needs of individuals and the requirements of the service in a much more systematic manner. A training budget which had been about 60 per cent underspent in the previous financial year was spent to the last penny in 1987/8 as staff saw a personal and service investment in training and supported and covered for one another as people went off on courses or groups got together to work on set tasks. The individual forms enabled the service manager to compile a profile for each establishment which showed, not only needs, but what the staff member could offer to others - ask not what the SEC can do for you but what you can do for the SEC. We often fail to appreciate the sheer wealth of experience and expertise our colleagues bring to the work in hand.

It may seem a truism, but needs to be stressed in today's climate, that it is only through the use of traditional casework and groupwork active listening skills that the manager can effect valid and long lasting change. John Harvey-Jones (1988) agrees that *lasting* success is only possible "when you work with rather than against people". At the end of the first six months we took the "risk" of bringing the staff groups of the traditional SEC and the newly opened centre together, without managers, and with an outside training consultant to both team-build and look at ways of creating good practice. Out of that came new ideas about working with clients, and later, funds from the council to create a better environment within the centre and additional staff to make more use of community facilities. Staff supervision and support was requested and another trainer brought in to give basic training in this vital art to *all* managers and seniors within the group. To make the value of supervision explicit the service manager met with each member of staff at the long-established centre together with his or her senior to discuss the value and role of supervision in such a setting and take any flak from introducing a new system! Now that "whole establishment training" has taken place, new skills for staff can be introduced in a "cascade" format so that each member of staff can feel their natural talents are being enhanced.

The training audit took about eight months to complete and place into both a personal and service context for evaluation. Again, the combined spearhead and broad-front approach has been useful as we have learned of training requirements and been able to meet a number of them as we have gone along. People do not of course, always want what you think they want or need. Peter Gilbert envisaged that one senior day centre officer would want to do a CSS or CQSW ultimately, and was interested to find that he felt a Certificate in Management Studies would be more appropriate for himself and more useful for the service, as he already had a professional qualification in the Dip.TMHA. An underspent fieldwork training budget was raided and the officer sent on the Certificate in Management Studies course at Croydon College. Later a colleague from the other centre followed him onto the specialist social services CMS at Bromley College.

Group needs right across the service were easy to identify from the audit and issues like working with people with challenging behaviours, and personal and sexual development are being addressed. Because the audit was essentially one of self-identification by staff some vital issues were inevitably left out. Racial equality was not highlighted by staff yet the proportion of people from ethnic minorities was rising within the borough. It was made clear from the start, however, that management reserved the right to introduce training on issues which were an organisational priority.

The hallmark following the initial period will be that staff training will include people from all parts of the service and relevant staff from the NHS and other agencies, so as to team-build through learning together.

"When service systems do not explicitly support values and beliefs", writes Ann Shearer (1983) "people are left to discover their own . . . These values can be precarious and easily challenged by societal values and structures." The aim of staff and service development should be one of constant revaluation and renewal: harnessing service values, individual enthusiasm, consumer experience and views, multi-disciplinary expertise, departmental commitment, managerial energy and clout, staff desire to learn and multi-agency desire to move ahead.

In late 1988 a training forum was set up with trainers, managers and a top grade psychologist from Merton personal services department, Sutton SSD, the health authority and St Ebba's Hospital in-service training unit. The result was that training arranged by any one body was made available to the others (self advocacy being a major topic) plus local voluntary organisations such as MENCAP Homes Foundation. In early 1989 a co-ordinated series of workshops was set up (with some financial support from the Association of Professionals in Mental Handicap) to inculcate the necessary values and skills to provide a successful care in the community programme at a local level.

When Peter Gilbert left Merton he was fortunate enough to see the exercise being taken forward by an able and energetic colleague, rather than left in midstream as it might have been. Arriving in Kent in February 1989 he was glad to see another training forum in existence and a development manager compiling a training audit across NHS and social services staff. Whether one organisation becomes a "lead agency" or there is a joint service or any one of many alternatives takes root, the need for people to share a common vision and learn to communicate and work together is paramount.

These kinds of initiatives can only work if both staff and agencies set a desire to learn and to co-operate as primary objectives and managers accept responsibility for staff and service development. As Lesley Bell (1989) writes: "Line managers need to consider staff training and development as an integral part of managerial responsibility, contributing directly to effectiveness, efficiency, team building and service provision". Only the *partnership* of operational managers and developers and trainers can ensure that, as in Plato's *Phaedrus,* the two steeds are kept in harness and moving forward to a common objective.

Striving to be "trainer" as well as "manager" is never easy but the generating of new ideas is always rejuvenating and it may be worth remembering President Eisenhower's words to Harold Macmillan: "Remember the old adage: 'Now abideth faith, hope and charity - and greater than these is a sense of humour'".

L. Bell (1989), *The Need for a Systematic and Coherent Approach to Staff Development and Training,* Local Government Training Board.

A. Fowler (1988), *Human Resource Management in Local Government,* Longman.

R. Goffee and R. Scase (1988), *Women in Charge,* Allen & Unwin.

J. Harvey-Jones (1988), *Making it Happen: Reflections on Leadership,* Fontana.

J. Mansell, "Training for staff development", in D. Towell ed. (1988), *An Ordinary Life in Practice,* King's Fund.

T. Meeajun, B. Spooner and P. Gilbert, "Jay walking in the community", *Nursing Times,* 23 October 1985.

T. Peters and N. Austen (1985), *A Passion for Excellence,* Fontana.

A. Shearer (1983), *Issues and Strategies for Training Staff in Community Mental Handicap Services,* King's Fund.

Parents speaking (1)

Premonitions prior to diagnosis

"I felt the uneasiness spread. Where was I in those early months? Going unconsciously with Zach from feeding to feeding, from nap to nap, feeling slightly disconnected, something monstrous and dark hidden from me, waiting."
Fern Kupfer, *Before and after Zachariah,* Gollancz, 1982

"I kept telling my family doctor that Michael couldn't be right. He wasn't happy, he wasn't feeding properly and his high pitched cry was driving us mad. None of us slept at night. My doctor had known me for ages. He knew I had two older children, but still he didn't seem to believe a word I was telling him. It was only when we had a Locum doctor that we got somewhere. He said immediately there was something wrong with Michael and had him taken into the hospital. They told us there that he had cri du chat syndrome. I knew there was something wrong right from the first."
Mother talking to Peter Gilbert

"We went into intensive care. He looked so tiny, wired up to all those complicated machines. The nurses were busy doing things we didn't understand. We felt large and in the way. It was hard to believe that he was the same boy that was running about full of life just a few hours before. Even before the doctor told us, somehow we knew that the old Donald had gone forever."
Quoted in S Hollins and M Grimer, *Going Somewhere,* SPCK, 1988

Reactions to the diagnosis

"Talking to other parents who have been in the same situation as we were, I am aware that we have all felt a sense of bereavement. We were denied our hopes of a normal baby. Yet it was different from my mother's death, although just as sudden. When she died it was final, and I had to come to terms with that abrupt end. Having a handicapped child meant beginning to adjust to an ever-changing situation, as new difficulties or challenges presented themselves."
J M Lloyd, *Jacob's Ladder,* Costello, 1986

"Our doctor told us ... 'Your child is severely mentally handicapped, a mongol' - I still hate that word, I think it is the ugliest word in the English language ... We both cried our eyes out, this couldn't be happening to us, what could we tell relatives, friends and neighbours? I felt I had produced faulty goods, I felt ashamed and as if it was all my fault. Many times I asked, 'WHY ME?'"
Quoted in Brian Stratford, *Down's Syndrome: Past, Present and Future,* Penguin, 1989

"For four months I never went out of the house, not even to the

shops. I just cut myself off from everybody. If it wasn't for my health visitor, coming in almost daily, I might have gone on like that forever."
Mother talking to Peter Gilbert

"When the full nature of his problem was revealed, shock, puzzlement and some anger were the first reactions ... I remember going for a walk on the Gog Magog hills with a friend and being overwhelmed by the sense that I had failed in every aspect of my life - there seemed no career prospects and I had failed as a mother . . . No-one could really gauge how handicapped he was, or what his future development would be. Consciously or unconsciously all parents have dreams for their children. We had to accept we would dream no dreams."
Frances Young, *Face to Face,* Epworth Press, 1985

"One day, I was browsing round our local Woolworths store with Cathy in her pushchair, when I met an old friend who I had not seen for years. After exchanging greetings and swapping news of our respective families, she glanced down at Cathy.

'And this is your latest, is it?' Her expression altered slightly, then she said in a bright but casual manner: 'Oh she's a little mongol, bless her.'

I stared at her, shock, like an icy hand, clutching my heart.

'No - she's not', I heard myself stammering.

'Oh but she is, love. I've worked with them for years and there is no mistaking' - she evidently read and understood the expression on my face. 'Oh, lord! haven't they told you? I am so sorry . . . ' "
Joan Hebden, *She'll Never Do Anything, Dear,* Souvenir Press, 1985

The first years

"Having a handicapped child is the best assertiveness-training course there is."
Fern Kupfer, *op cit*

"Joseph was scared stiff of the tractors, but made friends with the animals. Jacob hugely enjoys any new experience. There are occasions when his lack of inhibitions is a positive advantage."

"News is rarely about ordinary people doing ordinary things in ordinary settings. On the other hand, it is Portage's very ordinariness that is its greatest triumph."
J M Lloyd, *op cit*

"I felt very nervous because it was the end of one era and the beginning of another. This was the moment we had all waited for - her starting at normal school and we felt that it was the end of all we had worked for and yet it was just the beginning of another long fight."
E Byrne, C Cunningham and P Sloper, *Families and Their Children with Down's Syndrome,* Routledge, 1988.

17

Ensuring quality

"Quality improvement is a never-ending journey."
Tom Peters

Services for people with learning difficulties are experiencing profound changes, with the continuing run-down and closure of long-stay hospitals and establishment of community-based services. Similarly new values, based on positive views of the potential for people with learning difficulties to lead ordinary lives in the community, are achieving a growing acceptance. These values are steadily informing the core principles that should guide future developments, and are held by an increasing number of managers and staff, who are striving to build services that are relevant to users who desire a better quality of life.

It is in new services that quality is most frequently discussed. Planners, managers and staff do not want to repeat the mistakes of the past, where service provision was concerned primarily with coverage and minimum standards, but rather to design and deliver services that offer options and opportunities for users to realise their potential to lead valued lives in the community.

But, in spite of the enthusiasm and commitment that can successfully launch new service initiatives, these features can be lost as staff move on, and the resources and support that are available at the beginning of a project are focussed on initiatives elsewhere. To avoid the weakening of the commitment to innovation, and the risks to new models of care, with the consequence that practice will come to resemble that of traditional services it was designed to replace, ways have to be found to counteract this decline. Means of developing a culture of quality in services that can maintain and continually improve and adapt the model of care, as aspirations and expectations change is critical for the long-term success of services.

Quality also needs to be on the agenda of well-established services. These services are likely to have been established with little attention paid to discussion and agreement on the value base of the service, and as a consequence, have poorly defined service objectives or criteria of success. In working to improve such services, the introduction of quality assurance measures, based on agreed values and guiding principles, with explicitly stated service objectives and outcomes for users, is an important activity for managers and staff.

What do we mean by quality?

It is helpful in exploring quality in services to start with the distinction between the quality of life and the quality of care.

Quality of life can be defined in personal and subjective terms, and can refer to the users' experience of the service they receive, and the extent to which they feel their needs are being met (though, of course, quality of life is not only about what services provide). These perceptions of the quality of life will be influenced by factors such as, the values society attaches to the provision it makes for people using that service, the arrangements and opportunities made by the service to meet the unique need of the individual, and lastly by the abilities and personality of the individual.

Quality of care can define the opportunities offered by a service for the people who live or work in it, and can be examined in terms of what is achieved for the individual. Measuring the quality of care could mean assessment of service provision against service guidelines, or assessment using a checklist of standards, or more rarely, users' achievements. (See for example Raynes (1988)) for an annotated directory of measures of environmental quality.)

In an attempt to define quality in services it is important to develop a clear understanding of what constitutes quality of life. This can then be used as the basis for examining service outcomes and how much they promote or hinder the achievement of a high quality life for the users of the service. Beswick *et al* (1986) suggest that a high quality of care could be defined in terms of the quality of life of the users of a service. Good quality care could also be seen in terms of what people with a learning difficulty would want for themselves and/or what we would value in our society for ourselves.

Aspects of the quality of life

In attempting to explore quality of life it is helpful to identify those things that most of us would value for ourselves. Williams and Tyne (1988), list 11 statements, that they believe everyone is likely to value (see chapter 4). These are everyday expectations that most of us would recognise, and could form the basis for an exploration of a quality lifestyle.

Moving on from the broad statements of valued options to a more individual focus, Blunden (1988) describes four factors that can be said to influence the quality of life.

Physical well-being, means the presence of good health, fitness and the absence of disability. Where the person has a chronic illness or disability, this would be minimised by the provision of treatment or prosthetic devices, with particular emphasis on maintaining or extending the person's independence.

For people living in the community arrangements would exist to enable them to experience a high standard of physical well-being, and where necessary medical and other practitioner services are promptly available.

Material well-being includes an adequate income, appropriate accommodation, private transport and personal possessions. For people living in residential services, the level of disposable income available and under their control, the quality of the living environment and the quantity and quality of personal possessions would all be factors to consider.

Social well-being is particularly important as it is concerned with the degree to which people value their social networks, both for personal and survival reasons. A detailed approach to social well-being is provided by O'Brien's five accomplishments for a valued social life (O'Brien, 1987). These are:

- ☐ *Community presence:* including contact with the community, particularly non-segregated settings.
- ☐ *Choices:* which is concerned with opportunities for people to make decisions about major and minor matters which affect them.
- ☐ *Competence:* which is concerned with people being provided with opportunities to learn and develop skills.
- ☐ *Respect:* which is concerned with the experience of being valued by other people.
- ☐ *Participation:* which is concerned with involvement in a network of people, and developing relationships, particularly with non-handicapped people.

(See Chapter 4, for a more detailed description of the five accomplishments related to people using a day service.)

Cognitive well-being relates to the person's perception of his or her life situation. Here the emphasis is placed on the person's own views of the extent to which his or her needs are being met. This will be a subjective judgement, but it is important to listen to the views of users of services, or those that represent them, where the person is unable to speak for himself. A particularly useful approach to learning more about the life situation of people is to use the concept of "wounds", or "super-imposed handicapping experiences" described by Williams (1988). We have encouraged staff to use this list of experiences when attempting to develop a greater sensitivity to how people with learning difficulties view their past and present life experiences.

Taken together the descriptions of quality of life experiences can help begin the process of examining those aspects of the service that are providing opportunities for users to develop high quality lifestyles, or alternatively, those aspects of the service that fall short of these requirements, and fail to support a high quality of life, and require corrective action.

Traditional approaches to quality assurance

Turning to the quality in services, where this has been on the agenda, it has traditionally been concerned with monitoring procedures initiated by managers, or other advisory staff external to the service. This approach has placed emphasis on checking service features which are routinely available against defined standards, and taking remedial action when deficiencies are identified. The problem with this approach is, that standards set tend to become the norm for a service, and in turn define minimum acceptable standards. These standards are likely to fall well short of what would be recognised as a high quality service, and may not even focus on the most important issues to users (or their advocates), whose opinions are rarely sought, or front-line staff who have intimate knowledge of service delivery issues.

A further problem is that monitoring of standards can be seen as a threat by staff (catching them out when things go wrong), or of little importance except at times of monitoring activity. A recent example of the pitfalls of setting up external monitoring is described by Abbott *et al* (1990), where staff of a house felt resentful of this procedure, and raised the following questions: Where will information be going? What about confidentiality? They were also concerned with "us" inside versus "them" outside, and invasion of privacy.

Information collected from such monitoring exercises tends to be one-way, with data sent up the system, and little returned in a form that staff can use to improve services. This can be exacerbated by senior managers who may not be skilled in providing feedback for staff, and as a consequence staff are likely to perceive such exercises as time consuming with little return.

An alternative approach to quality assurance

An alternative approach to improving quality in services focuses on action in the service itself, with all those with an interest in the service (the stakeholders) playing a part. Mansell (1986) has described quality assurance as "the creation of a climate of innovation and development, in which staff feel motivated to assess the quality of their service and improve it" (p.42).

Taking this statement as a basis for action, the Independent Development Council publication on quality (1988) offers a wealth of ideas for managers and staff. These could be used as the starting point for introducing quality measures into day-to-day practice. But before taking action, the manager and staff need to consider the consequences of introducing ideas on quality which can mean a considerable shift in management and practice in the service. This change is a result of raising fundamental questions about how people using the service are seen by the organisation, and how much their opinions are sought and valued, and how much staff are encouraged to take responsibility for the development of quality in the service. These and other issues will need to be considered by the manager, who will need to respond and support users and staff whose expectations will be increased by the potential to achieve higher standards of care through the introduction of quality assurance measures.

The following ten areas from the IDC publication could be used as topics for discussion in staff groups as a first step in the development of quality assurance in the service.

Spending time with service users. Finding out what customers want from a service is a central part of a successful commercial organisation's operation. If we are to provide a high quality service to people with learning difficulties, then similarly we need to find out how they view the service they receive. This is a grossly neglected issue in services, but with the advent of approaches based on normalisation, advocacy and individual planning, the views of users are at last beginning to be heard.

Focussing on results rather than process. Services tend to concentrate on issues concerning delivery. For example, staffing levels, management structures, and building maintenance, rather than outcomes, which are concerned with the impact of services on the lives of people who use them. Outcomes are important because they can grow out of explicit statements by a service about what it intends to achieve for users. Quality of life statements can then be used to review outcomes for users. None of this is intended to mean that issues concerned with the processes of delivery are unimportant. Rather that services need to be driven by outcomes for users, as this will then begin to guide what service processes are necessary.

Concentrating on a small number of specific areas where substantial development is possible. When working to develop quality services, it is important to concentrate the efforts of staff on one or two key aspects, that if successful will have a significant impact on the lives of users. Concentration of effort is also important in terms of getting early success from specific actions that reinforce staffs' motivation and willingness to develop further initiatives on quality. A start could be made with one of the five accomplishments, whereby staff could involve stakeholders in a quality action group (Blunden, 1988), to work on specific service accomplishments. See below for a detailed description of the quality action group.

Developing a common vision and common values. A service needs to have a clear vision of what it is trying to achieve for users. This vision is based on values that are shared by people working in the service about how they view the place of people with learning difficulties in society. This would suggest what a quality service needs to do to create opportunities for these values to be translated into practical outcomes that benefit users. To achieve a strong and unwavering commitment to values requires considerable effort, with staff spending time together exploring how they can individually and collectively take action that leads to outcomes and real achievements for service users. (See Hoskins and Mansell (1988) for helpful material on developing a common vision for a service.)

Building on strengths and supporting achievements. Because staff so often see monitoring as people external to the service checking on their performance, and focussing on things that go wrong, other more supportive and creative ways need to be found to engage staff in the process of building and maintaining quality in services. Good management practice tells us that it is important to support people's strengths, and identify ways of celebrating those things in services that genuinely meet the needs of users, rather than demonstrate adherence to bureaucratic demands. Hout's and Scott's famous statement - "Catch your staff doing something right" - sums up the approach needed so succinctly. Recent work by Porterfield (1987), and again Hoskins and Mansell (1988) offer ideas on how to support staff who are striving to meet the needs of service users, that involve staff, with their manager, in developing joint approaches to improving quality.

Practical activities for developing quality services. Developing creative forms of quality assurance and putting them into practice is a key role for the manager. A systematic approach to introducing these ideas could take the following form:

Developing the mission of the service. Staff need an opportunity to meet together with users to explore the value base of the service, and where this is unclear or in opposition to the needs of users to establish through discussion and common agreement a "mission" statement that states clearly and succinctly what the service intends to provide for the people who use it. Developing a common value base for the service, that everyone involved feels they have contributed to creating and as a consequence feel committed to support is an essential first step on the quality road. In creating a mission for the service staff must consider the views of people who use the service, their advocates, and their own understanding of what users need. A consumer viewpoint is central to any development of quality measures in a service, as so often what staff believe users want does not accord with how the person with a learning difficulty sees his or her life. Here skilled and sensitive approaches to exploring users' needs, hopes and wishes is a key activity.

Identifying service objectives. Once the mission of the service is agreed, then this can be translated into practice, ideally through a number of key service objectives. These objectives and the resulting activities of staff should focus on those processes and outcomes that are desired by users and their advocates. A systematic approach that makes the goals of the service (ie, outcomes for users) explicit will enable quality activities to be planned around them.

Regular meetings to review quality in the service. Because staff need to work together to deliver effective programmes of care and training, good teamwork is vital. Mansell *et al* (1987) state that "the opportunity for staff to work out what they are going to do together is probably the single most important contribution to developing a good quality service". Mansell and colleagues suggest regular weekly meetings, arranged so that most staff can attend, which are used to explore practical issues, such as progress with individual plans, and with time set aside to discuss how the service can be improved. This meeting is seen as the major focus for quality assurance, and could take on a quality action group role as described by Blunden (1988). A quality action group would include staff and users, and other key stakeholders, and is formed with the specific aim of examining some aspect of the service, and to take action to improve service quality.

Beyer (1987), describes a quality action group based on a home support service that met over a considerable period of time, and sees such groups that focus on fundamental objectives, such as values, individuals' experience and user outcomes, as unique and vital, and one important part of monitoring service quality.

Giving users a voice. An important part of any quality assurance system is the consumers' viewpoint. Service providers need to find ways of enabling people with learning difficulties to voice their opinions of the service they receive. This is not easy for either staff or users, particularly where there has been no involvement by users in decision making, even of the most token kind. It is also made more difficult by the restrictions on users created by services, as well as their own lack of knowledge about options available to them. They may also have spent a lifetime dependent on others, and have become used to falling in with the wishes of parents and staff. There can also be the risk that users feel they run if they are heard to voice criticisms of the service which controls much of their day-to-day life.

One way forward is for staff to support the development of participation events and self-advocacy groups. There is now an increasing understanding of the importance of finding ways of giving users a voice, and staff who are willing to support individuals and groups can develop their own discussion groups based on the advocacy concepts. These activities can offer users opportunities to develop confidence in expressing their views, take control over matters discussed, and grow in self-respect as others begin to listen to their views. None of this should ignore the real difficulties that both staff and users can experience where the involvement of users is encouraged for the first time: the recognition that both parties will be faced with a novel situation, with staff having to share some of their power with users, and users needing to overcome the limitations of their experience on issues that concern them. Readers are directed to Gathercole (1988) who has described fully, both the importance, and the difficulties of involving service users. A detailed list of resources on advocacy can be found in the resources section.

Independent review of the service. Finally we need to consider the role of the independent review of a service as an additional feature of a quality assurance system. The independent review has a number of important aspects. First, it provides the staff of a unit with an evaluation of their work by people who are not connected with the service, and can look at the service with a new set of eyes, and question some of the ways of operating that are taken for granted. Second, an independent review could use one of the evaluation tools, such as PASS (Wolfensberger and Glenn, 1975), or simpler tools, such as the questionnaire of the quality of life, developed by a local CMH group (Cragg and Harrison, 1986). Third, the service can use methods of consultation with service users, their advocates or advocacy groups to express their views about the quality of the service. One approach could be to use the "Whose Lifestyle?" package (Brown, 1988), which has been designed to enable people with learning difficulties to express their views about their lives and the service they receive. Last, the external review could be combined with internal self-monitoring, as described by Abbott *et al* (1990). This approach uses the staff of a unit who have detailed knowledge of the service, assisted by outsiders who can help staff see afresh the quality of life offered.

The manager's role in quality assurance

The manager's role in supporting quality assurance will draw on many of the skills described in this book. For example, leadership is important in promoting a vision of the service, and clearly communicating service objectives to staff and others who are working to achieve desired outcomes for users. Staff also need to work together cohesively, and here the manager has an important role in building and maintaining an effective team, so that they are encouraged to contribute to the improvement of the service. These and other management activities will contribute towards building a culture within the service that demonstrates a commitment to the staff as a precious resource, and by a participative management approach, harness their full potential in order to gain a commitment to the mission of the service. Finally, the manager needs to promote training and development for staff, if they are to meet the current and future demands in the service. These activities are part of a manager's responsibility for providing the highest quality of service available within given constraints. It combines the strategy, with its vision of the future for people with a learning difficulty, and the creation of a culture of quality based on the potential of staff to work for the common purpose of the service.

Resources for developing quality in services

Self Advocacy

D. Cooper and J. Hertsov (1986), *We Can Change the Future,* Pavilion Publishing (Brighton) Ltd. Freepost, 42 Landsdowne Place, Hove, East Sussex BN3 2Z.

H. Brown (1988), *Whose Lifestyle?,* Pavilion Publishing (Brighton) Ltd. Address as above.

P. Williams and B. Shoultz (1979), *We Can Speak for Ourselves,* Souvenir Press.

Values Into Action (formerly Campaign for Mentally Handicapped People) (1988), *Learning about Self-Advocacy Pack,* and other publications on advocacy and participation events. VIA Publications, 5 Kentings Comberton, Cambs CB3 7DT.

Evaluation Materials

R. Cragg and J. Harrison (1986), *Living in a Supervised Home (Staffed or Unstaffed),* Birmingham Campaign for People with a Mental Handicap.

N. Raynes (1988), *Annotated Directory of Measures of Environmental Quality - for use in Residential Services for People with a Mental Handicap,* University of Manchester.

W. Wolfensberger and L. Glenn (1975), *Programme Analysis of Service Systems,* National Institute on Mental Retardation, Toronto.

Royal College of Nursing (1987), *Assuring Quality in the Private Sector: Residential Services in the Community for People with a Mental Handicap.* The Royal College of Nursing and Ruislip Press.

Quality Assurance

S. Hoskins and J. Mansell (1988), *What Matters Most: Quality Assurance for Front-Line Staff,* South East Thames Regional Health Authority.

K. Abbott, J. James and H. Howell, "Quality matters 2. From the inside looking out: How to tackle monitoring", *Mental Handicap,* Vol.18, March 1990.

S. Beyer, "Pursuing quality through a quality action group: Experiences in a CUSS home support service", in L. Ward ed. (1986), *Getting Better All The Time, Issues and Strategies for Ensuring Quality in Community Services for People with Mental Handicap,* King's Fund Project Paper Number 66.

R. Blunden, "Safeguarding quality", in D. Towell ed. (1988), *An Ordinary Life in Practice, Developing Comprehensive*

Community-Based Services for People with Learning Disabilities, King Edward's Hospital Fund for London.

R. Cragg and J. Harrison (1986), *Living in a Supervised Home (Staffed or Unstaffed),* Birmingham Campaign for People with a Mental Handicap.

C. Gathercole, "Involving people with learning disabilities", in D. Towell ed. (1988), *An Ordinary Life in Practice, Developing Comprehensive Services for People with Learning Disabilities,* King Edward's Hospital Fund for London.

S. Hoskins and J. Mansell (1988), *What Matters Most: Quality Assurance for Front-Line Staff,* South East Thames Regional Health Authority.

Independent Development Council (1986), *Pursuing Quality: How Good are your Local Services for People with Mental Handicap?*

Kent Social Services (forthcoming), *A Guide to the Good Care of People with Learning Disabilities.*

J. Mansell, "The nature of quality assurance", in J. Beswick, T. Zadik and D. Felce eds. (1986), *Evaluating Quality of Care,* British Institute of Mental Handicap.

J. Mansell, D. Felce, J. Jenkins, U. de Kock and S. Toogood (1987), *Developing Staffed Housing for People with Mental Handicaps,* Costello.

J. Porterfield (1987), *Positive Monitoring: A Method of Supporting Staff and Improving Services for People with Learning Disabilities,* British Institute of Mental Handicap.

N. Raynes (1988), *Annotated Directory of Measures of Environmental Quality, for use in Residential Services for People with a Mental Handicap,* University of Manchester.

P. Williams, "Evaluating services from the consumer's point of view", in J. Beswick, T. Zadik and D. Felce eds. (1986), *Evaluating Quality of Care,* British Institute of Mental Handicap.

P. Williams and A. Tyne, "Exploring values as a basis for service development", in D. Towell ed. (1988), *An Ordinary Life in Practice, Developing Comprehensive Community-Based Services for People with Learning Disabilities,* King Edward's Hospital Fund for London.

P. Williams and B. Shoultz (1979), *We Can Speak for Ourselves,* Souvenir Press.

W. Wolfensberger and L. Glenn (1975), *Programme Analysis of Service Systems,* National Institute on Mental Retardation, Toronto.

PART III

Service models

[Our aim is] "to bring about, stage by stage, an improvement and an aspiration to the Utopia which we know can never come but which we must never cease to search for".

Harold Macmillan

"Amateurs built the Ark, professionals designed the Titanic!"

Lord Rix

Consumer's view: What next?

Stephen Jones is 19 years old and lives with his parents and younger sister. An elder brother lives and works in a neighbouring county. Peter and Stephen know each other through shared social activities in their local community. He was talking to Peter Gilbert in Spring 1990.

Over the last years I went to the [school leavers] unit. We did computer work, travel training and woodwork. We went and got our lunch and cooked it. Some mornings I went to the children's home. Chris showed me what to do. I enjoyed it - the best thing was hoovering, but I didn't get a job there. Travelling to the unit was hard work. Up at 7.30 to get there at nine. Two changes of buses. Yes, you're right, when I get a job I'll need to travel on my own. Yes, good experience.

The Pathway got me a job at the hospital. In the kitchen. Not the whole week. Cleaning cupboards, washing dishes. They were friendly there but I needed more time. What next? Back to school, waiting for a job. Odd jobs for the headteacher, chopping logs, gardening. I get paid. We're having a group of people who went to school. I'm the chairman.

Next week I'm starting at the college on a course [YTS assessment]. I've tried the train journey. There are two stops. I get £29 per week from the college if I work hard.

I like discos, watching football. I went to Lourdes. I liked pushing the wheelchairs. In the evening we went out. No, no wine - Pepsi. My girlfriend likes discos. She is working in a playgroup. We go to each other's homes. We go to the Gateway Club together. On my own I go to yoga on Mondays [adult education], it's enjoyable. At the club we're putting on a show - *Opportunity Knocks* - I'm doing Scott from *Neighbours*.

I'd like to be a hospital porter or pushing trolleys at the Co-op. I can do a computer course at college. I don't want to go to the centre [SEC]. I want to get married and I need some money. I'd be bored at the centre. The best thing would be to stick to my jobs.

18

A comprehensive service

"We want to see something new. Forget what's happened in the past, because you can't change the past but we can change the future."
Gary Bourlet, Chairperson, People First

Although Part III focuses on only a limited number of service models it is vital that any one model is part of a comprehensive service - built up either on an integrated service system or through the Griffiths mode of commissioning (purchasing) and providing as set out in *Caring for People* (see chapter 19). Service should be based on agreed values and clearly stated principles. Most organisations nowadays, however large or small, attempt to set out the philosophy underpinning the service structure, or at least a "mission" or "value" statement denoting the immediate goals to be achieved. An example of such a statement could be: "The services provided by Wooltown District Health Authority reflect the belief that people with learning difficulties have a right to be treated as individuals, to be fully consulted in all decisions, and to enjoy normal patterns of life within the community."

Service principles

In general the following principles should be observed so that services:

- ☐ Affirm and enhance the *dignity, self respect* and *individuality* of people with learning difficulties and their direct carers.
- ☐ Promote a positive image and increase *public awareness* and *acceptance.*
- ☐ Engage individuals and their carers in a *partnership* within the planning process.
- ☐ Engage the local neighbourhood's acceptance to being about *care by,* as well as in, the community.
- ☐ Build in *flexibility* so as to respond to current individual needs and changing needs.
- ☐ Ensure that services are *locally* based in natural communities.
- ☐ Place the *consumer* in the centre of the service.
- ☐ Recognise each *individual* as having a past, a future and a wealth of experience.
- ☐ Ensure that *race* and *gender* issues are properly attended to and embedded in service design and staff training.

- ☐ Utilise *generic* services first but build in specialist services as necessary.
- ☐ Provide the appropriate *specialist skill* input for people with additional special needs.
- ☐ Base the service on patterns of *culturally valued* normality in everyday living.
- ☐ Enable service users and carers to have access to *independent advocacy* schemes and empowerment through *self-advocacy.*
- ☐ Bring about *ownership* by staff of the changing orientation of services.
- ☐ *Assess* individual needs and make future services consumer-led.
- ☐ Take *services to people* and not people to services.
- ☐ *Co-ordinate* the varied services necessary to give a *comprehensive* service.

Evolving services

Services must be evaluated against the value-base and service principles. An aggregation of individual needs and assessments, consumer surveys and pilot schemes, will lead to a general service model. This model is not an end in itself but should be subject to constant review and renewal.

A comprehensive service

Preventive

In recent years Britain has fallen behind its European partners in pre- and antenatal care resulting in a higher than average incidence of temporary or permanent disabling conditions.

A sound comprehensive service must start with a health education programme, including special attention to cultural groups within society, and go on to provide genetic counselling to those at risk and a high standard of prenatal and antenatal care. Just as much of British industry has a reputation for short-term planning which has led to markets being dominated by countries like Japan, so infant care in the UK has lagged behind other European Community countries creating a much higher cost in human and financial terms in the future.

Children's services

Building a comprehensive service in the future will be affected considerably by how the various agencies and their staff co-operate in an increasingly fragmented service environment (see chapter 19); and how services are shaped in response to the new policy context of the *Children Act* 1989, the need to interact sensitively with ethnic minorities, and the challenge to assessment and provision of those individuals with extra special needs.

The Children Act "provides", in the words of the guidance

document, "a legal framework for a new approach to provision of services to a child with disabilities" (DoH, 1991). Rather than, as in the past, legislating separately for disabled children under NHS legislation, such children are now officially "children first" as proposed by the Court report in 1976.

Part III, Section 17(10) defines a category of children "in need" for whom the SSD should provide services, if necessary, to safeguard and promote their welfare. A child is defined by the Act as being "in need" if:

- it is unlikely to achieve or maintain, or to have the opportunity of achieving or maintaining, a reasonable standard of health or development without the provision for him of services by a local authority;
- its health or development is likely to be significantly impaired, or further impaired, without the provision for him of such services; or
- it is disabled.

("Development" means physical, intellectual, emotional, social or behavioural development, and "health" means physical or mental health.)

The *Children Act* mirrors the *National Assistance Act* 1948 definition of disability, stating that "a child is disabled if he is blind, deaf or dumb or suffers from mental disorder of any kind or is substantially and permanently handicapped by illness, injury or congenital deformity or such other disability as may be prescribed". Thus a person with a disability qualifies for services before and after the age of 18.

In terms of services for children with disabilities the Children Act contains specific provisions:

- Section 23(8) requires that "where a local authority provides accommodation for a child whom they are looking after and who is disabled, they shall, so far as is reasonably practicable, secure that the accommodation is not unsuitable to his particular needs";
- Schedule 2, paragraph 2 separates out the requirement on local authorities to open and maintain a register of children with disabilities in their areas;
- Schedule 2, paragraph 3 provides that a local authority may assess a child's needs for the purpose of the Children Act at the same time as any assessment under certain other Acts;
- Schedule 2, paragraph 9 requires local authorities to provide services for children with disabilities which are designed to minimise the effects of the children's disabilities;
- Schedule 2, paragraph 6 requires that services should be so designed as to give children the opportunity to lead lives which are as normal as possible (DoH, 1991).

The intention to integrate children with disabilities into mainstream legislation and services is very clear, and, as Philippa Russell has pointed out "the Children Act . . . . restores the leadership role to the local authority" (P. Russell, 1991). The challenge for children, families, pressure groups and social services will be one that has faced services throughout history, namely does integration bring services for those with special needs up to the standard of the best or does it create an unintentional neglect? After the vicissitudes of children's services over the past few years parents and carers have a trust gap to leap. Local authorities have a massive task to build up the right sort of service in accessible locations and bridge the gaps in, for instance, respite care as highlighted by the recent NCH survey (NCH, 1991), and also to promote consultation, a positive image and the dissemination of information so that services are taken up appropriately (see C. Robinson, 1988).

The DoH guidelines stress the need to listen to children and their carers and allow for them to "exercise choice"; the essential element of good liaison with other agencies in the light of the *Education Act* 1981 and the *Disabled Persons Act* 1986 (see appendix); the value of a range of credible and assessable services; and the imperative "to ensure by early planning that a seamless transition to adult services takes place". This latter is to facilitate the *Children Act* and the *National Health Service and Community Care Act* complementing each other.

Figure 18.3.1 *Planning strategy for children's services*

The following service initiatives should be in place in a comprehensive service for children:

- Information concerning diagnosis and prognosis given at the parents' pace, and repeated when necessary (see M. Plank, 1987, and *Shared Concern: Breaking the News to Parents that their Newborn Child has a Disability*, Kings Fund Video, 1987).
- Written information on local and national services (see P. Gilbert and J. Hollingdale, 1985).
- Information on parents' support groups and specialist societies.
- Primary health care team, with paediatric and other specialist back-up.
- Keyworker to co-ordinate assessment and service provision.
- Portage home teaching service.
- Integrated playgroup provision.
- Integrated education (see Education Act, 1981).
- Short-term care based on child care principles (see Oswin, 1984).

Transition

Most carers report a sense of crisis at the time their offspring leaves school: part of "the lost child lives on" syndrome (see Gilbert, 1985). There is a great necessity for the education authorities to communicate properly with parents and other agencies and not merely through the often cumbersome procedure of the statementing process.

Both the 1981 Education Act and the 1986 Disabled Persons Act place great emphasis on assessment of need and planning ahead. This is again a time when customers require access to detailed information to enable them to make informed choices. As the decade develops services will need to reflect the changing perspectives and expectations of school leavers.,

Preparation is required for both individuals and carers in the transition from the more protected world of schooling to the world outside. Sensitive but realistic discussion at this stage will pay dividends later on. Services offered could be further and adult education in integrated settings; vocational assessment and flexible care support and training as a natural successor to home teaching in childhood. Special attention at this time has to be paid to people with additional sensory impairments.

Adults

To have any meaning assessment has to be carried out in real, rather than artificial settings with an impetus towards achieving the aspirations that are held by an increasing number of people with learning difficulties. Recent research by the University of Kent reinforces the findings of other studies that "there is a substantial unmet demand" for paid work in either sheltered or open employment and that in terms of accommodation "many people aspired to a more independent life" (S. Le Touze and J. Pahl, 1990). Leisure opportunities and a social network with close friends was a real gap that was identified (see also chapter 3).

Day opportunities should include open employment; work/community care/training placements; sheltered employment; co-operative schemes; specialist activities (for example, horticulture); social education, in a broad sense, in integrated neighbourhood settings; adult education in local colleges and adult education centres; leisure and sporting opportunities in integrated centres; and supported befriending schemes.

While group home living has served a purpose for some people, it is not a lifestyle valued by many people in our society except perhaps college students, and is prone to the kind of personality clashes identified in the NIMROD research (see K. Lowe and S. de Parva, 1987). Living opportunities should include the possibility of a home of one's own; supported living; carer's home with intervention towards greater independence, or perhaps own home with a paid carer living in; small group-living; adult family placement, community living.

Elderly people

Support will be needed for both individuals and carers in another era of transition. Carers require specialist advice on legal and financial matters (see G. Sanctuary, 1985), while individuals should have an opportunity to retire but not be abandoned at a time when they and/or their carer(s) have need of skilled assistance. This is a time when bridges can be built towards an alternative living situation while parents are still able to give moral support. Counselling should be available at times of change and loss.

Figure 18.3.2: *A comprehensive service: A planned contact strategy*

AGE	LIAISON WITH OTHER AGENCIES IN ADDITION TO INDIVIDUALS AND CARERS
Birth/Diagnosis	Paediatrician and paediatric social worker Health Visitor
3 years	Paediatric service Health visitor Playgroup Educational psychologist
5 years	School (special or integrated)
13/14 years	School Special education counsellor - "Statement of education ability" (1981 Education Act) - First review of "level of disability" (1986 Disabled Persons Act)
18 years	School/further education Special education counsellor Careers service Multi-disciplinary school-leaver conference held to determine the key agencies for each young person
21 years	SEC, residential training centre, employment agency etc.
25 years	With relevant agencies to ensure appropriate services are in place and nobody has slipped through the net
50 years	And at two yearly intervals after that to forestall crises

(Derived from E. Wallace, 1989 and P. Gilbert, 1983)

Black and ethnic minority communities

Unfortunately, the need for cultural sensitivity is not a major feature of the Act and some directions are a late addition following case law (see R. White *et al*, 1990, p.61). Guidelines indicate that short-term care should be "compatible with the child's family background and culture, racial origin, religious persuasion and language". Agencies are still very poor at understanding cultural differences, however, and as one commentator has pointed out, research into the needs of ethnic minorities has often had a problem orientation and a "homogeneous categorisation" (Bandana Ahmed in B. Kahan ed, 1989). Ahmed quotes a poem by Margaret Parr ("Black and in care") whose middle stanzas are

Here I am in a black community
I've grown up "white" but they can't see.
Which do I turn to — white or black?
I daren't step forward, I can't step back,
Help me someone please
To find my culture and identity.

Carol Baxter and her colleagues (C. Baxter *et al*, 1990) reinforce Ahmed's point that, while we live in a multi-racial society most of the key literature on developing services ignores this fact. Most plans for people with learning difficulties at a national, regional and local level, state the authors: " . . . show a similarly 'colour blind' approach". The theory of "normalisation" which is the basis for much service development in the USA and UK, while a positive force, can also fall into the trap of making unwarranted assumptions as to what is "normal" or "valued" in society in general or in local communities.

Baxter *et al* quote three definitions of normalisation. The first is from Bank-Mikkelson (1969) which is people with learning difficulties having "an existence as close to normal as possible . . ." The second (Nirje, 1970) is about enabling people with learning difficulties to enjoy "patterns and conditions of everyday life which are as close as possible to the norms and patterns of the mainstream of society." Last is Wolfensberger's definition (1983): "The most explicit and highest goal of normalisation must be the creation, support and defence of valued social roles for people who are at risk of social devaluation."

But Baxter and her colleagues then pose three questions:

☐ "In our multicultural society, can professionals be sure that they know what is 'normal' or 'valued' for *all* their potential clients?

☐ "Can we be confident that service planners and managers, who are largely white, know how to interpret and implement the principles of normalisation in ways that are positive and meaningful for black and ethnic minority people with learning difficulties and their families — whose life circumstances and aspirations may differ fundamentally from their own?

☐ "If the goal of normalisation is to create and defend 'valued social roles for people who are at risk of social devaluation', how can we use these principles to challenge the dual devaluation experienced by black and ethnic minority people with learning difficulties in our society?"

Sudhaker's continuing research shows that service planners and managers are required to make a special effort to identify and meet the needs of different ethnic groups. Where this does not happen then whole cultural groups and the individual family units within them remain isolated. Baxter *et al* (chapter 4) give an example, in their section on respite care, of an Asian widow with a son with severe learning difficulties. Soon after her bereavement a social worker visited and offered a respite care placement for her son. The offer was refused because it was misinterpreted as an attempt to take the son away. No further offer or attempt to work together was made and the mother was left unsupported until a voluntary agency became involved four years later.

These individual experiences add up to a major gap in understanding and provision between planners, managers and cultural groups with special needs. C. Baxter *et al* recommend the following "checklist for action" for agencies to conduct a systematic approach:

The local black and ethnic minority population

get to know the *whole* community

demographic profile

contact with all local black and ethnic minority organisations

charting unmet need

engaging staff from minority groups or key people to articulate needs

Current services

ascertain whether they reflect the needs and concerns of the local black and ethnic minority communities

ensure policies, procedures and practices are flexible and responsive

gauge social and physical accessibility

monitor take-up

staff reflecting multi-racial make-up of the community

multi-racial groups of users and carers

Racism

clear policy on racial prejudice

commitment to changing attitudes

changing practices to avoid imposing white, professional norms and values

Communication

employing trained interpreters and bilingual staff and advocates

target information in relevant languages and using the appropriate media

set up home-liaison services

Activities and curricula

curricula to reflect the everyday customs and practices of black and ethnic minority people

single sex activities provided, as appropriate

assessment procedures to be relevant to the everyday life of other cultures — activities to positively reflect and cater for black and ethnic minority leisure pursuits

links with local ethnic minority employers and organisations so to promote employment and activity opportunities

Everyday care

accent on individual needs and preferences

catering for dietary requirements

religious requirements attended to

agencies to adopt formal anti-racist and racial equality policies
local black and ethnic minority organisations to be active participants in policy formation and change
awareness of and commitment by all staff to the policy
senior management responsibility and a specific action plan to target change.

Challenging behaviour

Cultural sensitivity is of prime importance in the area of challenging behaviour. Where individuals are dysfunctioning to a great extent the dangers of misunderstanding and cultural alienation are at their greatest. This is particularly significant with most authorities reporting growing numbers of people with challenging behaviour moving into adult life.

The impact of the policy of hospital closures, and the steady growth of alternative services in the community, means that people with challenging behaviour are increasingly found in community-based services. Similarly people with behavioural problems living with their families, are less likely to be admitted to hospital as these limit admissions as part of reducing their services, and this is also increasing the number of people with challenging behaviour present in community services.

Challenging behaviour has been defined as " . . . behaviour of such intensity, frequency, or duration that the physical safety of the person or others is likely to be placed in serious jeopardy, or behaviour which is likely to seriously limit or deny access to the use of ordinary facilities" Emerson *et al*, (1988).

The numbers of people who require services can be based on estimates from findings in a Bristol study (Russell and Hall 1980). This study suggested that among adults with a learning difficulty, seven per cent of those living with families compared with 18 per cent among those in residential care had severe behaviour disorder. Extrapolating from the Bristol figures Maher and Russell (1988) suggest within a population of 100,000 there would be 10 children and 30 adults exhibiting behavioural disturbance on a daily basis.

Reporting on services for people with learning difficulties who have additional special probems the DHSS (1984) stated that, although there had been a substantial advance in the development of knowledge and skills in services generally, the position for people with additional behavioural handicaps had been slow.

The report stated that there was growing awareness on the part of managers of the importance of ensuring that people with behaviour handicaps are included in the progress now being made in services as a whole. Managers responsible for services need to develop policies that enable people with these problems to be helped in ways that meet individual needs, but also safeguard the person's rights. Providing services for people whose behaviour presents particular problems requires planning that is based on clearly thought out approaches. People with challenging behaviour can present unique problems to staff, who need support in constructing appropriate strategies for meeting needs.

The Special Development Team at the University of Kent has described a model of intervention that has demonstrated that high quality services can be offered to people with challenging behaviour (McCool *et al*, 1989). Central to their approach like much good practice reported elsewhere, is through the system of individual planning. The work of the Special Development Team has focussed on supporting services that are responding to a person's needs and assisting those services develop detailed and comprehensive intervention techniques. Similarly Maher and Russell (1988) are also firmly committed to a community-based model of service provision that nevertheless recognizes that there will be occasions when challenging behaviour cannot be managed at home, or fellow residents will no longer tolerate someone damaging their environment. Here the lack of comprehensive services may mean, where it still exists, admission to hospital. To provide support for families and services Maher and Russell describe a mobile workforce of staff who can assist, supplement and if necressary take over in the person's own environment, in order to avoid admission to a special unit or secure facility.

This approach has been seen as an alternative to the small special unit (DHSS, 1984), which provides an environment which is secure and offers facilities that provide a wide range of resources, and segregates residents from other living situations where their behaviour may have adverse effects on other people. Although these units may appear an attractive service alternative when staff are unable to cope with challenging behaviour in community settings, they have many disadvantages.

Particular problems (DHSS 1984) include, the small number of people needing such services and the resulting large catchment area with risks of dislocating the person from their local community staff becoming professionally isolated and inward looking. Once people are referred to such units they may find it difficult to move back into more integrated services. Lastly, is the risk that the existence of such units may lead to the tendency to refer all people who are "difficult" as an easy option rather than consider what other ordinary non-specialist services could be provided. Special units as a policy response could repeat the problems that hospitals experienced, with people living in environments that restrict their freedom, and separate them from valued experiences, and where the opportunity to learn skills in the least restrictive possible setting is denied.

People with challenging behaviour are increasingly less likely to be admitted to hospital, and as a consequence community-based services need to develop comprehensive alternatives so that people can be managed in ordinary settings. Special units may appeal as an institutional solution, but their weaknesses make services in ordinary settings the logical answer. To convince concerned parents, and staff in residential and day settings, means having the service structures described by McCool and her colleagues, and Maher and Russell. This would enable families and staff to feel confident that the service can respond to the needs of the person with challenging behaviour and support them in helping the person continue to use ordinary services, rather than risk segregation.

B. Ahmed (1989), "Child care and ethnic minorities", in B. Kahan ed., *Child Care Research, Policy and Practice,* Hodder and Stoughton.

Audit Commission (1987), *Personal Social Services for People with a Mental Handicap,* Audit Guide.

N.E. Bank-Mikkelson (1969), *Changing Patterns in Residential Services for the Mentally Retarded.* President's Commission on Mental Retardation, Washington DC.

BASW (1989), *Not So Much a Programme, More a Way of Life,* British Association of Social Workers.

C. Baxter, K. Poonia, L. Ward and Z. Nadirshaw (1990), *Double Discrimination: Issues for People with Learning Difficulties from Black and Ethnic Minority Communities,* King's Fund Centre/Commission for Racial Equality.

E. Byrne in E. Byrne, C. Cunningham and P. Sloper (1988), *Families and their Children with Down's Syndrome,* Routledge.

A. and D. Brandon (1987), *Consumers as Colleagues,* MIND.

M. Craft, J. Bicknell and S. Hollins (1985), *Mental Handicap: A Multidisciplinary Approach,* Bailliere Tindall.

I. Cocking and S. Athwal (1990). "A special case for special treatment", *Social Work Today,* 8 February.

D. Cooper and J. Hersov (1986), *We Can Change the Future,* NBHS.

H. Davis and P. A. Choudhury, "Helping Bangladeshi families", in A. Brechin and J. Walmsley (1989), *Making Connections,* Hodder and Stoughton.

Department of Health and Social Security (1984), *Helping Mentally Handicapped People with Special Problems,* HMSO.

Department of Health (1991), *The Children Act 1989 Guidance and Regulations, Volume 6, Children with Disabilities,* HMSO.

E. Emmerson, R. Cummings, S. Barrett, H. Hughes, C. McCool, A. Toogood, (1988), "Challenging behaviour and community services: 2. Who are the people who challenge services?" *Mental Handicap,* Vol 16, March.

P. Gilbert and J. Hollingdale (1985), *Coping with Mental Handicap in Horsham, Crawley and Mid Sussex,* West Sussex County

Council.
P. Gilbert (1985), *Mental Handicap: A Practical Guide for Social Workers, Community Care*/Reed Business Publishing.
P. Gilbert (1983), "New services, new strategies", *Community Care,* 31 March.
S. Hatch and T. Hinton (1986) *Self Help in Practice,* University of Sheffield/*Community Care.*
J. Hogg *et al,* "Ageing and mental handicap" in A. Leighton ed. (1988), *Mental Handicap in the Community,* Woodhead Faulkner.
S. Hollins and M. Grimer (1988), *Going Somewhere,* SPCK.
IDC (1982), *Elements of a Comprehensive Local Service for People with a Mental Handicap,* Independent Development Council.
S. Le Touze and J. Pahl (1990), *A Survey among People with Learning Disabilities,* Kent County Council/University of Kent.
K. Lowe and S. De Parva (1987), *Canvassing the Views of People with Mental Handicap,* Mental Handicap in Wales Applied Research Unit.'
J. Maher, and O. Russell (1988), "Serving people with challenging behaviour", in D. Towell (ed) *An Ordinary Life in Practice,* King Edward's Hospital Fund for London.
C. McCool, S. Barrett, E. Emmerson, S. Toogood, H. Hughes, R. Cummings, (1989) "Challenging behaviour: 5, Structuring staff and client activity, *Mental Handicap,* Vol 17, June.
MENCAP, *Care in the Community,* Stamina Paper No. 7. 1986.
NCH (1991), *Sharing the Caring,* National Children's Home.
B. Nirje (1970), "The normalisation principle — Implications and comments", *British Journal of Mental Subnormality* 16.
V. Nzirz (1989), "Race: The ingredients for good practice", in T. Philpot ed., *The Residential Opportunity, Community Care*/Reed Business Publishing.
M. Oswin (1981), *Bereavement and Mentally Handicapped People,* King's Fund.
M. Oswin (1984), *They Keep Going Away,* King's Fund/OUP.
J. Pahl and L. Quine (1984), *Families with Mentally Handicapped Children: A Study of Stress and Service Response,* University of Kent.
M. Plank (1987), *Begin at the Beginning,* Campaign for Mentally Handicapped People (now Values into Action).
G. Sanctuary (1985), *After I'm Gone,* Souvenir Press.
O. Russell and V. Hall (1980), *Mental Handicap and Functional Disability: A Survey of Disablement of Mentally Handicapped People in One Health District. Research Report No.6,* Mental Health Department, University of Bristol.
P. Russell (1991), "A better working relationship", INSIDE supplement, *Community Care,* 26 September.
C. Robinson (1988), "Pride and prejudice, *Mental Handicap* Vl 16, December.

A. Shearer (undated), *A Community Service for Mentally Handicapped Children*, Barnardo Social Work Paper No. 4.
A. Shearer (1986), *Building Community*, King's Fund/Campaign for Mentally Handicapped People (now Values into Action).
D. Sines ed (1988), *Towards Integration: Comprehensive Services for People with Mental Handicaps*, Harper & Row.
S. Sudhaker (forthcoming research thesis on the needs of Asian families in the UK).
L. Ward (1982), *People First: Developing Services in the Community*, King's Fund Project Paper No. 37.
R. White *et al* (1990), *A Guide to the Children Act 1989*, Butterworths.
W. Wolfensberger (1982), "Social role valorisation: A proposed new term for the principle of normalisation", *Mental Retardation*, December.

19

Integrating services

"Unfortunately the present management arrangements do not promote the essential integrated service and operational planning . . . The structure of local community-based services is confused, with responsibility and accountability . . . fragmented."
The Audit Commission, (1986)

"Bureaucracies are not about doing things. They are about explaining why they couldn't be done in the first place!"
Sir John Banham, director-general of the CBI

The Audit Commission (1986) severely criticised the organisational fragmentation of care services. One of its diagrams depicted the principal agencies involved in community care (reproduced in Figure 1.3.2. in this book) - a maze of interlocking lines. "These services", the commission stated "must 'mesh' if community care is to work."

The commission highlighted a number of barriers to the effective delivery of services. Responsibility and accountability for elements of the services are fragmented between different tiers of the NHS and local government. Joint planning arrangements are complex and time-consuming. There are very different styles and ways of thinking between different organisations. There are few incentives to encourage co-operation in planning. Regional health authorities "have only a limited contact with local authorities and they play a more direct role in the closure of hospitals than in the build up of alternatives in the community." There is a perverse incentive towards residential care through DSS benefits and the obligations on local managers to support services they have no control over. There are widely differing priorities within each agency, eg, acute services for the NHS and child protection for SSDs. The commission also cited overlapping roles of staff from various agencies, and the "culture shock" between agencies.

Since 1982 health authorities have operated the Griffiths style of devolved general management, whereas local authority managers must look over their shoulders to see which way their local councillors are inclining - or some would say "wobbling" in the wind of public opinion!

In an attempt to tackle this tangle of confusion the commission recommended that, first, people with learning difficulties and physical disabilities should be the responsibility of the local authorities except those who require "medical supervision". There should be a transfer of resources. Second, people with a mental illness should primarily be the responsibility of the NHS which would buy-in social care services from SSDs. Third, services for elderly people should be under the control of a single manager in each locality with a budget provided from NHS and SSD funds.

When the Audit Commission published its Occasional Paper No. 4 in November 1987, it singled out three authorities - Hillingdon, Somerset (see below) and West Sussex (see chapter 2) - where health and social service authorities had reached agreement over service direction. It also affirmed that "the first step should be the integration of the service".

In 1989 the commission's survey of local authorities' services in the learning difficulty field found that 60 per cent had no agreed joint strategy with their health service counterparts. As the hospitals run down the pressure on the health authorities coping with the most dependent people left in the long-stay hospitals, and on local authorities not equipped to cope with those who would have received NHS care in the past, has become acute.

In an effort to react positively to the 1986 report a number of authorities developed specific organisational models along four main lines.

- *Lead agency model.* A single agency steers and develops the new service, but not in isolation from the other agencies involved. The lead agency is responsible for budgets and resources overall, and may buy in resources from other agencies (*à la* Griffiths). There may be full or partial transfer of funding (most usually from health authority to social services), accompanied by a contract detailing the conditions of transfer. Overall management of the service will be by the lead agency. (Examples: Brighton HA/East Sussex SSD Foremost scheme, Hillingdon MESH).
- *Multi-agency model.* Different parts of the service are run by different agencies, with separate management and financial accountability but in accordance with an agreed joint plan. Responsibility for different services and categories of client are clearly defined between the agencies involved. There is broad collaborative consensus, but each agency also has its own agenda (Example: Plymouth HA/Devon SSD (West).
- *Joint agency model.* Agencies operate together (for example, by appointing a joint service manager) and accountability for a jointly agreed set of services is shared. Financial resources are to all intents and purposes pooled (Example: Isle of Wight).
- *Semi-independent agency model.* A third party organisation (typically a private company or charitable body) takes responsibility for service delivery, including management and financial accountability, according to criteria set by the statutory agencies involved. Funds are transferred by the responsible statutory authorities (Example: Bexley SSD).

The alternative to these four models is a pluralistic agency model, in which separate agencies deliver separate services without necessarily having commonly agreed goals and principles, ie *not* a joint service.

Throughout this chapter when we reflect on a number of practice models it is important to bear in mind some of the injunctions that management writers like Peters and Waterman have made about organisations (see chapter 6) eg, that they should have a "lean, fit" management structure, be "tight" on essential values but "loose" to allow management autonomy, and they should "stick to the knitting" - ie, do what they are good at and not attempt to be all things to all people.

Ticket to Ryde? — A joint agency model on the Isle of Wight

In the late 1970s planning for learning difficulty services was merely part of a wider mental health planning group. Current managers recall that it was shortly after a specialist sub-group had been set up that a health authority manager presented a proposition to close the long-stay hospitals and set up in their stead an 80-bedded unit. It was a reaction against this proposal that sent the members of the planning group off to Cardiff to view the NIMROD service and produce in June 1982 a policy document which proposed the establishment of an inter-agency management team; a plan for CMHT development over three areas; devolved services to be set up on a localised basis; services to offer a range of options to service users; and a pilot project set up in the Ryde area.

Moving towards a joint service

Following the policy statement the joint management group was established consisting of the community unit manager (health) and community service manager, the deputy director and assistant director (SSD), the chairperson of MENCAP and the manager of the joint service (appointed 1987). This was designed to be at the right level to formulate policy and financial decisions, but in retrospect JMG members believe it would have been wise to include the director of social services and the district general manager.

Between 1982 and 1987 long-stay mental handicap hospitals on the island were closed — St. Mary's (55 beds), Longford (40 beds) and Castle View (25 beds for children only) - and residents transferred to community units or ordinary housing. Capital was released from the closures but although the island planners were committed to ordinary housing and an eventual transfer of responsibility and resources to social services, the regional health authority was wedded to local hospital units and had no system for the transfer of monies via the dowry system.

Despite Wessex Region's health-orientated approach, the mid-1980s saw a momentum towards a single-agency model which came to a juddering halt over the cost of service transfer which would have meant both agencies finding an additional £100,000 a year to satisfactorily transfer NHS staff into the social services. In 1987 a joint manager was appointed to conduct both services in tandem, and shortly afterwards the group homes were transferred to MENCAP Homes Foundation so as to take advantage of the DSS allowances in the independent sector.

Current service provision

Notwithstanding a "lean/fit" command structure, the Isle of Wight is proud of its ability both to set up services and develop them in response to the challenge of change.

In residential terms services range from support in people's own or family home (with each CMHT having a small budget to buy in support, plus sitting, tucking-in and laundry services), to ordinary housing schemes, staffed houses, residential training units etc. The CMHTs with their care programmes devised around individual needs, local knowledge and support budget, have combined some of the best features of the Care Management and multi-disciplinary approaches. Children's services offer support in the home, link families and residential short term care when needed.

Day care has developed from the day hospital (health) and large adult training centre (social services) to a very flexible, individualised service where users have options in further and adult education, therapeutic rehabilitation, open employment and sheltered work. Nowadays only about 40 people attend the 100 place Medina Centre in Newport, while a number of limited companies are being developed to tap into local industries. There are active voluntary groups and local support and a developing self-advocacy movement.

Current challenges

Although a market leader a few years ago the Isle of Wight service has now hit a few snags. As in so many things local managers seem to have to expend their greatest ingenuity trying to double-guess the intentions of central government.

The JMG believes there are four challenges. First, the DHA feels that they've "done their bit". The targets in the original plan have been met and there is little recognition of the new needs now surfacing. Second, most of the financial savings made by the housing transfer to MENCAP have been siphoned off to meet the demands of the new district general hospital and the acute sector. Third, MENCAP are finding a tension between their traditional advocacy and their new provider roles. The management strain on a small infrastructure is stressful and they are frustrated at the clawback of financial savings into acute medicine - only £15-20,000 was retained for the service out of about £200,000 savings. Last, the joint service leaves too many different groups of staff on varying grades who leapfrog each other as the various pay awards and regradings come into force.

Proposals for the future

To respond to the challenge the island is considering setting up a new company which would have staff seconded to it with protected conditions of pay, but new staff would come in on one of a small number of grades based on specific levels of responsibility. Bricks and mortar would be managed by a housing trust.

A higher level of revenue would be aimed for than at present with surpluses ploughed back into service development.

In the spring of 1990 financial and management officers were seconded by both authorities to work out the steps towards a new agency arrangement. The lesson the JMG members stressed was: be innovative but at the same time be quite clear about contractual agreements.

Hillingdon - leading the way

When Ian White, the former director of social services, spoke of the Hillingdon prototype at a CCETSW conference in 1986, he was disarmingly modest about the scale of Hillingdon's achievement in producing a coherent service for people with learning difficulties and their carers in this outer London borough (see Francis 1987a). Part of the impetus appears to have come from an acknowledgement by the health authority that without the encumbrance of a long-stay hospital within its boundaries and a much smaller service component for this client group than their social services counterparts, it was sensible for social services to run the entire service.

Hillingdon had other advantages: coterminous agency boundaries; good working relations at all levels between DHA and SSD; nurses already shedding some of their traditional roles, and social services valuing their skills; and considerable investment in learning dificulty services by the SSD over many years.

No such change is ever easy and it took 18 months of careful negotiation before the agreement was signed in a public ceremony. The transfer of staff within a relatively small area with previous close working appears to have been far more successful than in the case of Somerset (see below) where there were long-stay hospitals and a considerable change of emphasis for staff. When Peter Gilbert met members of Hillingdon's CMHTs in 1988 he found them very positive about the changes, and as Francis (1987a) put it: "The benefits to clients are clear: there is one door rather than two and the people behind it know exactly what is available and where, rather than having to liaise with another body."

Making it work

When Brunel University undertook an independent evaluation of the mental handicap services in Hillingdon (MESH), it found that first, with hindsight some of the legal delays could have been overcome. Second, different NHS/SSD accounting systems are problematic in service transfers. Third, the transfer of staff requires considerable personnel expertise. Fourth, communication between agencies, and, with consumers, carers and staff needs to be continuous (See E. Spencer and I. Macdonald, 1990).

According to Hillingdon (personal communication with the authors and conference at Wye College, 12 March 1990) these difficulties are being worked through and the major strength of the lead agency model is that now planning is simpler and more effective; the service has a single manager with increased speed of decision-making and better communication; and the service has a unified value base and a common agenda.

The manager for the service is part of the social services departmental management team but also has direct access to the district general manager. Money for the service has been ringfenced and neither authority has creamed money off for more "glamorous" priorities.

Somerset – A pilot project

The Somerset Mental Handicap Strategy was launched in 1985 as one of the DHSS-sponsored Care in the Community demonstration programmes, specially funded between 1984-88 (see Chris Smith *et al* in P. Cambridge and M. Knapp 1988, and Francis, 1987b).

Somerset SSD and DHA had largely coterminous boundaries; a director of social services (John Chant) with a personal commitment to developing learning difficulty services; a good working relationship (officers from both authorities shared the same building in Taunton); and a history of placing residents from the three long-stay hospitals into community settings (see Dorothy Atkinson's research in chapter 3).

In November 1985 they produced a joint strategy document which gave a lead role to social services. As the district general manager pointed out (Francis, 1987b): "There really is no point in running services side by side. It inevitably creates conflicts and grey areas. If people are going to be looked after in the community, then that is Social Services' job."

The plans involved the closure of all three hospitals by 1995, with the movement of 355 long-stay residents with a budget of £4.8m, plus £60,000 a year development money for the years 1985-95. The service model was for there to be a "core and cluster" network set up in each of the ten social service team areas and under a single community care manager. In 1986 a joint management team was established to oversee service development and later a series of policy reviews investigating the needs of service users and carers in *separate* studies so as not to confuse what could be two very different agendas.

When Alison Wertheimer, former director of CMH, visited Somerset in 1988 she was impressed by the way that "staff ... talked a lot about working with individuals not for 'a service' such as a day centre". Self-advocacy was very much part of the picture (Wertheimer, 1988).

One major stumbling block has been the conditions of service in the new model and although many of the problems have been ironed out, with nursing qualifications recognised and trades union representatives added to the JMT, senior nurses have still been reluctant to apply for community-based posts. Possible reasons may include marginally inferior local authority salaries; no enhanced payments for unsocial hours; and disincentives associated with status. (Local authority posts may not be viewed as prestigious as those in NHS.)

But while the strategy fell behind schedule in 1987-8 because of industrial troubles, by the end of 1988-9 it had exceeded its target with 163 people leaving hospital and entering the scheme (JMT progress report).

Current Challenges

First, cost increases in NHS facilities due to the diseconomies of scale have meant a rise in unit costs from £17-£35,000 per bed. Only 50 per cent of variable costs are released until whole units are closed, whereas the maximum demand for funds is in the middle of the transition period. The second challenge concerns the difficulties in attracting qualified staff (see below). The third challenge for staff is as service users "expect more out of life" and "expect more out of their support" (C. Smith *et al*).

Service Groups - Integrated services at a local level

While the Audit Commission has, since 1986, been urging a greater integration of the different agencies involved in providing care in the community, one of the major stumbling blocks has been the lack of managerial integration within the different authorities themselves.

In 1986 the London Borough of Merton moved from a traditional model where there were fieldwork team leaders and residential home advisers to one where day, residential and fieldwork services (social workers, occupational therapists and so on) were managed in specialist service groups.

This had the considerable advantage of a single manager, with a devolved budget and good information systems, being able to draw services together to produce packages of care adjusted to individual needs. The grouping of different elements gave a considerable flexibility - what Napoleon called the "orde mixée". The fact that Merton's personal services department contained both housing and social services under one directorate and in the same locality offices also helped in the formulation of community programmes.

Structures after the NHS & Community Care Act

Ironically the rediscovery of specialist work in many social services departments in the late 1980s will be radically altered by the White Paper of November 1990, *Caring for People: Community Care in the Next Decade and Beyond,* and the consequent NHS and Community Care Act. The White Paper placed a very clear emphasis on separating the management of services that the local authority provides from those that carry out the purchasing function. This gets away from the collusion which could easily operate if purchasers and providers were managed by the same person (see N. Warner, 1990(b)).

The kind of organisational structure which Kent SSD is moving into in 1990 looks superficially as though it is a return to the earlier "functional" model which prevailed immediately after the 1971 Seebohm reorganisation. In fact, however, the integration of services results from the aggregation of care managers' individual assessments and service packages in a "bottom up" integration - rather than it being imposed by management from above. Both health and social service authorities will have a "commissioning" role from 1993, that is, buying services from the independent sector and their own provision to meet the needs identified by the care purchasers. Internal provision will need to be inspected by the same inspection units which apply a uniform standard to the independent sector and managed as "direct service organisations", contracting with the commissioning unit to "provide a certain volume of service of an agreed quality and at an agreed price" (N. Warner, 1990(b)). This should provide a demonstration of cost-effectiveness to counter allegations of preferential treatment for the in-house providers.

Housing associations are more likely to take on the management of the "bricks and mortar" of local authority and NHS provision, though most associations themselves have expressed reservations against taking on the care element as they are no more care experts than social and health services are housing experts.

The keys to success

Many people probably feel like the Roman soldier and writer Petronius when he wrote:

> "We trained hard - but it seemed that every time we were beginning to form up into teams we would be reorganised . . .

I was to learn later in life that we tend to meet any new situation by reorganising, and a wonderful method it can be for creating the illusion of progress while producing confusion, inefficiency and demoralisation."

The health service has experienced the advent of general management and the abolition of area health authorities. From 1991 the district health authorities, which were given many of the area functions, will find themselves too small to carry out the commissioning role envisaged by the acute sector White Paper *Working for Patients,* and some sort of area authority may need to be restored.

The Audit Commission and Sir Roy Griffiths saw distinctly the need for clear accountability between the agencies and simplified structures. In his *Agenda for Action,* Sir Roy stated: "I emphasise responsibilities; collaboration, joint planning, joint finance are admirable provided that in the first place responsibilities are clear and, in the absence of collaboration, authorities can be held accountable. Of course, this would be helped by restructuring at the local level with health authorities, social services authorities and family practitioner committees enjoying co-terminosity, or even being brought within a common structure. To make restructuring mandatory would be enormously disruptive and would create turmoil under a semblance of action. I believe that there is a diversity of response at local level which is appropriate and would be forthcoming in the planning system proposed. Some clarification has inevitably, however difficult the task, to be sought between the role of health authorities and social services authorities."

Unfortunately the White Paper *Caring for People* did not adequately clarify the roles and responsibilities of health and social services, and much of the message was one in tune with the *laissez faire* economic theory of the government think tanks (see chapter 6 of *Caring for People*). In the event the result may either be greater diversity or more chaos as no one is left with the responsibility for a long-term view.

The schemes portrayed in this chapter are only some of many that have been developed across the country in an attempt to provide organisational coherence and accountability. In Bexley a consortium was established from health and social services provision. Press coverage suggested that this particular scheme ran into difficulties ("The perils of Griffiths", *Social Work Today,* 29 March 1990) and was fortunate to be bailed out financially. One particular lesson is that the health authorities do not have the same flexibility to raise additional income as service demands change, and the central government allocation for inflation tends to be substantially lower than reality.

Plymouth DHA and the West Devon division of social services have developed a successful multi-agency strategy with a wide consultation of interests on its joint management group. Conversely, East Devon division and Exeter DHA have developed a looser planning structure based on identified needs in six separate localities. Clwyd also has local planning groups involving service users alongside local managers and carers' representatives (G. Harper, 1988). Fortunately, the All Wales Strategy gave Clwyd four years to develop community services *before* the long-stay hospital run-down began.

The keys to success would appear to be a number of factors. These are strong and committed "champions of change" (Audit Commission) in both mainstream authorities and the independent sector; a shared vision and clear objectives; identification of a model which suits local conditions; and a focus on action following sound planning. There are also integrated management arrangements; and an ability to change tactically in response to environmental changes (for example, changes in benefit rules) without sacrificing the essential values of the scheme. Last, there has to be attention to consumer choice and individual needs; and partnership between statutory and voluntary organisations.

Conclusion

When Aneurin Bevan introduced the National Health Service Bill to the House of Commons in April 1946, he stated: "Our hospital system has grown up with no plan, with no system; it is unevenly distributed over the country."

The greatly expanded range of choices open to people with learning difficulties and their carers and the examples of good practice at an organisational and practice level demonstrate that there is no lack of imagination and practical application in community care services.

When Judy Renshaw *et al* (1988) considered the DHSS pilot projects their conclusion was hopeful but they also cautioned that: "The stickiest problem for the future is perhaps that bright examples of innovation and enterprise remain outnumbered by others which exhibit a singular blend of confusion and inertia. The continuing challenge for public policy, therefore, is to find effective means of harnessing the talent and goodwill of those resourceful individuals and agencies who - given the opportunity - have proved they can make care in the community a reality."

The question, perhaps, is whether central government will give this radical restructuring of services the time and finances to work or whether its best option at a time of growing demand and limited resources is to keep moving the goalposts and changing the rules so that both players and spectators are confused and the rule-makers don't get the blame if the game doesn't work out!

Despite the general satisfaction with local government services (*Which?* report, March 1989) - "key services such as education and social services attracted high levels of satisfaction among people who'd used them" - there is a suspicion that the government is only using local authorities as a "temporary home and potential scapegoat for community care" ("From the front line", *Insight,* 11 April 1990). The government may well abolish county councils and if there hadn't been conflict with GPs over their contracts then primary care might have been where community care would have been located.

Watchdog organisations like the Independent Development Council have already begun to warn that learning difficulty services are sinking in the priority ranking list (IDC, *Cinderellas Again? The Impact of Current National Policies on Opportunities and Services Available Locally to People with Learning Difficulties and Their Families,* IDC, January 1990) and the National Development Team has pointed out that for the market to deliver the goods and not to descend into Dickensian chaos, a complex set of relationships must be created and nurtured.

Specifically, the government will need to work on its own service integration and create a framework where one department (for example, the DSS) is not undercutting the policy of another (for example, the DoH).

Even more than before, the 1990s will see a need for leaders (D. Towell, 1988) to orchestrate the vision of new services; gain and maintain support for the vision; stimulate effective action at all levels of the organisation and across the interface of different agencies; make change stick; and continue, as one statesman maintained, to aspire to a state of things which we know can never be fully attained but which we must never cease to strive for.

Audit Commission reports (1986, 1987 and 1988) see reading list in chapter 1 for details.

Association of County Councils (1990), *Caring for People: Meeting the Challenge.*

BIMH (1981), *Making Things Happen: Top Management and the Mental Handicap Services.*

P. Cambridge and M. Knapp (1988), *Demonstrating Successful Care in the Community,* PSSRU/UKC.

M. Craft, J. Bicknell, S. Hollins ed (1985), *Mental Handicap: A Multi-Disciplinary Approach,* Balliere Tindall, Part I.

W. Francis (1987a), "Making services mesh", *Community Care,* 13 August.

W. Francis (1987b), "Setting wheels in motion", *Community Care,* 27 August.

G. Harper, "Community-led service planning", *Community Living,* March/April 1988.

P. Healy ed (1989), *Innovatory Management Practice in Social Services Departments,* Local Government Training Board.

MENCAP Stamina Paper No. 8 (1987), *Better Joint Planning.*

J. Renshaw et al (1988), *Care in the Community: The First Steps,*

Gower.
E. Spencer and I. MacDonald (1990), *MESH: A Report of the Development of Services in Hillingdon*, Brunel University.
D. Towell (1988), "Managing strategic change", in D. Towell ed. *An Ordinary Life in Practice*, King's Fund.
N. Warner(a), paper to Social Services Inspectorate conference, 18 January 1990.
N. Warner, "Kent hops to it", *Insight*, 31 January 1990 (b).
"Town hall ratings", *Which?* report, March 1989.
A. Wertheimer, "Leaving long-stay hospitals", INSIDE supplement, *Community Care*, 27 October 1987.

Parents speaking (2)

"The daily grind"

"With our other children it was different. Helen and James were often bloody, but I knew they would grow out of it. With Frankie it's different, the problems go on and on."
Mother talking to Peter Gilbert

"He has been throwing things at the electric light and breaking many other things in the house. He is shouting and waking the neighbour's baby."
quoted in Elizabeth Browne, *Mental Handicap: The Role for Social Workers, Community Care*/University of Sheffield, 1982

"There are no myths about the maddening eternity of babydom, the suffocating effect of constant need. And of course, I can talk about what this life is like for me, for our family. Sometimes I tell it to professionals, always well-meaning, who offer advice but have no idea what my family life is really like."
Fern Kupfer, *op cit*

"I can maybe have a good day, but if you had caught me yesterday I could have just sat down and cried all day long . . . It's there every minute of the day, you just can't get it out of your mind."
quoted in Caroline Glendinning, *Unshared Care: Parents and Their Disabled Children*, RKP, 1983

"He won't stop in bed, he is in and out of bed all night, so he's been sleeping with my husband, and I sleep in his bed."
quoted in M. Bayley, *Mental Handicap and Community Care*, RKP, 1973

"He cries invariably, and it makes it more difficult. It's so much better if he doesn't cry for me. Just occasionally he doesn't and then it's terrific . . . I feel it's a shame that when I get him up the first thing I do is to brutalize him."
quoted in Lindy Burton, *The Family Life of Sick Children*, RKP, 1975

Daily joys and changing perspectives

"This is not a path we would have chosen, but it has brought unexpected joys. It has increased the quality and dimension of our lives and we live in the certain knowledge that she is a whole and complete person in the eyes of God."
quoted in P. Gilbert *et al*, *We are One People*, Diocese of Arundel and Brighton, 1988

"I think she is really funny. She makes you laugh. It's funny. I'm very reserved. I am not a toucher and yet with her it doesn't bother me, but sometimes it does with the others . . . She hates it when I shout at her. It really upsets her. Then she'll say, 'Come and give me a love, I'm sorry', and so you have to give her a cuddle then, you know, so that everything's alright . . . She's great really."
quoted in E. Byrne *et al, op cit*

"I've re-evaluated what is important. Before, I would have thought that someone with little academic ability was less of a person."
E. Byrne et al, *op cit*

"After being told one's child would be a 'lovable cabbage', I watched her swim and wanted to shout that even one small talent can achieve something, and that our children can give something back, however small."
quoted in A. Worthington, *Coming to Terms with Mental Handicap,* Helena Press, 1982

Relations with professionals

"He [the doctor] explained that doctors were taught not to tell parents, but to respond to questions; in the post-natal period there is a danger of the mother rejecting the baby, and it is better to wait until bonds are formed. So did it have to be eight months? Did he have to duck the task of telling me and let it all happen so impersonally, without preparation? . . . Did he not realise that he was dealing with an intelligent and self-sufficient person who had struggled for months rather than run for help? . . . I felt increasingly angry and let down. Doctors pay dearly for losing a patient's trust."
Francis Young, *op cit*

"I felt really heartened when I came down to Sussex and the manager of the training centre gave me a social services booklet on what's available to handicapped people in the local area. It was really encouraging to see that people had taken the trouble. It was like a real hand of friendship."
Parent talking to Peter Gilbert about a social services information handbook

"I am a little bit against generic social work, because it is far too much to expect any one person to remember all the facilities appertaining to all the various groups in the community. You'd have to have a head like Einstein to remember everything . . . It will be better to have specialised social workers for specialised needs."

"We've often found that we are better informed than the social worker."
quoted in Caroline Glendinning, *op cit*

"She (the health visitor) was a nice lady, but she was in a tizz as much as I was, that was the time I most needed someone."

"She's [the health visitor] great, makes sure I get everything I need."

"He's (the social worker) a decent bloke. He's available and he gives his time. He's helped us to get grants and benefits."

"She (the portage home teacher) taught me how to teach, how to break tasks down, and she came every week."

"I can never get hold of her (the social worker), and when I do it's too late."

"You knew you weren't alone."
quoted in E. Byrne, *op cit*

"All social workers should equip themselves with more knowledge of mentally handicapped children to enable *sound* advice to be given."
quoted in P. Gilbert, *Mental Handicap; A Practical Guide for Social Workers, Community Care,* 1985

Relations with other parents

"The biggest support is other mums. You must have a mentally handicapped child to understand and really know the thoughts and problems a mother has."
"I tend to steer clear of parents with handicapped children, which is a bit weird, but I think if you are living with the problem, why make your life revolve around other people's handicapped children . . . I think the best thing is to lead as normal an existence as possible."
quoted in E. Byrne et al, *op cit*

"My social worker is helpful, but I tend to get information quicker from other parents. It was one of the mums who told me about how to get hold of a maxi-buggy during one of the playgroup coffee mornings."
Mother talking to Peter Gilbert

20

Community mental handicap teams and beyond

"The families themselves are the first and best resource a child can have . . . the family must therefore be assisted to do all they can to improve their child's functioning and development ... support can best be developed by the operation of a multi-disciplinary community mental handicap team drawing its personnel from both the NHS and local authorities."
National Development Group (1977)

"Multi-disciplinary teams have the advantage of putting different skills and perspectives to work on a problem, thus enabling a fuller picture of the individual to emerge, including their needs and possible solutions."

J. Renshaw *et al* (1988)

The impetus towards multi-disciplinary teams

When the Court committee on child health services reported (1976) its findings showed that most parents experienced a lack of service cohesion. It discovered:

- "Parents . . . find the existing pattern of services confusing."
- "There is a prevailing but unacceptable lack of urgency in providing adequate assessment in the community."
- "Parents understandably want a single door leading to assessment, explanation and treatment."
- "They [parents] need a co-ordinated service of care, therapy and education, with regular reviews of the child's progress leading to advice and support."

A year later the policy team set up by the government, the National Development Group stated that, in its view: "Domiciliary support can best be developed by the operation of a multi-disciplinary community mental handicap team drawing its personnel from both the NHS and local authorities" (Pamphlet 2).

The NDG was clear that to describe a good service was "to describe a co-ordinated service", and the DHSS, which was urging the need for joint working between health and social services at a strategic level, also asserted the benefits of multi-disciplinary work at the point of assessment and service delivery. In its circular LAC(78)2 of January 1978 it spurred authorities to set up district handicap teams (DHTs) for children along the lines advocated by the Court report and also recognised the value of community mental handicap teams (CMHTs).

Co-operation and conflict

The DHSS was, in fact, recognising a phenomenon which had started to appear in many districts. When Morag Plank of CMH published her study paper in 1982 (M. Plank, 1982), she found that out of the 158 health districts covered, 87 already had DHTs and 71 had a CMHT. Further multi-disciplinary teams were at an advanced planning stage.

The aims for CMHTs, defined by Pamphlet 2, were to act as a first point of contact for parents and to provide advice and help with problems related to learning difficulty; co-ordinate access to services; and establish close working relationships with local voluntary groups.

In its *First Report, 1976-1977* (1978) the NDG laid most emphasis on the first of the three aims, promoting the need for specialist advice and support for carers and guidance on practical management. In fact, most teams *had* to concentrate on these aspects as they were mainly small in size, with members who had a relatively low status within the health and social services hierarchies. When one of the authors visited the Wandsworth CMHT in the mid-1980s, however, that team had drawn in social services managers so that decisions could be taken on the allocation of resources from both a health care and social care perspective.

In 1982 when CMH published its research on CMHTs (M. Plank, 1982), a number of issues were identified and many are still alive today:

The age group served. Philosophy dictated the CMHTs should work with people from the teenage years so as to preserve the "people first, disabled second" leitmotif of the Court report. In fact, however, 60 per cent of CMHT teams in Plank's survey were working with children, probably for the two reasons identified by the Mid Downs team (see below) that the district handicap teams were large (some would say over-large) bodies co-ordinating the clinical contribution but not making direct interventions as a team, and parents with dependent offspring of all ages often desired a specialist service which would intervene quickly and effectively.

Team base. "A major shortcoming of CMHTs", wrote Plank, "is their close identification with mental handicap hospitals and the health service." This is not surprising in that the resources needed for release into the community teams were often locked up in the long-stay hospitals and isolation could be combated by good liaison in the setting-up stage. When one of us visited a CMHT in a large coastal town in 1982, however, he found they had been in operation for six months but had made no contact with either the local education or social services departments!

Team membership. Pamphlet 2 envisaged the community mental handicap nurse (CMHN) and specialist social worker as the core members of the team and this was reinforced by G. B. Simon (1981), Dr. Simon being the then director of the National Development Team. Other professions could also usefully be team members but might have other responsibilities outside the CMHT.

In fact, Plank (1982) showed that not every team had this core component.

Table 20.1.1: *Core membership*

Profession	No of CMHTs having one or more of each profession	% of CMHTs replying
Social worker	66	81
Community nurse	65	80
Psychologist	54	67
Consultant in mental handicap	52	64
Doctor (other than consultant in mental handicap)	25	31
Therapists	16	20
Educationalists	9	11
Health visitors	4	5

(From M. Plank, 1982)

When one of the authors and his community nursing colleague, Barry Spooner, gave a talk to a conference on CMHTs at West London Institute in 1986 they were disappointed to discover that in many parts of the country social services and health service managers were still blocking the development of CMHTs with remarks like: "We've got social workers, so we don't need nurses", or *vice versa.*

Membership would appear to be balanced most productively when there is a core team of nursing, social work, medicine and psychology; with the group in its own discrete team base; and with access both to a variety of therapies and to health and social care resources (see M. Craft, J. Bicknell, S. Hollins, 1985). One rather eccentrically staffed CMHT had seven speech therapists as its entire team, not only a strange balance but peculiar use of speech therapists at a time of national shortage!

Leadership. In 1982 the most likely convenor of a CMHT was a consultant psychiatrist or community medical officer but already Plank had identified the use of a rotating convenor which showed the way many teams would move during the decade. Teams with an eye to practical politics might wish to have a doctor of some complexion on the team so as to liaise effectively with the GPs and specialists, and bargain for NHS resources. It would be naive to think that professional status is no longer important. One respondent to Plank's questionnaire told of no convenor and no meetings. As the researcher pointed out: "It is hard to understand how a team can operate as a team without meeting each other"!

Team roles. Simon (1981) warned that in newly developing services there could well be interdisciplinary rivalry, but that "there must be interprofessional trust in each other if CMHT members are to function to the complete satisfaction of their clients."

Certainly in some areas social workers have felt threatened by the arrival of community nurses, psychiatrists have been under professional pressure from clinical psychologists, and OTs have overlapped with physiotherapists. In the well-run team, however, especially one that has taken the trouble to undertake team building (see *First Things First* pack, 1989), there are considerable benefits to consumers in a rich skills mix.

In teams that work well the attitude has been one of "there is plenty of work for everybody and we'll work most effectively if we consider both our professional and personal strengths." The Tunbridge Wells District CMHT has both a co-ordinator, an internal management group, with a senior representative from each discipline, and an external support group of social service managers and representatives of the voluntary organisations.

Partnership with carers. As Gordon Grant *et al* (1986) indicate, CMHTs have led the way in involving parents and carers in partnership and in the "effective interworking" of voluntary and statutory services. For many families the appearance of CMHT workers in the late 1970s and early 1980s was the first glimmering of domiciliary support since the demise of the mental welfare officer in 1971 with the Seebohm reorganisation.

A developmental CMHT

When Nottinghamshire developed its CMHTs in the early 1980s (see G. Wiston and K. Wray in Grant *et al*, 1986), its approach was informed by the idea that there was little point, and, indeed, it could be counterproductive in going out to families as a caseworker if you had nothing to offer. The formula was, therefore, to set up teams of specialist social workers across the county who would have a primary task to develop services. Each team had its own small budget to pump-prime new ventures.

This way of working came under criticism from the National Development Team, the local health authority who argued for practitioners to provide "hands on" support to families, and some of the generic social services teams who perceived the specialists as having a "cushy number". Despite these initial differences in perspective and some tensions within the SSD as to management arrangements, the teams pressed ahead and by 1986 there was clear impetus towards service development. In describing a number of their enterprises and general approach (see S. Almey, 1989) the teams' work is seen to have many similarities with the Wells Road Service described below.

Inevitably the Nottinghamshire teams did undertake casework with families while preserving their initial drive to develop services. As one senior social worker asked: "How can we retain high credibility with parents if, when they approach us for help, we pass the case over to the area and it ... doesn't get allocated?" (Wistow and Wray, *op cit*). But by that time the department's commitment to give the teams a breathing space away from reacting to crises had borne fruit.

A practice-based CMHT

When the Mid Downs CMHT formed in 1981 West Sussex had no community teams despite the example and encouragement of the department of the psychiatry of mental handicap at St. George's Medical School. The inspiration for the team came from a senior community nurse, Barry Spooner, who immediately made himself unpopular with his senior management by insisting on forming a multi-disciplinary team when he had been engaged to form a community nursing team only, and he approached the newly appointed head of social work (Peter Gilbert) within the Forest Hospital to join him.

Initial challenges

- ☐ Resourcing for the team had to come from within the staffing of the long-stay hospital.
- ☐ The hospital management team was implacably opposed to multi-disciplinary working and the consultants felt that there was a team already in existence as they told other disciplines what to do!
- ☐ There were only three specialist social work posts in the county.

Positively, there were staff outside the management group who were receptive to the concept of a CMHT; the resident psychologist and social worker had already broadened people's ideas about the needs of the wider community outside the institution; and the nurse training school (RNMH) was crying out for community placements.

Formation

With perseverence the team gradually formed during the summer of 1981 and built up over the next few years to five community nurses and four social workers (both social work and community nurse leaders being practitioners as well as managers). The reluctance of the consultant to join was overcome by offering him the chair! In fact, having a doctor as the first chairperson was useful in opening discussions with GPs, consultants (for example, in adult psychiatry and the clinical medical officer chairing the district handicap team). Later the CMHT split into three sub-teams, serving three distinct geographical areas: Horsham (population 67,000), Crawley and East Grinstead (population 114,000) and Mid Sussex (population 81,000), with some overlap between East Grinstead and Mid Sussex because consumers from East Grinstead had to look to Crawley and Haywards Heath for their services. The team had a rotating chairperson, (from each profession in turn), leading the combined CMHT.

An operational policy was produced by the CMHT (*Working Together*, 5 September 1985), with a clear referral system and defined roles for each profession with flexibility and encouragement towards joint work and learning new skills. One of the community nurses became something of an expert on welfare rights, while a social worker became a trained portage home teacher. Some of the management and liaison problems experienced in Nottinghamshire were avoided in Mid Downs where a principal officer (health) from social services managed the social work part of the team and good links were quickly established with the area social work officers. With the CMHT prepared to take on cases, especially those with a multi-agency complexion, there was little of the "soft option" slings and arrows thrown at the Nottinghamshire specialists. Any such comments were dealt with politely but robustly!

Both children and adults were seen as the district handicap teams were essentially co-ordinating bodies rather than agents for intervention.

Extending the role

Despite the predominantly casework nature of the team's role initially it gradually began to take on a developmental perspective.

The social workers had to balance their commitment to community work with their responsibility to hospital residents, especially after the closure plan had been agreed (see chapter 2) and priorities were set out with care.

Team members became involved in identifying individual and group needs; helping people move into independent living; setting up and running summer playschemes and a sitting service; producing a very successful community placement scheme for student nurses on the RNMH course (see V. Meeajun, B. Spooner and P. Gilbert, 1985); and creating an adult family placement scheme in response to the desire of a significant number of service users to experience family life (especially those from long-stay hospitals).

The social workers developed what was termed a "specialist patch" system (see P. Gilbert, chapter 8, 1985), where specialist workers were attached in a liaison role to special schools, playgroups, centres and so on. A considerable body of knowledge was built up both about service users (and those who had opted out of current service provision) and community resources in the patch, and workers had in addition the specialist knowledge to bring to bear on the challenges identified. Increasingly, parents would approach the social worker for informal advice and recommend the team's service to other parents. Typical was the carer who asked for help with DSS benefits saying: "I need some help, but I can't stand the hassle of ringing up the local social services and all that paper work", or another who said: "My mother was the rock for 'Jane' and me over the years. I didn't ask her to do much but I always knew she was there. Since her death you and the CMHT have been our network of support."

Community nurses also joined the liaison system, and in the case of the special schools the tasks of the liaison workers were to:

- ☐ visit the school regularly to get to know children and staff and to discuss current concerns with the headteacher and her staff;
- ☐ accept referrals from the headteacher that involve time-limited intervention, and personally refer others to the relevant social work office if necessary;
- ☐ attend case conferences (for example, so as to be a "known person" and an informal point of contact);
- ☐ collate needs that would have to be met by policy changes in own and other agencies - which was aided by working in a multi-disciplinary setting;
- ☐ attend case conferences (for example, those introduced under the 1981 Education Act), meetings for pupils entering the further education centre and discussions designed to foster inter-agency links;
- ☐ be "the human face" of the service.

The liaison role, even when carried out by a designated specialist, is essentially facilitating: fostering rather than truncating links between agencies, and hopefully avoiding the pitfalls of specialism - tunnel vision and professional imperialism. As the right grows of people to receive generic as well as specialist services in health care, and services such as adoption and fostering, the worker must have skills other than those of the traditional specialist.

The liaison role should aid communication by:

- ○ creating confidence in the service by giving immediate access, and by reinforcing goodwill in the belief that each agency wants to communicate;
- ○ giving parents the opportunity to ask advice without going through the area office referral procedure;
- ○ stimulating other social workers' interest in casework with people with learning difficulties and their families;
- ○ not monopolising or causing bottle-necks in communication,

and relaying the need for direct contact on specific issues;

- giving information about working patterns, times and places where people can be contacted;
- interpreting the difference in outlook, pace of action and priorities between different agencies;
- presenting a consistent and familiar face for parents and education staff.

Themes in practice

Open referral system. Although the original consultant wanted a doctor-to-doctor referral pattern, other team members insisted on it being open to everybody. In the first year of operation the main referrers were generic social workers with only two parents making the initial contact with the team. By 1985, however, the percentage of referrals from carers had risen to 23 per cent along with a small number of self-referrals by service users themselves.

By 1987, 24 distinct referring agents had been identified ranging from GPs, MENCAP, the special education adviser, hostels and centres, to a new general psychiatrist who was prepared to open up her service to people with learning difficulties who had psychiatric problems, and would refer to the CMHT those individuals who were on the borderline between learning difficulty and mental illness and could benefit from the team's particular skills.

Early intervention played a large part in the success of the team's operation. If a clear diagnosis of learning difficulty was made by the paediatric team at birth, then a keyworker from the CMHT (usually a social worker in this instance) would offer the family a visit. The worker's counselling skills, specialist knowledge, and community contacts, not least with other parents, were found invaluable by the parents at this stage. The CMHT found that the "new generation" of parents were thirsty for knowledge and tended to look constructively at the future. The workers were able to help the parents through what Cunningham (1979) calls the "psychic crisis" and, as Byrne and Cunningham have recently pointed out, skilled early intervention can lead to very positive outcomes for both parents and their children (E. Byrne *et al,* 1988).

The CMHT operated a planned visiting system which offered contact to families at times of likely decision-making over life-events (see Figure 18.3.1).

Co-ordination of services was vital both for those people with multiple disabilities and for all consumers in the early years. For parents with young children a package of services and information could be constructed; visits could be made with parents to playgroups etc; links were made with other parents whose child had the same disability and groups were formed to meet specific needs.

The team found that when discussions took place with GPs

they often had on their lists middle-aged clients living with frail elderly parents and the CMHT was able to provide a safety-net in conjunction with the primary health care team.

Referral was for a wide range of reasons, but assessment and co-ordination and the treatment of behavioural difficulties were prime examples.

The collation of information was something that the CMHT was able and keen to do. The *Coping with Mental Handicap* series (produced by West Sussex SSD), originated in the Mid Downs District and was then compiled by the CMHTs set up in the two other West Sussex DHAs. In an area with so many new residents arriving in the London commuter belt, sound information was most important. As one carer recalled: "When I moved into the area I didn't know a soul and I felt really encouraged to get the handbook. It was like a real hand of friendship" (see J. Munro and P. Gilbert, July 1985).

Diverging or converging?

At first sight the developmental and practice CMHTs look quite different. But as Wistow and Wray (Grant *et al*, 1986) point out, the Nottinghamshire teams needed to move into casework while the Mid Downs team set up some specific developments (for example, the family placement scheme) when they observed a consumer need and a service vacuum. Both models, in effect, converge, though it is important that the original ethos of the team is preserved if it continues to meet the needs of the consumer.

Alternative models

During the 1980s while some areas were trail-blazing CMHTs, others were making progress towards a different type of service. This was often because health and social services could not agree on the kind of service they wanted; personalities clashed; or a less professionally defined service was seen as desirable.

One example of an alternative model was the Wells Road Service set up by Bristol and Weston Health Authority in 1982 (see L. Ward, 1987 and L. Ward, "Alternatives to CMHTs", in G. Grant *et al*, 1986). This project serving a small, discrete population of 35,000, had two interrelated components. There was a residential service providing the opportunity for local people to gain access to ordinary housing in the locality; and a community support service initiating a more innovative process of enhancing the quality of life for those people already in the community, usually living with their families.

In the latter role staff started by offering practical help (for example, transport, a sitting service) but broadened out into projects such as a Manpower Services Commission community programme employing neighbourhood workers to operate on a one-to-one basis with service users, creating leisure and work opportunities. As one mother stated to the evaluation team: "Instead of an introvert, it has made him (her son) realise the outside world because he never used to go out . . . If you sum it up in one word, I would say it has put confidence in him" (quoted in L. Ward, 1987).

A number of other modes of working exist, some within a CMHT model like South Glamorgan's Flexicare Service (T. Newman and S. Cox, 1987), but Linda Ward (1987) stresses some lessons from the Wells Road experience:

- A flexible, localised service is greatly valued by its users.
- The lack of a professional identity for support workers encourages responsiveness but can leave the workers vulnerable.
- Projects need to inform the value base of managers especially when structures change so rapidly.

Beyond CMHTs?

Where CMHTs have worked as they were designed to, they have provided the "one door" entry to service provision which many consumers sought. In 1990, however, a new "one door" has opened and this is care management (or case management), which the Audit Commission (1989) describes as "the lynch-pin of an individual client needs-led service" (see chapter 10).

Just as in the late 1970s CMHTs were increasingly proposed in government and academic circles and enacted in localities, so care management, as concept and practice, is now gaining ground. By providing a single worker with his or her own budget at the client level there is a chance to "provide a solution to the fragmentation of the system" (see David Challis *et al* in P. Cambridge and M. Knapp, 1988 and chapter 10 above). Up until now care management has been mainly employed in services for elderly people. However, there would appear to be no good reason why it would not work just as well in regard to people with learning difficulties, with its accent on assessing individuals in their social context; identifying the service elements they need in individual service plans; and securing the provision of the appropriate packages of services, as long as it is recognised that normalisation for elderly people might be to live supported in their own home while for people with learning difficulties it may be to move away from the family home in adulthood.

The CMHT with its multi-disciplinary make-up, is a more complex animal and the success of teams has often depended on the leading individuals at the time of formation. Unfortunately a number of teams have been a compilation of talented individuals, what Payne and Scott call their "network" or "athletics team", rather than the more unified and cohesive "team" or "football team" (C. Payne and T. Scott, 1982). Some others have become too much of a self-regarding clique. In both cases it is vital that outside evaluation is harnessed, clear goals stated, the CMHT's members concur as to what it is about, and performance indicators are developed to ensure that consumer needs are being served.

As the legislation on community care moves into the 1990s, care managers are likely to become the "all-singing, all-dancing answer" (King, 1990) to complex problems which the CMHTs were presented as in the eighties.

CMHTs will have to evolve to survive, but their specialist skills will almost certainly be vital to care managers in the assessment process and to the flexible, user-centred and domiciliary-orientated service of the nineties. The ultimate verdict will remain with consumers as to what services they require and articulate the need for. Will CMHTs be seen as the help to individuals and families they were designed for, or merely how George Bernard Shaw saw all professions - as "conspiracies" against the laity"? But while the jury is out, the effective CMHT is building bridges between health and social services which are often divided by barriers of their own making.

S. Almey (1989), "Moving towards independence", *Social Work Today,* 27 April.
APMH (1988), *CMHTs: The Way Forward.*
Audit Commission (1989), *Occasional Paper No. 9,* October
BASW (1985), *Towards Extraordinary Services for People with a Mental Handicap.*
H. Brown and A. Craft (1985), "Getting a team to pull together", *Health & Social Services Journal,* 19 September
E. Byrne *et al* (1988), *Families and their Children with Down's Syndrome,* Routledge
P. Cambridge and M. Knapp (1988), *Demonstrating Successful Care in the Community,* Personal Social Services Research Unit, University of Kent
M. Craft, J. Bicknell and S. Hollins (1985), *Mental Handicap: A Multi-Disciplinary Approach,* Balliere Tindall
C. Cunningham (1979), "Parent counselling", in M. Craft ed., *Tredgold's Retardation,* Balliere Tindall
Court committee, (1976), *Fit for the Future,* HMSO
P. Gilbert (1983), "New services, new strategies", *Community Care,* 31 March
P. Gilbert (1985), *Mental Handicap: A Practical Guide for Social Workers, Community Care,* Reed Business Publishing Group
P. Gilbert and B. Spooner (1982), "Strength in unity", *Community Care,* 28 October
G. Grant, S. Humphreys and M. McGrath (1986), *Community Mental Handicap Teams,* British Institute of Mental Handicap
J. King (1990), "A helping hand", *Community Care,* 22 February
V. Meeajun, B. Spooner and P. Gilbert (1985), "Jay walking in

the community", *Nursing Mirror*, 23 October
J. Munro and P. Gilbert (1985), "Extending the hand of friendship", *Community Care*, 4 July
National Development Group (1977), *Mentally Handicapped Children: A Plan for Action*, HMSO
T. Newman and C. Cox (1987), "Your flexible friend ...", *Social Work Today*, 2 March
J. Ovreteit (1986), *The Organisation of Multi-Disciplinary Community Teams*, Brunel University
C. Payne and T. Scott (1982), *Developing Supervision of Teams Part 1*, National Institute for Social Work
M. Plank (1982), *Teams for Mentally Handicapped People*, Campaign for Mentally Handicapped People
J. Renshaw *et al* (1988), *Care in the Community*, Gower
G. B. Simon (1981), *Local Services for Mentally Handicapped People*, British Institute of Mental Handicap
L. Ward ed. (1987), *Getting Better All the Time?*, King's Fund
K. Webster (1989), "pioneering a personal approach", *Community Care*, 27 July
G. Wistow and K. Wray (1986), "CMHTs, service delivery and service development: The Nottinghamshire approach", in G. Grant *et al*, *Community Mental Handicap Teams*, British Institute for Mental Handicap
A. Woolych (1988), "Community mental handicap teams: Is management the answer?", *Social Work Today*, 7 September.

Parents speaking (3)

Brothers and sisters

"When we met I was struck by Lily's unhappy clouded face.
'Tell Doran I'm sorry, Mummy'.
'What for, my darling?'
'Because it's my fault he is like he is, I was first'.
'Darling, it's nothing to do with you, it's biology'.
'I can't face Doran'."

"Lily reported developments.
'Boys can't actually marry their sisters can they? Because Doran just said "I love you" and pinched my bottom. 'It's alright' she said 'He isn't a problem. He's my younger brother and he is bound to be a pain at times but he's my very good friend, too'."
Linda Scotson, *The Other Child,* Collins, 1988

"I used to think how nice it would be if I had a normal brother and our family was 'normal' like all my friends' families, but after a while I realise that everyone thought their families were weird!"
14 year old sibling quoted in Pauline Fairbrother, *I Was the Lucky One,* Mencap, 1988

"Then they are amazed at how grown-up I can be and start expecting too much from me. After all, I am only six, I can't be sensible all the time."
Mother quoting her six year old son in Pauline Fairbrother, *op cit*

"Paul and Amy were playing ludo and Amy was losing. Suddenly she smacked her hand hard on the table and said 'I can't play this game. You can't expect me to play this game, I'm a Down's!'. Paul looked her straight in the face and said: 'What's being a Down's got to do with anything? Just get on with the game and stop whingeing'."
Parent talking to Peter Gilbert

"There is a great cry of: 'If he were normal you wouldn't dream of doing that' . . . We wouldn't dare put him for a holiday because they adore playing with him on the sands".
quoted in C. Hannam, *Parents and Mentally Handicapped Children,* Penguin/MIND, 1975

Facing the future

"If you have a child, you have to let go, don't you? It is very tough if you can't. It's a measure of your love if you let them go, but it isn't easy, believe you me. It isn't. It's very difficult."

quoted in Ann Richardson and Jane Ritchie, *Letting Go*, Open University Press, 1989

"The relief of knowing that if anything happens to me, he is alright, and that is worth all the grief, all the tears, all the sadness."
Ann Richardson and Jane Ritchie, *op cit*

"Your family isn't it? You get married, you have your children, they grow up and go, but, you see, the pattern doesn't happen here. One doesn't go . . . So now we're saying: 'He's 29, now he must have a life for himself.' It's something we can't provide. It's something he can't provide on his own, so he is going to need help from the social services. Now it's trying to find the right thing for him."
quoted in Ann Richardson and Jane Ritchie, *op cit*

"They (her parents) still won't let me get my own place. I look after them too well. I do all the shopping and tidying. They would be lost without me."
28 year old woman with Down's Syndrome, quoted in C. Cunningham, *Down's Syndrome: An Introduction for Parents*, Souvenir Press, 1982

Last word

"I would have said she has drawn us more together. As years have gone on she has been a great comfort to me and I am never lonely, I always have Kathleen. We have found something in Kathleen that there seems to be a great bond of love and affection. We've made a lot of friends by having her . . . I don't feel I have given any part of my life up for her. We are her parents. She is our child. I feel it is our duty to look after her and treasure her and in return she has given us a great deal of joy and happiness in life. What I have enjoyed about Kathleen is how she appreciates everything, life in general . . . There's always been this great love and affection between us."
quoted in D. May ed, *Living with Mental Handicap: Transitions in the Lives of People with Mental Handicaps*, Jessica Kingsley, 1988

21

Living in the community

"One day, I remember talking to a man in my ward who had been in hospital for 39 years. I remember thinking that life wouldn't be worth much if the same happened to me. I began to think about a flat of my own, a job, a girlfriend, how I wanted those things for myself."
Quoted in D. Atkinson and F. Williams (1990)

Since the publication of *An Ordinary Life* (1980) which stated that it wished to see people with learning difficulties living "in the mainstream of life, living in ordinary houses in ordinary streets, with the same range of choices as any citizen, and mixing as equals with others, and mostly not handicapped members of their own community", the movement towards a community-based service has become more clearly articulated.

In 1980 this statement may have been seen as wildly idealistic, but in a few short years it has been demonstrated that the basic principles stated in the report have become accepted wisdom. It is, though, still not reality for considerable numbers of people who live in hospitals and large-scale residential services in the community that still effectively segregate them from ordinary community opportunities. This philosophy also needs to be extended to work, where considerable change is still needed for community integration to take place. In spite of slow growth in many areas, the movement is now firmly rooted as a result of some of the pioneering examples described below. These developments have shown that community-based services can begin to provide the potential for a lifestyle and opportunities that the authors of *An Ordinary Life* dreamed of for the future when their report was published.

Designing community services

Some essential elements of service design have been identified that point to some of the features that can assist people become socially integrated in the community. These have been described in a wide range of publications (for example, see Carle, 1984; Atkinson and Ward, 1986; Humphreys *et al*, 1987) and are now well established. Briefly they are:

- ☐ a service is comprehensive, and provides for all those people in a neighbourhood regardless of the severity or type of disability.

- the service uses ordinary houses from the local housing stock in ordinary residential neighbourhoods, with the houses blending into the neighbourhood and not calling attention to themselves as "homes".
- if the house is in an ordinary street, near facilities it is likely to be a lot easier for residents to become integrated into the neighbourhood. Similarly, if the houses look ordinary, people are less likely to start off with assumptions about the people being different.
- the number of people living in a house should be small, ideally not more than four people. A key factor in keeping the size of house small, is that local people do not feel overwhelmed by large numbers of people with learning difficulties moving into the neighbourhood.
- people living in houses in the community should be taught skills that will enable them to participate in community life. Living in a house in the community does not automatically mean acceptance by local people (see below).
- how homes are set up is important in how quickly people become accepted as part of the neighbourhood. Initial fears can be overcome by low key intervention, which focusses particularly on the new residents of a neighbourhood undertaking ordinary household duties, participating in ordinary daytime activities and behaving and relating appropriately to local people.
- providing people with integrated and valued day activities that offer opportunities for community presence and participation that is denied in segregated day centres (see chapter 22).
- supporting people to use sports and social clubs in order to develop friendships and broaden social contacts. This means finding alternatives to segregated leisure facilities where opportunities to meet non-handicapped people are limited.

Ensuring an "ordinary life"

The developments influenced by the model of residential services described in *An Ordinary Life* have demonstrated that locally-based services, using ordinary domestic housing and placing emphasis on the use of local community facilities, are a powerful starting point for providing the potential for an ordinary community life. But as Ward (1987) points out, high quality residential services are not enough. People with learning difficulties want more than that. Good services closely integrated into local communities are the first step, not the last. Once such services are established the people living in residential facilities and using day time services want an opportunity to "belong" to their neighbourhood and become "valued" in their communities.

Ward (1987) describes how many of the ordinary activities

which are the key to a good quality of life are essential if people are to integrate into their community, rather than be in the community but still segregated for much of the time because professionals have tied them into services that reduce their opportunities for integration, or where it is assumed that people will develop their own neighbourhood links.

Atkinson and Ward (1986) describe the interventionist approach which assists service users become more involved and accepted in their neighbourhood. The purpose is to promote integration, but also to avoid the limitations of the non-interventionist approach that according to Wertheimer (1983) can leave users "isolated, friendless and lonely". Atkinson and Ward describe a threefold strategy as follows:

Social skills training, where someone, such as a friend, advocate or social worker, uses their relationship with the person to enable the person to develop a range of social skills that increase the opportunity for relating to others who are met in day-to-day contact in the community, and establishing long-term relationships through awareness of social norms and conventions.

Building and maintaining social networks, is important when people are moving to a new neighbourhood or returning to somewhere they lived in the past. To avoid the risk of isolation the key helper can do much to create or support new links, or revive original relationships. Much of this work will be in those activities that begin to build up links with friends, neighbours and acquaintances. In addition to new relationships, the helper can be sensitive to the need to maintain social links, and undertake repair work where the network is at risk.

Neighbourhood involvement, is about becoming part of the local neighbourhood. If we are known by our actual involvement in social activities, joining classes or attending clubs, then this suggests where the helper needs to assist. Not in choosing what the person does, but giving them the choice, with appropriate help, and supporting their involvement through introductions, visits, enlisting the help of others, and support where needed to enable the person to ease their way into situations that increase their recognition and acceptance by the community.

Community-based services - Some examples

Services that have been established to take account of the ideas described above are becoming increasingly commonplace. Early examples are NIMROD and the Wells Road, Bristol, services. It is useful to examine these as they display many of the features that are essential if people living in the community are to receive services that are sensitive to their needs, and are deliberately designed to enable people using a service to remain within their community and integrate within their local neighbourhood.

NIMROD (New Ideas for the Care of Mentally Retarded People in Ordinary Dwellings) began life in the mid 1970s following an initiative by South Glamorgan Health Authority. A subsequent working party, which included health authority, local government and research interests, resulted in a pilot project commencing in 1981 and intensively researched over its five year life and then integrated into social services in South Glamorgan in 1986.

NIMROD was established as a comprehensive service for people with learning difficulties, regardless of age or severity of handicap, and their families in the west of Cardiff. It aimed to offer a range of community-based services to all people in its catchment area. Its stated objectives were: "To promote the health, safety and rights of each handicapped client and to ensure that each is helped to live and behave in as normal a way as possible". The catchment area was divided into four sectors or "communities" with the purpose of offering a service that enabled people to remain living with their families or to live locally in ordinary houses in their neighbourhood.

Shearer (1986), in her account of NIMROD, highlighted some of the key factors that need to be considered when developing community-based services. The project had a clearly stated philosophy, with a service model understood by everyone involved. A small, committed staff team working from their own identifiable base, and a supportive management group who were committed to the success of the project, were also noted.

The project was able to maintain high standards through regular monitoring by the research team, and regular staff meetings and consultation with service users. Careful staff selection, induction and on-going training reinforced the high standards. Staff were committed to the development of individual plans for users, drawn up in conjunction with user, family and service practitioners.

The major components of the service include, a resource centre, where managers and domiciliary teams are based, but which also provides an advice and information service, and a meeting place for volunteers. There was also provision of residential accommodation using existing, ordinary houses, where up to five people are accommodated, with the aim of increasing opportunities for people to live as normal a life as possible. Also included are community care workers who support people in staffed houses and group homes, and also supported families.

What Shearer's account makes clear is that in spite of problems, for example, scarce staffing resources that stem from providing an individually tailored service that addresses peoples needs, the paucity of appropriate day services, and the need to create more supported housing, the project demonstrated that it is possible to build a community-based service that is genuinely comprehensive and does not need to reject any of the people it is designed to serve.

Like NIMROD the Wells Road Service started with the aim of offering a comprehensive community-based service for adults with a learning difficulty who live in a defined area of south Bristol. The health authority funding the service recognised the case for the development of ordinary housing as the basis for new community services rather than hostels, and was influenced by local university research which had detailed the shortage of services in this area of Bristol.

The service which started in 1983 is named after the street where its first two staffed houses are sited. The service is funded by a health authority and has two interlinked parts - a residential and community service. The residential service has been developed along the lines suggested by *An Ordinary Life* and relies entirely on ordinary domestic housing in the local area. The community component of the service is a feature not found in all services, which tend to focus on residential provision exclusively. Here the service is concerned with supporting people in their own homes, in preparing them for a gradual and planned move to a home of their own, and providing a flexible service that supports users, and evolves according to their needs. In this sense the service is not pre-planned but responsive to individual and changing need.

The Wells Road Service started with a clear commitment to the principles of normalisation, with users helped to live as normal and full a life as possible. Like NIMROD, the presence of a clear service philosophy was seen as a key factor in enabling the service to strive to develop opportunities for users to use integrated neighbourhood facilities, rather than segregated services. Again, as in South Wales, the lack of appropriate day activities is commented on by Ward (1986) in an early description of the progress of the service, with the suggestion that alternative integrated day activities would be necessary. However, day services were not part of the remit of Wells Road, which was health-funded. Day services were a local authority responsibility.

Other features include the use of individual programme plans, with keyworkers, family (where appropriate) and other relevant people planning for current and future needs with individually tailored action plans.

Another crucial factor in developing and maintaining high quality services was the emphasis on extensive induction training for staff underpinned by an understanding of the principles of normalisation, and a commitment to on-going training to consolidate the initial training, and to prepare staff to respond effectively to the changing needs of users.

As with NIMROD, this service was monitored and evaluated by a university department, in order that lessons could be learned about new service developments, and this could be disseminated in order to inform other service planners.

Wells Road, like NIMROD, set new standards for community-based services, but still faced many challenges. Ward (1988) has described the difficulties in establishing new homes for people where the local community is sceptical, where delays in opening houses means pressure on prospective residents, their families and staff who need to support them, and where regulations can result in residences having to be substantially modified to meet the requirements of fire officers and other regulatory authorities. Ward (1989) also described how the quality of life of people living in the community can still fall short of the ideal. In particular, the lack of close personal relationships within their neighbourhood, with the need for staff to act as "bridges" into the local community is seen as one way forward. The use of volunteers to introduce individuals to neighbourhood activities on a one-to-one basis has been developed as one way of avoiding group outings, with all the risks of segregating and reinforcing the difference of people with learning difficulties.

In looking at service models it is easy to focus on the schemes which have already attracted national attention. The Tonbridge Staffed Housing Scheme or TOSH started in 1988 as a response to people from the Tonbridge area in Kent, who needed new homes as Leybourne Grange Hospital underwent a closure programme. A co-ordinator for the scheme was appointed in May 1988 and worked closely with the steering group as the preparatory work progressed. The co-ordinator was already a trained nurse within the hospital, with a commitment to people with learning difficulties living in ordinary housing. Her contacts within the health service and her relationship with those residents proved invaluable in bridging the transition from hospital to community.

The issues prevalent during the setting up period have connections with issues identified elsewhere:

- Gaining the necessary finance to fund people who had been living in an "economy of scale provision" and were moving to a dispersed housing scheme.
- Staff transferring from Health into a social services-run service lost prized conditions of service such as mental health officer status and unsocial hours payments.
- Negotiations between health and social services were carried forward on a predominantly verbal agreement basis. When staff changed, previously "understood" arrangements were thrown into the melting pot again.
- Because of financial constraints not enough staffing was funded to cover leave and sickness, in fact not as high a proportion as that funded within the hospital.
- The local MENCAP group were concerned that the focus on ex-hospital residents ignored the needs of people already

living in the community. Two "non-hospital" people were admitted to the scheme, but this led to funding difficulties later on.

The project co-ordinator and hospital social worker worked with the discharge panel to ensure that both individuals and carers were fully aware of the implications of change. A number of the service users did not wish to use the conventional social education centre, so there was considerable use made of sessional places in adult education, clubs, the farm (see chapter 22), with two people in part-time employment with local firms and two others in work experience. "Gareth" who surprised a number of people by gaining part-time employment with a nearby multi-store, has raised his confidence and horizons. One member of staff recalls: "He was always keen on drawing but they were very cramped. Now they are bolder and more expansive, reflecting his increased confidence." All arrangements for activities are based on individual planning which starts with the wishes of the service user.

As in other dispersed housing designs, staff turnover has been higher than hoped for because of isolation and pressure. Younger staff have considerable energy and ideas but some become disillusioned as progress slows. The service users' individual development and broadening of horizons puts up a positive challenge for staff to respond to. The hospitals from which service users and part of the funding originates do not always comprehend the vastly different nature of running a housing scheme based on individual need and dispersed provision. Just as NIMROD found, TOSH is discovering the need for an operational policy which is comprehensive, but not so monumental that it gathers dust!

An evaluation of the scheme has been carried out from various perspectives. The service users were positive about their new lifestyle. They liked the staff currently working with them and were positive about each other ("with one or two exceptions!", as the evaluator points out). Interestingly, a number of the residents expressed a desire to see some of the staff at the hospital again; their memories being very much coloured by individual experiences. All attached a strong value to real work (interestingly this included those over retirement age). They made it clear to the evaluator that as other people work and get paid for it, token work and token wages were not sufficient.

The staff were very committed to the scheme and its value-base, but were also frustrated by staff shortages and the domination of bureaucratic and financial issues over values-led service issues. Concerns raised were communication and support in a dispersed housing scheme, in which total isolation may alternate with claustrophobia: "One minute you're on your own and have to do everything, then you're not on your own and you're told you're too junior to do certain things . . . "

Carers were generally positive but had some incisive comments. They said things like: "This should have happened years ago. This year has been the best in 'X's' life ... she's really got a life now. But they also said: "What will happen when we die and there's no one left to fight to keep places like this running?"

Adult family placements

Recent literature has carried a number of descriptions of family placement schemes for children (e.g. chapters 7 and 8 in N. Malin, 1987) as a way of providing services in more integrated settings, but little or nothing on alternative families for adults (see Ward, 1982; and Atkinson, 1983).

As Malcolm May recalls in the case of children's programmes (see chapter 8 in N. Malin *op.cit*), there was some resistance to such a concept among a number of parents and voluntary bodies who felt safe with "more of the same" residential developments. There has been a growing recognition, however, that a significant number of people with learning difficulties, given the choice, wish to opt for the nurturing of a substitute family, or the relative independence, with on-site support, of a lodgings placement.

Some of the increasing numbers of successful schemes are mentioned below but there are also a number of unresolved issues and a sense of a Sword of Damocles over the concept as central government has never given these sort of ventures its whole-hearted backing, despite their appropriateness in a comprehensive community service and research evidence as to their success in the UK and USA (see R. Olsen, 1978). Some of the issues still pending are:

- *Registration.* Under the Registered Homes Act 1984 homes with less than four residents do not need to be registered with the local authority. This has created a problem over standards of care, but conversely has allowed carers approved under properly run placement schemes to retain a family atmosphere without the imposition of all the (often intrusive) regulations which registration imposes.

  In March 1990 the Health Minister, Virginia Bottomley, speaking at the report stage of the NHS and Community Care Bill, indicated that the government might bring three-bedded homes under the auspices of the Act but that they would not be subject to the full battery of regulations.
- *Finance.* Many DSS offices have been reluctant to pay more than the board and lodging rate for care in unregistered homes even if the service user has in effect been part of a family with a high standard of living, rather than a lodger.
- *Recruitment, evaluation, training and support.* In the child care field considerable thought has been given to these important areas and there are now national standards to relate to. This is still being developed in adult family placements.

Among a number of schemes operating at present, Wandsworth SSD's has been running for three years and by the autumn of 1989 had 13 people placed with 12 families (Pierce, 1989). Carers are recruited from a number of backgrounds and, while many have considerable past experience, attitude and personal characteristics are considered the most important attributes. Those adults being placed have their own social workers to avoid a conflict of interest for the scheme's project workers. A contract is drawn up at the beginning of the placement involving all concerned parties and this agreement is regularly reviewed. The local authority tops up DSS benefits to approximately £200 per week to reflect the quality of care within a caring family way of life.

The scheme's organisers have found considerable benefits for individuals, for example one young man is talking for the first time in his life. "Every one of them is blossoming as a result of the much closer care and more consistent handling they are able to receive in a family" (quoted Pierce, *op.cit*).

Hampshire's Adult Placement Scheme has been running since April 1979 and provides a service for a number of client groups. It is the largest scheme in the country. As in the Wandsworth design, adult placement officers were separate from the area social workers, who looked after the interests of individual service users.

At its inception the Hampshire scheme was joint financed by health and social services. Individual placements were funded by the DSS (then DHSS), with careful negotiations leading to a rate between the board and lodging and residential home's rate. Unfortunately, the change in DSS regulations after April 1988 has meant that a higher level can only be paid if there are more than two carers in the home. If one of these is employed outside the home this can be for no more than 24 hours per week. This has limited the numbers of potential carers willing to come forward. The success of a placement is sometimes dependent on the carer's family network becoming involved and occasionally this wider family will take on the main caring role when the original carer is incapacitated.

Hampshire recognises that there is an anomaly between regarding carers as staff and allowing a natural homely set-up to develop. As one organiser put it: "Clients don't want to be trained all day every day - they may come back from their day centre or job and just want to get away from 'staff'."

The People to People programme in Medway began about five years ago as a response to the needs of residents in long-stay hospitals. Funded by Medway DHA and managed by Kent SSD, the current team consists of a manager, two placement officers, two social workers, two support workers and a team clerk.

The recruitment, assessment, training and support of carers is primarily the work of the placement officer, with the scheme's manager providing an overall quality control of the recruitment procedure. As in some of the other schemes across the country, work with carers and service users is separated so as to pay careful attention to the needs of both and provide a clearer perspective. The social workers create links with hospital residents and use community resources to assess their strengths and needs.

In April 1990 the scheme had 14 full time carer families and one respite carer. Five of the full-time carers have a respite bed as well. Of the 24 people placed with families, four have a physical disability, while six have a severe sensory impairment as well as learning difficulties. Ages range from 35-83 years. Eleven of the 24 are over 60, and although some older people find a move from institutional care difficult to face, placement workers across the country have found many older residents yearning for a more domestic setting in which to live.

Appropriate day settings that complement the family placement are hard to find but the workers have arranged a broad range of options from work experience to community arts groups, sports, leisure, adult education and community facilities for elderly people. To fill some gaps the scheme has set up its own club to help during the transition period.

Training, support and respite is offered to carers who have regular support group meetings and are able to partake in training such as the Open University "Patterns for Living" course.

The scheme has been hit by changes in DSS regulations, with the scheme having to top-up a number of families who have lost money on the direct benefits from the DSS.

Reviews are held regularly, based on individual planning principles, with particular attention paid to emotional needs and integration within the community.

Looking forward

These small-scale examples of applying the "ordinary life" in practice demonstrate what can be achieved where service planners, operational staff and service users all contribute to the development of service models that begin from the needs of people with learning difficulties, rather than service systems that do not "fit" what individuals need and want for themselves. In spite of their admitted limitations, they nevertheless instruct us in what we should aim for when developing community-based services in the future.

The King's Fund has spelt out the agendas facing service planners in the future. Services will need to focus on what community means to people with learning difficulties and their families. This will mean finding ways of involving and empowering service users. Services will need to be designed to meet the needs of individuals. Last, safeguards on quality will need to be built into services.

All the planning, management and financing of services will

take place against the backcloth of the service structures developed in response to the NHS and Community Care Act, where local authorities have lead agency responsibility for community care, where there will be new arrangements for joint planning between SSDs and health authorities, where services will be provided in a diversified market place of social care, and where the response to individuals' needs will be determined by care management arrangements.

D. Atkinson, "They just have to muck in", *Community Care,* 4 August, 1983.
D. Atkinson and F. Williams (1990), *Know Me as I am*, Hodder & Stoughton
D. Atkinson and L. Ward (1986), *A Part of the Community: Social Integration and Neighbourhood Networks,* The Campaign for People with Mental Handicaps
N. Carle (1984), *Key Concepts in Community-Based Services,* The Campaign for People with Mental Handicaps
L. Davies (1987), *Quality, Costs and 'An Ordinary Life' - Comparing the Costs and Quality of Different Residential Services for People with a Mental Handicap,* King's Fund
G. Evans, S. Todd, R. Blunden, J. Porterfield & A. Ager (1985), *A New Style of Life - The Impact of Moving into an Ordinary House on the Lives of People with a Mental Handicap,* Mental Handicap in Wales Applied Research Unit
S. Humphreys, G. Evans and S. Todd (1987), *Lifelines: An Account of the Life Experiences of Seven People with a Mental Handicap who use the NIMROD service,* King's Fund
S. Humphreys, K. Lowe & S. de Paiva (1986), *Long-Term Evaluation of Services for Mentally Handicapped People in Cardiff,* Mental Handicap in Wales Applied Research Unit
S. Humphries, K. Lowe & S. de Paiva (1986), *Long-Term Evaluation of Services for People with a Mental Handicap in Cardiff - Clients' Views,* Mental Handicap in Wales Applied Research Unit
S. Humphries, K. Lowe & S. de Paiva (1986), *Community Care Workers, Parts 1 and 2,* Mental Handicap in Wales Applied Research Unit
King's Fund (1980), *An Ordinary Life - Comprehensive Locally Based Residential Services for Mentally Handicapped People,* King's Fund
N. Malin ed (1987), *Reassessing Community Care,* Croom Helm
R. Olsen (1978), *Alternatives to Hospital Care,* BASW
J. Pierce, "Providing an ordinary home life", *Social Work Today,* 16 November 1989
A. Shearer (1986), *Building Communities with People with Mental Handicaps, Their Families and Friends,* Campaign for People with Mental Handicaps and King's Fund

A. Shearer (1983), *An Ordinary Life - Issues and Strategies for Training Staff for Community Mental Handicap Services*, King's Fund
L. Ward (1982), *People First - Developing Services in the Community for People with Mental Handicap*, King's Fund
L. Ward, "An ordinary life", *Community Care*, 10 November 1983
L. Ward, "Changing services for changing needs", *Community Care*, 22 May 1986
L. Ward, "An ordinary life - The early views and experiences of residential staff in the Wells Road Service", *Mental Handicap*, Vol. 17, March 1989
L. Ward, "Thwarting ordinary lives", *Community Care*, 21 January 1988
L. Ward and J. Wilkinson (1985), *Training for Change - Staff Training for 'An Ordinary Life'*, King's Fund Centre
L. Ward, "Developing opportunities for an ordinary community life", in D. Towell ed (1987), *An Ordinary Life in Practice - Developing Comprehensive Community-Based Services for People with Learning Disabilities*, King's Fund
A. Wertheimer (1983), *Leisure*, Campaign for Mentally Handicapped People

22

Day services: From occupation to real work

"It does not matter what work you do; if you are in work, you have dignity and you have worth."
Martin Luther King

Day services for people with learning difficulties - adult training centres and social education centres - are currently the main day resource to approximately 50,000 users, and provide a service that is increasingly recognised as no longer meeting the daytime needs of those users. These services have evolved through a series of changes from the concern to occupy users, to one where the range of activities, in theory, is so wide as to provide no real focus as far as the needs of people using the service are concerned. The main problem is that the services remain segregated and fail to offer the one thing the majority of people who attend centres would like - a job.

Changing expectations

Survey after survey has found that the majority of people want employment in ordinary jobs (Wandsworth SSD (1976), Flynn (1987), Brandon (1988), Jahoda *et al* (1989), King (1990)). This perception is at odds with the main purpose of many centres, which have not placed emphasis on getting people jobs, even though this is what many users think they are being prepared for. For example, Brandon (1988) reported that at two centres he surveyed, where 200 people attended, only 12 users had found employment in five years, yet work was what most people using the services wanted. The main difficulty is that the real purpose of day services has not been made explicit. Whose need is the service meeting? Gathercole (1988) states that the main purpose of the service is to meet the needs of parents, and this view is reinforced by Seed's research (1988) which suggests that the majority of parents see the service in social and respite terms, even though their sons and daughters believe it is about work.

These conflicting views of whose needs the service is meeting highlight the difficulties facing day services, as they move into the future where expectations are rising for a number of reasons:

- the impact of improved educational provision since the early 1970s;
- a new generation of parents with higher expectations about

what services will provide for their children when they become adults;

- the developments in habilitation technology (Gold, 1980, Bellamy *et al*, 1979) which demonstrate the success in teaching severely disabled people work skills;
- the growing demands of users themselves (articulated strongly through self-advocacy groups);
- the success of employment schemes such as Pathway, Shaw Trust, Blakes Wharf and numerous individual initiatives in centres up and down the country where users have successfully moved on to open, or supported sheltered employment.

But in spite of these developments new centres are still being built in some parts of the country at a time when other areas are taking the first steps towards eventual closure, and developing alternative services based on the identified needs of users to what they wish to do in the community which may be to work, attend classes or a number of other things.

Redeveloping day services

Re-developing day activities in order that they can provide support for users who wish to move into open or supported employment should be a priority for services. A first step could be to develop a vision of what the future might look like. This then becomes the guiding light as the service develops initiatives in response to users' needs. The concepts of socially valued roles (Wolfensberger, 1983, and the five essential accomplishments of O'Brien, 1987) constitute a valuable starting point for service development and would enable a day service to monitor whether changes are promoting desirable futures for users.

The next stage would be to establish service principles that can inform the service as it redevelops its role. The King's Fund Centre (1984) identified five principles to guide service design. Gathercole (1988) describes these principles in his discussion of employment services:

- *Employment services should not exclude people who are thought to be too disabled to work.* This is a particularly important principle, as services need to be designed on the assumption that everyone should be given a chance to work, with the service challenged to explore what might be needed to make this happen. As Gathercole (1987) states: "In the past services have been designed on the self-fulfilling assumption that severely disabled people will never work. Since they then do not get the chance, of course they never do."
- *Whatever support is needed to enable the person to work should be provided.* This includes all the resources, both in human and practical terms needed to support the person in employment. This is in absolute opposition to the traditional readiness model,

whereby the person would have to achieve a standard of performance in a segregated setting before being given the chance to work. This approach focused almost totally on preparation for work, with extensive use of checklists, rating scales and tests. The alternative is to provide the necessary support in real work situations, where the training and preparation is done on the job, with someone working alongside if necessary teaching the required skills (see King, 1990 for a description of a supported employment scheme in Thameside SSD). This approach is considered by Gathercole to open up enormous opportunities in the future.

● *The personal choice of the worker should be the priority determinant in the search for work.* In the past emphasis has been placed on what a person was thought capable of doing, based on assessment by staff of skills and work readiness. The views of the person were not necessarily a consideration. This approach was based on a number of premises, including, doubt about the person's ability to make decisions, fear of failure if the person aimed too high and overprotection, with concern that the person might be damaged by disappointment.

Shifting the emphasis towards personal choice means enabling the person to take responsibility for their own life, increased opportunities for learning, and increased motivation. This shift also means rejecting assessment as a means of trying to measure skills and performance, and finding out what the choice of the person is, and what opportunities and support they have had in the past to make decisions about work, and what they will need in the future in relation to their preferences.

● *The service should maximise contact between a disabled worker and non-disabled people.* Integration is a major theme of normalisation, with work an important opportunity for developing relationships and participating in the life of the community. Being segregated in a setting with people who have nothing in common but the label of disability, reduces the potential for contact with non-disabled people, and is very damaging. Experience of non-segregated settings was a major reason why people interviewed in Jahoda *et al* (1989) were disenchanted with segregated day services.

● *The service should ensure an adequate income.* When developing work opportunities services need to ensure that safeguards are built in to schemes so that people are not exploited. This is a particularly difficult area with rigid rules on earnings levels and potential loss of benefits, which currently penalise rather than encourage movement into work. As far as possible jobs should pay wages that free people from reliance on state benefits and enable them to live an ordinary life.

Essential tasks of an employment service

An Ordinary Working Life (King's Fund 1984) identifies some of the essential tasks which an employment service would need to perform:

- *Assessment and individual planning.* Identifying the person's employment preferences so that the appropriate support could be provided.
- *Co-ordination and monitoring of individual programme plans.* Co-ordinating the means of meeting the person's vocational needs, and monitoring the implementation of means to meet those needs.
- *Guidance for service users.* Providing guidance and support to enable service users to understand how their disabilities may affect their employment (for example epilepsy), and to enable them to overcome personal difficulties that affect job performance and retention.
- *Transport assistance.* Transport can be a critical issue in getting and retaining a job. Learning to use public or other forms of transport is therefore a useful part of any vocational programme.
- *Help in getting vocational training.* This includes work with employment services, firms' own training departments and colleges of further education who provide appropriate training, and supporting people to use these services.
- *Links with employers.* To establish links with local employers and to facilitate job placements for users.
- *Guidance for employers.* Providing advice and support to employers in order that suitable work situations, training, supervision and rights are available.
- *Job development and placement.* Spending time with users discussing their job preferences, and learning what job openings exist and matching people to the work they would like. Providing support and training for users as necessary.
- *Job retention.* Follow-up support to help people keep their jobs, by support and sorting out difficulties that may arise.
- *Arranging co-workers.* Providing workers with guidance, supervision and modelling by co-workers or job coaches at the job site. Either workers employed at place of work or appointed to take part in job-sharing scheme.
- *Work experience.* Provides people with unpaid opportunities to experience jobs first hand, and learn about their capabilities.
- *Job skills training.* Teaching specific job skills at the work site, either by employers or staff or employment service.
- *Job design.* Tailoring a job to make it possible for a worker to perform it adequately, where strength, dexterity, judgement, speed or co-ordination create difficulties.
- *Improving community and professional acceptance.* Public relations work with parents, instructors, teachers, lecturers and any other individuals who can facilitate vocational development.

Employment schemes

The following examples of employment services organised by

voluntary organisations and SSDs demonstrate forcefully that the pessimism about the potential for people with learning difficulties to work in ordinary jobs is both ill-founded and inaccurate. They confirm that services based on the assumption that people with learning difficulties want to work, and are seen as valued workers by employers, counteract the traditional view that employment is for the few "most able" users of day services, and that extensive training, often lasting many years, is necessary before users are ready to take ordinary jobs.

The Pathway Employment Service

The Pathway Employment Service is a national service run by MENCAP and operates in many parts of England and Wales. This service was started in 1975 in South Wales. Pathway is established in a borough or county when the local authority "purchases" the service, agreeing a service package, which is offered on a three or five year basis. The package includes the cost of running the service, including salaries of staff and administration, and the reimbursement of wages paid to people placed in jobs.

Once the Pathway officer has found a job for a person with a learning difficulty, the employer receives a reimbursement of wages paid for up to 12 weeks, which takes account of the person's need for supportive training to enhance their employment prospects. A weekly gratuity is also paid to a nominated "foster worker" who provides the Pathway employee with supervision, instruction and support. The Pathway officer provides a follow-up service once a placement is made, to meet the needs of the worker, employer and foster worker.

Pathway accepts referrals from a wide range of professionals, parents and people with learning difficulties themselves. People supported range from 16 to 60 years of age, and jobs have been found in a wide range of employment settings, including, industry, domestic and hotel services, supermarkets, farms and gardens.

Contact: Pathway Employment Service, 169a City Road, Cardiff CF2 3JB.

The Shaw Trust

The Shaw Trust was established in 1982 "to promote the education, training and rehabilitation of persons who by reason of mental or physical handicap or otherwise are in need of and are unable to gain employment". The trust operates under the model of "sheltered " employment, with the worker employed by the trust ("the sponsor") with the firm where the person works the "host". The "host" pays a proportion of the person's wage based on his or her productivity, and the trust makes up the wage to the full amount through re-imbursement by the Department of Employment. The proportion of wages paid by the "host" is negotiated with the sponsor based on the output of the person.

The trust is gradually extending its work throughout the country, with a growing number of development officers, whose main role is to identify employment opportunities in the open employment sector and to match those with people with learning difficulties in the local community. Each development officer is supported by an administrative team.

Contact: Shaw Trust, Caithness House, Weston Way, Melksham, Wilts SN12 8NZ.

Blake's Wharf

Blake's Wharf is an employment service for people with learning difficulties in the London Borough of Hammersmith and Fulham SSD. It started in 1984, funded by health and social services, and was developed as an alternative to a new training centre in the borough. Taking the traditional route was seen as inappropriate with the needs of users better met by an employment service. The primary aim of the service is to prepare people for work, by providing work experience placements, on the job training, guidance about work and assistance in obtaining work.

Blake's Wharf is a service based on the principles of normalisation, and has developed a model of practice which is community-based, rather than centre-based. Training in work skills is not seen as a centre activity, but something that is more appropriately undertaken in the workplace. Users have an individual plan, with a supervisor who has keyworker responsibility. When employment is found users are provided with on-the-job training and support by staff from Blake's Wharf for as long as required, with the aim of achieving independence in work.

Contact: Blake's Wharf, 147 Stevenage Road, Fulham, London SW6.

Weir Road Employment Assessment Centre

Weir Road Employment Assessment Centre is based on an industrial estate in Wimbledon and organised by the London Borough of Merton personal services department. The centre was funded by joint finance with the district health authority, and provides 35 places for people with learning difficulties. It was originally conceived as a sheltered workshop managed by a nearby social education centre, but by the time it opened it was seen as a service primarily concerned with placing people into employment.

The centre opened in 1987, with the aim of assisting users who wished to work in open or sheltered employment. It provides assessment, and training in skills necessary to secure employment, a job finding service (in partnership with Shaw Trust), and supported work experience placements. A range of work in a variety of locations has been obtained since the centre opened, including retail shops, horticultural centres, factories, supermarkets, child care centres, hospitals, local government and British Rail. In addition the centre undertakes some limited contract work and has set up a community work scheme for a number of users who do not wish to move into open employment.

Since the centre opened the number of people found employment is considerably more than was originally anticipated. This has meant that the support role to people who are now in open employment has created greater demands, and the centre has had to hand over some of its outreach support role to the Shaw Trust.

Contact: Employment Assessment Centre, 9 Weir Road, Wimbledon, London SW19.

Employment projects

Agriculture and horticulture

In the 1950s and 1960s agricultural and horticultural schemes played a significant role in the "therapeutic approach" for people with learning difficulties. By the 1970s they had fallen out of favour, but then staged a comeback through the work of the rural communities, and as satellites to training centres. More recent projects have focussed on providing a wider range of choice for users, and increasingly a route into open employment.

West Sussex SSD is establishing the *Brinsbury Project,* which is based within the West Sussex College of Agriculture and Horticulture. This project is funded by social services, but managed by a voluntary organisation. Although the project will have its own facilities, students will have access to the college resources. Progress for students can be made through further study at the college, or into direct employment through MENCAP's Pathway Employment Service.

Princess Christian Farm, in Kent, was originally purchased by the SSD, from a long-stay hospital, and has been developed into a training farm for students from the West Kent area. The farm offers 35 places on a sessional basis, with opportunities for training in agriculture. The farm also has a shop, and is currently investigating a produce delivery service. The farm is also associated with Spadework, a grant-aided voluntary organisation providing complementary training in horticulture on an adjacent site.

Thrift Farm managed by Buckinghamshire SSD, and opened in 1978, is a rural training centre which offers training in livestock management, and horticulture for the 50 users who work at the centre. The focus is on activities that involve contact with the local community, whether through cattle shows, or gardening and landscape contract work that takes users into the community. For a description of the work of the farm, see Kelly (1989).

Service industries

As service industries become a higher percentage of commercial activity, with a decline in manufacturing industries, so the service sector is an increased source of employment for people with learning difficulties.

Dr. B's Kitchen is a Barnardo's-funded restaurant and coffee shop in Harrogate that opened in 1984, and trains 24 people with learning difficulties, who are instructed to professional level and work towards the Catering Base qualification recognised by the Hotel and Catering Training Company. After a period of training at Dr. B's trainees move on to work experience in local hotels, where previous trainees have acquired permanent employment. Hills (1989) reported that 61 trainees had completed the training, and moved into employment, with the majority still in work since the project began.

The Canterbury Oast Trust, founded in 1983, took over the Mariners' Hotel in Rye, where eight young people with a learning difficulty have made their home and run the next door restaurant and tea rooms. Joe Graham, the director of the Trust, believes public attitudes can only change appreciably "at grass-roots level" and therefore it is extremely important that people with disabilities are employed in situations which allow them to rub shoulders with members of the general public (correspondence with the authors). Over the next few years other catering ventures are planned.

In Liverpool the local MENCAP and the SSD have developed *a grocery delivery service* from a Tesco superstore. A team of people with a learning difficulty now deliver groceries to some 200 elderly people in South Liverpool. The workers wearing Tesco's uniforms and sharing facilities with Tesco staff are paid union rates, with some individuals working full-time and others part-time, dependent on their entitlements to benefits. John Darby, the project supervisor, sees the purpose of the scheme to train people for normal employment, developing numeracy, literacy and independence and to progress to normal employment (see Jervis, 1988).

Finally, advice from the well-known *Applejacks Cafe* project, developed by Camden Society for Mentally Handicapped People, is worth restating: keep it small; keep it real; keep it totally in the community; and have the highest expectations of the people with special needs who work with you (*Applejacks: Project Manual,* 1987).

Changing day services

Rethinking the role of day services means moving away from the model of service that places emphasis on the continuum of services, where users are gradually prepared for more demanding activities through training programmes. Callahan (1986) suggests that this idea is totally flawed. The continuum does not flow with sufficient speed to be meaningful to any but the fortunate few. In fact users rarely, if ever reach integrated employment. In reality traditional day services systematically deny access to regular employment for people with learning difficulties. The alternative is to move towards supported employment, where users can develop the skills they need in actual work experience, and where off-the-job training, if required, is directly relevant to needs identified in work.

Some of the changes needed to enable the many thousands of people with learning difficulties to move from occupation to real work is now beginning to take place in day services, with more and more centres recognising that users' needs are not met by the wide range of activities currently provided, and that a start can be made by listening to users and developing plans that are in response to needs identified by users, rather than the needs of the service. These developments can in turn motivate staff who are often frustrated in their desire to offer a service that is more closely related to the needs of users, and break out of the straight-jacket of traditional services.

It is clear from the guidance contained in *An Ordinary Working Life* that day services have the potential to develop an employment service, and our personal contact with a number of centres has demonstrated that many staff are enthusiastic about the opportunity to assist users to realise their dream of an ordinary job. Changes have been particularly effective where day centre officers have been redesignated as employment support workers and job finders. They have been able to set up work experience projects following contact with local employers and identifying placements for users. These initial steps have quickly led to users being offered full or part-time jobs, with positive effects on other people attending centres who are then motivated to request help in finding jobs.

Alongside this work day centre officers have involved parents in discussion about the changes, and to gain their commitment and support in developing an employment service. Even though many parents have been concerned about the new demands community-based day activities will make on their sons and daughters, very few parents we have spoken to have been opposed to such developments, once they are consulted and feel confident that a programme is well organised, and will lead to genuine work opportunities. In fact, parents have spoken with pride that their son or daughter is doing a "normal job" like other people. This was something they had often been led to assume would never be possible.

Tunbridge Wells: An evolving social education centre

It is nearly always easier to set up new projects than to change outdated services. A building spells safety to carers, service users

March 8 1990
King's Fund Centre (1984), *An Ordinary Working Life: Vocational Services for People with Mental Handicap,* King's Fund Centre
J. O'Brien, "A guide to life-style planning: Using the activities catalog to integrate services and natural support systems", in B. Wilcox and G.T. Bellamy (1987), *A Comprehensive Guide to the Activities, An Alternate Curriculum for Youth and Adults with Severe Disabilities,* Paul Brookes, Baltimore
P. Seed, "Salient practice issues", in G. Horobin ed (1987), *Why Day Care?,* Jessica Kingsley
Wandsworth SSD (1976), *Project 74: A Research Study in which Mentally Handicapped People Speak for Themselves.* London Borough of Wandsworth
W. Wolfensberger, "Social role valorisation: a proposed new term for the principle of normalisation", *Mental Retardation,* Vol. 21, 1983

Consumer's view: I enjoy life

Glenda Robinson

I have an illness. It is called Sille de la Taurette Syndrome. I sometimes shout and scream but I have got better.

I get exhausted. I behave myself. I am no trouble. I am very well-behaved. I am no trouble to my neighbours. I live in a flat on my own. But when I go down to the shops I meet people who help me. They help me get it and pack my bags for me and check it on the table. I bring it home and unpack it and put it away.

On Tuesday I go to the post office and draw my money. Toddie, the post-master, helps me with my money and gives me all fivers to make it easier for me. I go into the newsagents to pay for my papers once a fortnight.

On Mondays and Fridays I go to the playgroup. I love the children and the staff are very kind to me. We have a cup of coffee for 15 pence. Joyce is in charge of the playgroup.

I go down to the laundry on my bike twice a week with my washing. You can leave your washing and they will do it for you. I have friends round Arbury, and I go down to the chemist and fish shop. I go and see Dr. Gant every four weeks. We often have a chat. Dr. Gant comes and has a cup of tea with me. Dr. Gant says I am much better in myself and doing very well. He is pleased with me and so is Dr. O'Brien.

My next door neighbour Valerie helps me and I help her. She has two cats. I see Val at weekends. I also go to the supermarket and see Carole sometimes for a chat. I sometimes go for a walk and a bike ride. There are lots of shops round here. I quite enjoy life very much. People are kind. They help me and I help them. Muriel, my befriender, comes to see me. I go to her house and she comes to mine.

I go on the bus into town for 50 pence there and back. I go to Cambridge market or to the Thursday market. I get my cleaning things from Thursday market. I do all my own cleaning in my flat. I have a bath. I do not like it too full or too hot. I cope better in myself than I did when I first came to live here. I am on tablets. I have eight a day and I take them and they help me. If I take them I feel better. Dr. Gant has helped me a lot but I have also helped myself. I am very fond of Dr. Gant. He is kind and we are good friends.

Rachel and I are good friends and we go out for a meal together and go to the shops. I have known Rachel since I was at the Ida

Darwin Group Home. I stayed there at Christmas for two nights and had a nice time with Sue and her friend Debbie. It was a nice day on Christmas Day.

I wish Mum or Dad could see me now. My brother Desmond lives at Bottisham and he comes to see me when he can. My sister Cora lives in Kent. She comes up once a year and we have a day out. She has a car.

I am very happy in my flat. I like being on my own and trying to do everything on my own. It is hard but I do pull my weight and do most of it for myself. I have a little help with a light bulb - Mr. Swan or Val puts it in for me - but most things I do myself.

Judy lives upstairs at number 10. She has been in hospital. I go up at the weekends and see if she is all right. Judy is a kind-hearted girl. Mr. and Mrs. Harper live over the road. They help me. Mavis and John help me also. Carole helped me a lot when I came to live here. I am a lot better and I am grateful to all my friends.

I have lived in my flat four years - five years come this 19 August. I have a lot of friends. At the playgroup we play with the children. We put them all up on the table. They sit on a chair and have a drink and they sometimes have birthday cake. We sing and play with the children.

I am a happy person. I enjoy life. I do not like Saturday because it is a bit under the weather and you get sport on the television. I like Sunday because you get a lot of good music.

Mr. and Mrs. Harper are good friends and they have two children called Sherri and Charlie. Sherri is a dear little girl and she sent me a Christmas card. She is very sweet and I often talk to her. I am very happy and I make lots of friends.

Reprinted from Community Care, *(2 June 1988).*

23

Managing into the future: Power to the consumers

". . . if my aspirations are very high, my depressions are very deep, yet my pinions never loved the middle air".
John Milton

"When we got back from London, I said to the group that we would not be a self-advocacy group unless someone from the group took over . . . The tutor [Sue], stayed with the group for a while as an adviser . . .

"I felt I had enough tutoring and one day Sue said we should do something, I said, 'No, we don't have to do what you say'. After a while it was decided that Sue, the tutor, should leave the group. Now we meet and we have a new adviser who is quiet and doesn't keep talking like Sue!"
A consumer quoted on D. Atkinson and F. Williams eds (1989)

As we started by saying at the beginning of this book, the front line and middle manager may well feel as though they are the "meat in the sandwich", but they don't have to clip their wings to fly in the middle air or walk the middle ground any more than the poet Milton did. The increased use of information technology, devolved budget management, clear service specifications and greater responsibility for day-to-day management should allow the manager to be creative and concentrate on positive outcomes for consumers.

Services in the future are going to have to be more business-like, confronted as they are by increased consumer expectations, from both users, carers, policy makers and the public at large; the individual purchasing power of care managers; and the block purchasing power of large commissioning agencies. To survive and prosper organisations will need sound hard information on budget forecasts and activity levels, but also a feel for what will work in the market place. To remain creative and productive "the new leadership . . . must tap the energies and potential of talented subordinates whose skills and knowledge are vital for dealing with complexity and change" (D. Bradford and A. Cohen, 1984), and to develop a managerial style which is participative and transformational (J. Rosner, 1990) and energises and enables at all levels of the organisation (R. Kelly, 1988). Not only will the manager need to be constantly learning (B. Garrett, 1987) but so will everybody in the service, the aim being to promote the highest possible quality at the interface of service delivery. The quality test is what happens in the face-to-face interrelation between individual staff members and consumers, and managers need to reinforce this message by everything they say and do, values they espouse, the symbolism they employ, and, most importantly, how *they* interact with users, carers and staff.

To prosper in a world which is changing at a rapidly increasing pace, public as well as private services will have to become "totally responsive to the customer" both purchasers and users of the service (T. Peters, 1989). Some commentators, such as Norman Flynn, director of the Institute of Public Sector Management at the London Business School, go further and state that "the principle should be the users in control unless there are compelling reasons why they should not be" (N. Flynn, 1990).

In the field of services for people with a physical disability, the Isle of Wight's Riverside centre, for example, is managed by a user council. In services for people with learning difficulties progress is slower and less radical. A number of services encourage the involvement of users and carers in decision-making and it is clearly vital to ensure that the involvement of the latter does not infringe the rights of people with learning difficulties themselves. For real rather than token power to be handed to consumers attention needs to be given to the input of advocates, to the promotion of self-advocacy and the development of citizenship.

With the promotion of choice and independence underpinning the government's commitment to community care reforms, and the principle of partnership in the Children Act 1989, how can managers help turn these fine intentions into reality? With authorities beginning the task of redeveloping their services to meet the requirements of the reforms the voice of the user could remain peripheral in the process of change. Although the reforms offer opportunities for greater involvement of users in the decisions about services they require, this will mean authorities supporting initiatives that give a voice to people who have traditionally had little or no say in the decisions about their lives, and at the same time avoiding the tokenism that could so easily result. The examples of the advocacy movement suggest one way authorities could learn about the needs of people they are required to serve.

The growth of the self-advocacy movement through local People First groups, where people using services (often together with a facilitator in the early stages) meet together to learn to express their views and opinions, has been significant in the lives of many people with learning difficulties. This movement provides many examples of the sort of activity that will need to be greatly expanded, if there is genuine concern to listen to users' views in the reformed services.

Similarly citizen advocacy (Butler *et al*, 1988), although

independent from authorities, is a means of linking users to members of the community on a one-to-one arrangement to ensure that the person with a learning difficulty has someone with a voice to work with them. It is an arrangement where persuasive and supportive trained and selected volunteers work on behalf of users where those people cannot defend their own rights as citizens. Although both self-advocacy and citizen advocacy need to be independent of authorities, support for the development of these movements could be another way statutory services could commit themselves to listening to the voice of the users.

Involving people in planning their future requires services to use their imagination. There is a difference between being an information source for service planners, and a user of services who actually shapes policy and services. If users are to have a voice that is heard and influences how services develop, then policy makers need to become aware of the difficulties users face in moving beyond consultation to involvement. Lack of personal resources and organisation means that service providers need to offer support to users, their carers and their organisations, so that users can develop their own voice. There are a number of things that service planners can do to increase the involvement of users in the planning process — supporting outreach workers, or users' organisations own facilitators; funding groups so that vital campaigning work can be done; providing organisational skills and training so that people with learning difficulties and their organisations can confidently present their case to service planners.

Although people with learning difficulties have successfully challenged traditional assumptions about their ability to voice their viewpoint, for example through the self-advocacy movement, nevertheless users are weak and powerless in relation to service organisations. They also have low status and need sponsors in the form of committed managers who can fight for resources to be allocated for development work on increasing the power of users to voice their views and concerns about what they want. Users have opinions, but these opinions risk going unheard unless powerful interests find ways of supporting change. Advocates of change may want to bring about new forms of organisation, but they do not necessarily have the power to sponsor it themselves.

It is here that the manager can play a crucial role in using his or her knowledge and skills about service systems and sponsorship of the users' voices to help bring together resources and demands, with the intention of matching these for the benefit of people who depend on the services. It will be a matter of constantly finding new and novel ways of involving the users in order that their ideas actually influence service design which will be a mark of the effectiveness of services in the future, and a measure of how much the intention to increase choice and independence is turned into reality.

The transfer of power and responsibility from the top of the pyramid to the users of services and their direct carers (paid or unpaid) cannot take place, therefore, without a conscious and authoritative move from those in control of decision-making and resources. This is both a personal and political issue because the way power and influence are wielded at every level will have a profound effect on whether individuals' voices are heard and attended to. The nineteenth century essayist, William Hazlitt, once remarked that: "the love of liberty is the love of others, the love of power is the love of ourselves". The government, as a protagonist of disability rights Michael Oliver (1991) has pointed out, has been deeply ambivalent to the rights of users especially in its refusal to implement the whole of the Disabled Persons Act of 1986, but, as Oliver states, "disabled people are empowering themselves anyway", and indeed the logic of the government's own policy and rhetoric is propelling it towards a more consumerist stance, even for those with little political clout.

One of the major deficiencies in social welfare has been the inability to translate the effectiveness of successful initiatives into a wider strategy. This major shift in thinking is essential in services such as ours where the market will benefit some consumers, but is liable to leave others adrift. There are plenty of examples of excellent services which don't often gain the attention they deserve; users' views are being heard in some instances (Atkinson and Williams *op. cit.* and Bridges, 1991); and the brokerage concept developed in Canada and Denmark — where buying power is handed to users, is being researched by the Norah Fry Research Centre, Bristol University, and others. But as Brandon has argued there has been "too much portent and not enough real change" (Brandon, 1989; see also Oswin, 1991, chapter 5).

The transfer of power to service users and their carers must not be an abdication (see chapter 6) but a devolution where people are given the correct infrastructure and education. Firms, such as British Airways (Hampden-Turner, 1990) adopting a customer-orientated approach, deliberately considered social workers and hospice staff, and found that the staff who cared best for consumers of the service were those who were best cared for by their leaders. In our search for an excellent service we must be assiduous listeners to our customers and searchers after qualitative improvement. The people and organisations who are most successful in the 1990s and beyond will be those who learn fastest and most profoundly. Managing services into the future is not, therefore a destination, it is a journey, and we hope to meet many of you on that journey.

D. Atkinson and F. Williams eds (1989), *Know Me As I Am*, Hodder and Stoughton/Open University.

D. Bradford and A. Cohen (1984), *Managing for Excellence*,

John Wiley.
D. Brandon (1989), 'We can talk but can we dance to their tune?', *Community Living*, January.
Bridges (formerly APMH) (1991), *Talking Together: Views of People with Learning Disabilities and their Carers on Future Services.*
K. Butler, S. Carr, F. Sullivan, (1988) *Citizen Advocacy: A Powerful Partnership*, National Citizen Advocacy.
N. Flynn (1990), *Public Sector Management*, Harvester Wheatsheaf.
B. Garrett (1987), *The Learning Organisation*, Fontana.
C. Hampden-Turner (1990), *Corporate Culture*, Hutchinson.
R. Kelly (1988), 'In praise of followers', *Harvard Business Review*, November/December.
Kent Social Services Department (1991), *A Guide to Quality Management in Residential Care*, Kent County Council.
M. Oliver (1991), *Social Work: Disabled People and Disabling Environments*, Jessica Kingsley.
M. Oswin (1991, 2nd Edition), *They Keep Going Away*, chapter 5, King Edward's Hospital Fund for London.
T. Peters (1989), *Thriving on Chaos*, Pan.
J. Rosener (1988), 'Ways women lead', *Harvard Business Review*, November/December.

Appendix

Legislation and reports particularly relevant to services for people with learning difficulties

Date	Report	Legislation	Comments
1325		*De Praerogativa Regis*	Recognised the distinction between mental illness ("persons of unsound mind") and learning difficulties ("natural fools"), and legislated both for the protection of their property and to "provide for their necessities".
1601		Poor Law Act	Marks formal move from Christian charity provided by a nationwide network of monasteries to a secular poor relief based on local parish taxation.
1662		Act of Settlement	Poor relief restricted to people belonging to one's own parish.
1732	*An Account of the Workhouses in Great Britain in Year 1732*		"Very great number of lazy people, rather than submit to the confinement and labour of the workhouse, are content to throw off the mask and maintain themselves by their own industry" (Maidstone poor law authorities).
1774		Act of Regulating Private Madhouses	No person to take charge of more than one mentally disabled person for profit without a licence. Five commissioners appointed for London.
1801	*L'Education du Sauvage d'Aveyron by Jean-Marc Itard*		French physician's attempt to socialise a "wild boy" through educational/environmental means.
1808		County Asylum Act	Laid down detailed specifications for the construction and maintenance of county asylums. Only nine counties proceeded to erect asylums.

Date	Report	Legislation	Comments
1845		Lunatics Act	Each county to build an asylum. Inspection by statutory authority. Separation of certification of diagnosis from certification of consignment. Proper records of admissions and discharge to be kept.
1870,1876 and 1880		Education Acts	Introduction of compulsory education and, therefore, the identification of those with special needs.
1886		Idiots Act	Recognised special asylums for "an idiot or imbecile from birth or an early age".
1891		Lunacy Act	"The triumph of legalism" (Kathleen Jones). No distinction between mental illness and handicap.
1899		Elementary Education (Defective and Epileptic Children) Act	Permitted local authorities to set up special schools.
1908	Report of the Royal Commission on the Feeble-Minded		Argued for segregation to protect both the "mental defective" and society.
	Publication of the first edition of *Tredgold's Mental Deficiency*		
1913		Mental Deficiency Act	Created four categories: ☐ Idiots ☐ Imbeciles ☐ Feeble-minded ☐ Moral Defectives Obliged local authorities to ascertain the number of "defectives" in their area. Statutory supervision of "ascertained defectives".
1914		Elementary Education (Defective and Epileptic Children) Act	Obliged local authorities to provide special schools for those children who are "dull and backward" but not "imbeciles".

Date	Report	Legislation	Comments
1927		Mental Deficiency Act	Widened the definition of mental handicap and added the training and occupation of "defectives" to the duties of local authorities.
1939	Departmental Committee on the Voluntary Mental Health Services (Faversham report)		Favoured an all-purpose mental health social worker who would provide: ☐ supervision of early cases of mental and functional disorder. ☐ after-care of mental hospital patients. ☐ statutory and voluntary supervision of "mental defectives". ☐ follow-up of children presenting problems of behaviour.
1946	Report of Care of Children Committee. (Curtis report)		Children with a learning difficulty seen as a medical responsibility and recommended provision apart from other children.
1946		National Health Service Act	Transfer of mental handicap institutions from the local authority to the NHS. Creation of a unified mental health service.
1957	Royal Commission on Mental Illness and Mental Deficiency.		
1959		Mental Health Act	Introduced new terminology: "subnormality" and "severe subnormality". Allowed social services authorities to accommodate mentally disordered people in residential care. Created mental welfare officer to carry out supportive and statutory functions.
1959	Report of the Working Party on Social Workers in the Local Authority, Health and Welfare Services (Younghusband report)		Recommended improved training and a better career in the mental health setting.

Date	Report	Legislation	Comments
1968		Health Service and Public Health Act	Provision for local authority services (amended by the NHS Act, 1977).
1969	Report of the Committee of Enquiry into Allegations of Ill-Treatment of Patients and Other Irregularities at the Ely Hospital, Cardiff.		Revealed both specific instances of cruelty and general failings of the hospital system. Published in the same year as Pauline Morris's study of mental handicap hospitals, *Put Away*.
1970		Chronically Sick and Disabled Persons Act	Laid a duty on local authorities to inform themselves of the numbers of disabled people who might need their services, and in turn inform them of the services available. Some of the specific provisions in the Act have never been properly implemented by some authorities because no money was made available to the local authorities by central government.
1970		Local Authority Social Services Act	Created generic social services departments out of the children's, mental health and welfare departments (based on the Seebohm report of 1968).
1970		Education (Handicapped Children) Act	Brought children with severe learning difficulties into the education system, who had previously been classed as "ineducable".
1971	*Better Services for the Mentally Handicapped* - DHSS White Paper.		Laid down recommendations over the whole range of services and set target dates for the implementation of a move from hospital to "community care".
1972	Report of the Committee on Nursing (Briggs report).		Recommended changes in the training of nurses.

Date	Report	Legislation	Comments
1974	*Social Work Support for the Health Service* (Otton report).		
1974	Butler committee on mentally abnormal offenders.		Recommended regional secure units.
1974	Report of the Committee of Enquiry into South Ockenden Hospital.		Revealed ill-treatment of patients, overcrowding and poor levels of care.
1975		Children Act	Enshrined "the welfare principle" in law and gave an impetus towards looking at children in hospital in the same way as other children in residential care.
1976		Education Act	Looked towards the 1981 Act in its recommendations for integration.
1976	Report of the Committee on Child Health Services (Court report).		Stressed the need for handicapped children to be treated as children first. Proposed an integrated child health service with district handicap teams serving the needs of families.
1976	National Development Group, Pamphlet One, *Mental Handicap: Planning Together*		The NDG pamphlets set guidelines for service development and urged multi-disciplinary co-operation both in planning and in service delivery (e.g. setting up community mental handicap teams).
1977	Normansfield Hospital Enquiry report		Revealed a repressive hierarchical regime deleterious to the well being of residents.
1977	NDG Pamphlet Two, *Mentally Handicapped Children: A Plan for Action.* Pamphlet Three, *Helping Mentally Handicapped School Leavers.* Pamphlet Four, *Short-Term Care for Mentally Handicapped People: Suggestions for Action.* Pamphlet Five, *Day Services for Mentally Handicapped Adults.*		

Date	Report	Legislation	Comments
1978	NDG, *Helping Mentally Handicapped People in hospitals.*		Argued for a social work service in mental handicap hospitals.
1978	Report of the Committee of Enquiry into the Education of Handicapped Children and Young People (Warnock report).		Recommended the abolition of the categorisation of handicapped children and was the forerunner of the 1981 Education Act in its proposals.
1979	Report of the Committee of Enquiry into Mental Handicap Nursing and Care (Jay report).		Proposed a unified training for nursing and social services staff, but looked beyond this to propose a local model of care with a move away from segregated services
1980	*Mental Handicap: Progress, Problems and Priorities.*		Evaluated progress since the 1971 White Paper.
1981	*Care in Action: A Handbook of Policies and Priorities for Health and Social Services in England.*		Put forward the essential elements in a locally based service.
1981		Education Act (Implemented 1983).	Abolished the categorisation system. Pupils with special educational needs, in principle, to be educated in normal schools, contingent on certain considerations. Assessments to be carried out at certain ages and in partnership with parents (see chapter 18).
1986		Disabled Persons (Services, Consultation and Representation) Act	Some sections of the Act were implemented on 1 April 1987. These were: ☐ Section 4, the duty to assess the need for services; ☐ Section 8(1), the duty to take carers' abilities into account; ☐ Section 9, the duty to provide information about services; ☐ Section 10, the duty to consult with organisations of disabled people when making co-options on to committees; ☐ Sections 5 & 6, the identification and assessment of disabled

Date	Report	Legislation	Comments
			school leavers, were implemented on 1 February 1988. The "advocacy" sections — 1 & 2 — covering the "authorised representative" have not been implemented.
1986	Audit Commission, *Making a Reality of Community Care*		An in-depth critique of care in the community and proposals for future action (see chapter 1 for detail).
1987	Audit Commission, *Community Care: Developing Services for People with a Mental Handicap.*		A succinct critique of the challenges, and proposals for the next steps.
1988	*Community Care: Agenda for Action* (The Griffiths report).		Endorsed the criticisms made by the 1986 Audit Report. Proposed that local authorities should play the major role in ensuring that services met individual needs, though not necessarily providing the services themselves.
1989	*Caring for People: Community Care in the Next Decade and Beyond*		Government White Paper following the Griffiths report. It sets out six key objectives for service delivery: ☐ "To promote the development of domiciliary, day and respite services to enable people to live in their own homes wherever feasible and sensible. ☐ To ensure that service providers make practical support for carers a high priority. ☐ To make proper assessment of needs and good case management the cornerstone of high quality care. ☐ To promote the development of a flourishing independent sector alongside good quality public services.

Date	Report	Legislation	Comments
			☐ To clarify the responsibilities of agencies and so make it easier to hold them to account for their performance. ☐ To secure better value for taxpayers' money by introducing a new funding structure for social care."
1989		Children Act	Brings children in need including children with disabilities (Sect. 17(10)) into mainline children's legislation. Lays a duty on local authorities to: ☐ Promote the welfare of children. ☐ Keep a register of disabled children (Schedule 2, Part 1,2(1)) ☐ Tie-in assessment with assessments under disability legislation. ☐ Provide services to minimise the effect of disability. The Act seeks to shift local authority intervention towards a partnership with families. Implemented October 1991.
1989	*Working for Patients*		Government White Paper on acute health services. Proposed: ☐ Creation of self-governing hospital trusts. ☐ Development of an internal market. ☐ New contracts and cash-limited budgets for GPs. ☐ Restructuring of health authorities on business lines.
1989	Social Services Inspectorate, *Inspection of Day Services for People with a Mental Handicap.*		Drew attention to the shortfalls in: ☐ Joint Planning. ☐ The involvement of clients and carers. ☐ A clear policy of intent. ☐ Support, supervision and training for staff. Recommended a system of assessment - planning - activity - review.

Date	Report	Legislation	Comments
1989	Audit Commission, *Developing Community Care for Adults with a Mental Handicap.*		Results of the commission's national survey of local authorities.
1990		*Code of Practice* Under Section 118 of the Mental Health Act 1983	
1990		National Health Service and Community Care Act receives Royal Assent	On 18 July 1990 Secretary of State for Health Kenneth Clark told the House of Commons that the care in the community reforms would be phased in over three years: ☐ *April 1991:* arms-length inspection units and new complaints procedures. Specific grant for mental health services. Development work on care management and the separation of purchasers and providers within SSDs. ☐ *April 1992:* New planning arrangements for SSDs and district health authorities. ☐ *April 1993:* The new benefit arrangements.